Congenital Anomalies of Coronary Arteries

Gianfranco Butera • Alessandro Frigiola
Editors

Congenital Anomalies of Coronary Arteries

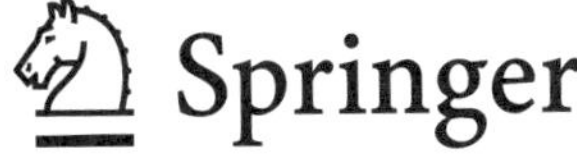 Springer

Editors
Gianfranco Butera
Pediatric Cardiology and Cardiac
Surgery
Bambino Gesù Hospital
Rome, Italy

Alessandro Frigiola
Cardiac Surgery Unit
Policlinico San Donato
SAN DONATO MILANESE
Milano, Italy

ISBN 978-3-031-36968-1   ISBN 978-3-031-36966-7   (eBook)
https://doi.org/10.1007/978-3-031-36966-7

This Springer imprint is published by the registered company Springer Nature Switzerland AG
The registered company address is: Gewerbestrasse 11, 6330 Cham, Switzerland

Acknowledgments

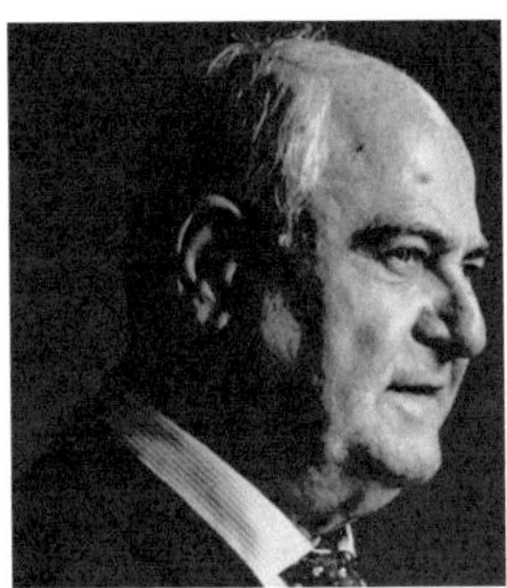

Paolo Angelini 1941–2023

Professor Paolo Angelini has been a true giant in medicine, particularly in the field of coronary artery anomalies, where he was a pioneer. He was always easy to reach and available to share his knowledge and wisdom when a difficult case came to the attention of colleagues from all over the world. He has been a true inspiration and also a strong force within this book, which he had been waiting for a long time.

Sadly, he will not be able to hold it in his hands.

His legacy will last and his contribution to this book is the last witness of his passion, knowledge and wisdom that will guide colleagues worldwide.

Gianfranco Butera and Alessandro Frigiola

The original version of the chapter has been revised. A correction to this chapter can be found at https://doi.org/10.1007/978-3-031-36966-7_23

Contents

Introduction

Anomalous origin of coronary arteries has been the subject of numerous studies trying to describe the embryology, anatomy, diagnosis, mechanism of myocardial ischemia, and treatment methods. With this book, the authors have focused their attention on such aspects and provided the most updated evidence and knowledge on coronary anomalies. However, the exact mechanism(s), the reasons for the occurrence of symptoms at a specific moment in life when the anomaly has always been there, and many other questions remain unsolved.

As is often the case, many discoveries are made by chance. During one such surgical procedure to correct an anomalous aortic origin of the coronary artery, one (the?) mechanism of coronary flow limitation was revealed to us! These images have been forever impressed in the memory!

A young patient with anomalous origin of the left coronary artery from the right coronary sinus complained of typical anginal chest pain. Surgical correction was indicated. The patient was prepped and anesthetized; following the opening of the chest, the left coronary artery appeared pink and well perfused. The patient suddenly developed a hypertensive crisis with systolic blood pressure that reached 200 mmHg and a heart rate of 180 beats per minute. On the monitor ECG there was evidence of Pardee waves (symmetric inversion of T waves), indicating acute ischemia. Suddenly the coronary artery appeared pale and collapsed, clearly hypoperfused. After normalization of blood pressure and heart rate within a few minutes, the ECG ischemic alteration regressed and resolved. The left coronary artery regained its initial macroscopic appearance and was pink and of full caliber once again. It was under our eyes that the hypertension-induced aortic root dilatation caused (1) narrowing of the ostia of the anomalous coronary artery, which appeared slit-like and, therefore, easily collapsible; (2) on the other hand, the adherence of the coronary artery to the aortic wall, because of the aortic root distension, caused the compression of the coronary segment between the ostium and the distal coronary segment (Fig. 1, left).

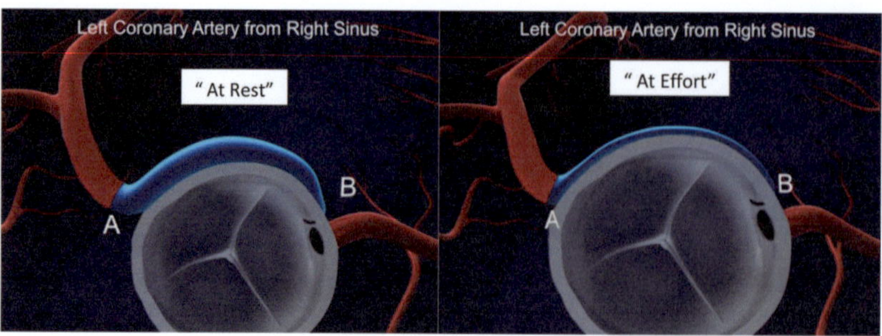

The AAOCA represents the third cause of sudden death in young athletes and often is not detected by routine screening. The effective rate of sudden death for AAOCA may be higher than what has been reported.

"We only see what we know!" Johann Wolfgang von Goethe

This is particularly true for AAOCA! Spreading the knowledge is then a must-do of our times in order to increase the detection of such anomalies and to reduce the burden of sudden death in particular in otherwise healthy young people!

Part I

From Embryology to Diseases

The Development of the Coronary Arteries

1

Robert H. Anderson, Timothy J. Mohun, and Deborah Henderson

Introduction

Our aim with this chapter is to provide an account of the development of the coronary arteries so as to help in understanding the malformations that afflict them in the setting of congenital heart disease. Many, if not most, of the controversies that continue to surround their embryological development are of limited significance when considered relative to the understanding of the variations found when the heart, or the coronary arteries themselves, are congenitally malformed. This is not to suggest that the knowledge of initial formation of the coronary vasculature is itself insignificant. On the contrary, it is vital to know how, and when, the endothelial linings of the developing vessels can first be identified, and whether they form by a process of angiogenesis or vasculogenesis. Knowledge of this early development, however, does not impact directly on understanding how the developing epicardial coronary arteries achieve their connection with the aortic root. Nor is it directly relevant to an appreciation of how the epicardial channels themselves extend so as to percolate through the so-called compact components of the ventricular walls. The manner of formation of the compact component of the ventricular walls remains controversial in itself. Those investigating the interaction between formation of the coronary arteries and the development of the compact portions of the ventricular walls have presumed that the compact layer is thinned in the presence of so-called "non-compaction" [1]. This is not the case. There is significant evidence to show that such "non-compaction" is better described in terms of excessive trabeculation [2]. As such, the presence of an extensive non-trabeculated meshwork is more likely to be an epiphenomenon rather than a discrete cardiomyopathy [2]. Irrespective of these potential disagreements, there can be no question that the mural coronary arterial circulation cannot be established without the appropriate formation of the compact ventricular wall. Once the circulation is established, the capillaries are able to return to the arterial flow from the aortic root into the coronary venous system, and eventually back to the cavities of the heart itself. It is the manner of connection of the epicardial plexus to the aortic root that provides the understanding of lesions such as anomalous origin of the coronary arteries from the pulmonary trunk, or anomalous origin from an inappropriate aortic sinus. Understanding the abnormal arrangements found in the setting of either the hypoplastic left heart syndrome or pulmonary atresia with an intact

R. H. Anderson (✉) · D. Henderson
Biosciences Division, Newcastle University, Newcastle-upon-Tyne, UK
e-mail: sejjran@ucl.ac.uk; Deborah.henderson@Newcastle.ac.uk

T. J. Mohun
Francis Crick Institute, London, UK

© Springer Nature Switzerland AG 2023
G. Butera, A. Frigiola (eds.), *Congenital Anomalies of Coronary Arteries*,
https://doi.org/10.1007/978-3-031-36966-7_1

ventricular septum, in contrast, is dependent on the knowledge of how the ventricular walls are converted from the initial pattern, which is a meshwork of trabeculations, with minimal formation of the compact mural component, to the situation in which it is the trabeculations which are of minimal significance. It is these two features, therefore, namely the connection of the epicardial arteries to the aortic root and the establishment of the ventricular mural circulation, on which we concentrate our attention. We begin, nonetheless, with a brief overview of the ongoing discussions regarding the origins of the different components of the coronary arterial walls.

Angiogenesis Versus Vasculogenesis

An elegant overview of this important topic, and its relevance to the understanding of the anatomy of both normal and abnormal coronary arteries, is provided in the document prepared by the Working Group on Cardiovascular Development of the European Society of Cardiology [3]. In that review, the authors base their analysis on the fact that the definitive coronary arteries are formed on the basis of their endothelial lining. This endothelial scaffold is subsequently surrounded by the wall of vascular smooth muscle, which itself is encased in a fibrous matrix continuous with the external adventitial layer. It is the endothelial primordiums that appear first during embryological development. And it is these components that continue to be the subject of debate with regard to angiogenesis as opposed to vasculogenesis. It was initially accepted that the overall coronary arterial endothelium was produced by angiogenesis [4]. This meant that new vessels were formed from pre-existing ones by a process of endothelial sprouting [5]. The initial "sprout" was presumed to grow out of the aortic root [4]. This notion fell from grace when it became accepted that the epicardial arteries, rather than sprouting out from the aorta, grew into the valvar sinuses [6]. There is now much evidence,

both molecular [7] and morphologic [8], to show that the initial arterial stems do, indeed, grow out from the aortic root to join with the developing epicardial vessels. But since the epicardial channels themselves are present prior to the emergence of the aortic sprouts, it remains appropriate to question the notion that the entire vascular network, including the coronary venous system, is generated by angiogenesis from solitary aortic primordiums. Indeed, much evidence has accrued to show that at least part of the endothelial network is formed by vasculogenesis [9]. In this latter process, it is presumed that angioblasts, which are the progenitors of the endothelial cells themselves, coalesce to form clusters, which then transform to become new vessels.

Irrespective of whether the endothelial linings are generated by vasculogenesis as opposed to angiogenesis, further debate has surrounded the origin of the endothelial cells themselves. Excluding the possibility that they all expand from original aortic sprouts [5], various investigators have suggested that they derive from the endocardial lining of the ventricular trabeculations [10], the liver sinusoids [11], or the epicardium [12]. Yet another theory has now achieved prominence. The channels, rather than sprouting from the aorta, are alleged to sprout initially from the systemic venous sinus. In this concept, the channels are then presumed to reprogram to become arterial rather than venous [13]. That the entirety of the coronary arterial network is derived by sprouting from the systemic venous sinus seems just as unlikely as that it would sprout from the aorta. And, if the initial channels are re-programmed to become arterial, a second parallel system will be required to form the veins. Subsequent molecular biological evidence, furthermore, has questioned the unitary origin of the endothelial cells. In this regard, it has been shown that a subset of epicardial progenitors, at least in the murine heart, make endothelial contributions [14]. It has then been shown that parts of the network, at least for the coronary arteries, are derived from the endocardial linings of the ventricular trabeculations [15]. Questions must now be posed regarding yet another piece of evidence advanced in favour of the formation of arterial endothelium from ventricular endocardium. This concept proposed that the endocardial cells became trapped during alleged coalescence of the ventricular trabeculations to form the compact parts of the ventricular walls [16]. Since there is no evidence that the compact ventricular wall is formed by so-called "compaction", this final piece of evidence must now be questioned. Intertrabecular spaces, nonetheless, can become connected to the epicardial coronary arteries when the heart is congenitally malformed. There can be little question, therefore, but that the endothelial linings of the developing coronary arteries within the ventricular walls originate, at least in part, from epicardially derived cells. And, in abnormal situations, endocardial channels from the ventricular cavities can make direct connections with these mural coronary arteries, and thence with the major epicardial coronary arteries.

In contrast to the debate regarding the origin of the endothelial lining of the coronary arteries, there is general agreement that the vascular smooth muscle is largely produced by epicardially derived cells. Molecular biological studies, nonetheless, have shown that not all the smooth muscle cells within the arterial walls are labelled by epicardially derived markers. Some of the myocytes in the arterial walls are derived either from the neural crest or from the second heart field [17, 18]. And significantly, it is the initial stems of the major coronary arteries as they originate from the valvar sinuses that have been shown to have an endothelial lining of neural crest origin [19]. The fibrous components of the arterial walls are almost certainly derived primarily from the epicardium [20], although the possibility remains that some fibroblasts could arise from bone marrow cells [21]. Combining all this data produces the notion that the coronary arterial network is a developmental mosaic [3]. In terms of the understanding of malformed coronary arteries, nonetheless, the key features are the connection of the epicardial coronary arteries to the aortic root, and the connection between the mural arterial vasculature and the epicardial arteries themselves. These processes, in turn, are intimately linked with the formation of the compact components of the ventricular walls. It is an understanding of these processes, therefore, that is our primary focus.

Development of the Human Heart

In their review of normal and abnormal coronary arteries [3], the Working Group of Developmental Pathology emphasises that much of our knowledge of development is driven by experiments made using the mouse. Evidence from murine development now serves to confirm inferences that can be made when with regard to the mechanism of connection of the epicardial coronary arteries to the aortic root [8]. When seeking to consider the relationship of developmental events to congenital cardiac malformations, however, it is important to concentrate on human cardiac embryonic development. The major changes span the fifth through the eighth week subsequent to fertilisation. These stages of development are usually described using the system developed at the Carnegie Institute, in the United States of America [22]. The key stages are those extending from 10 through 23. By Carnegie stage (CS) 13, when the embryo is around 32 days old, the initial heart tube has passed through the stage known as looping. It is then possible to observe the apical components of the developing right and left ventricles, which are forming from the inlet and outlet parts of the ventricular loop. The developing atrial chambers at this stage open exclusively into the developing left ventricle, with the developing right ventricle supporting the entirety of the outflow tract. The outflow tract is serpentine. Its walls, significantly, are myocardial to its junction, at the margins of the pericardial cavity, with the aortic sac (Fig. 1.1). At this stage of development, the ventricular walls are formed mostly by a meshwork of the trabeculations, with endocardium encircling each of the individual trabeculations. The compact layer of the ventricular walls is barely formed.

By CS 15, when the embryo is around 36 days old, the atrioventricular canal has expanded such that a direct connection is established between the right ventricle and the right atrium. The out-

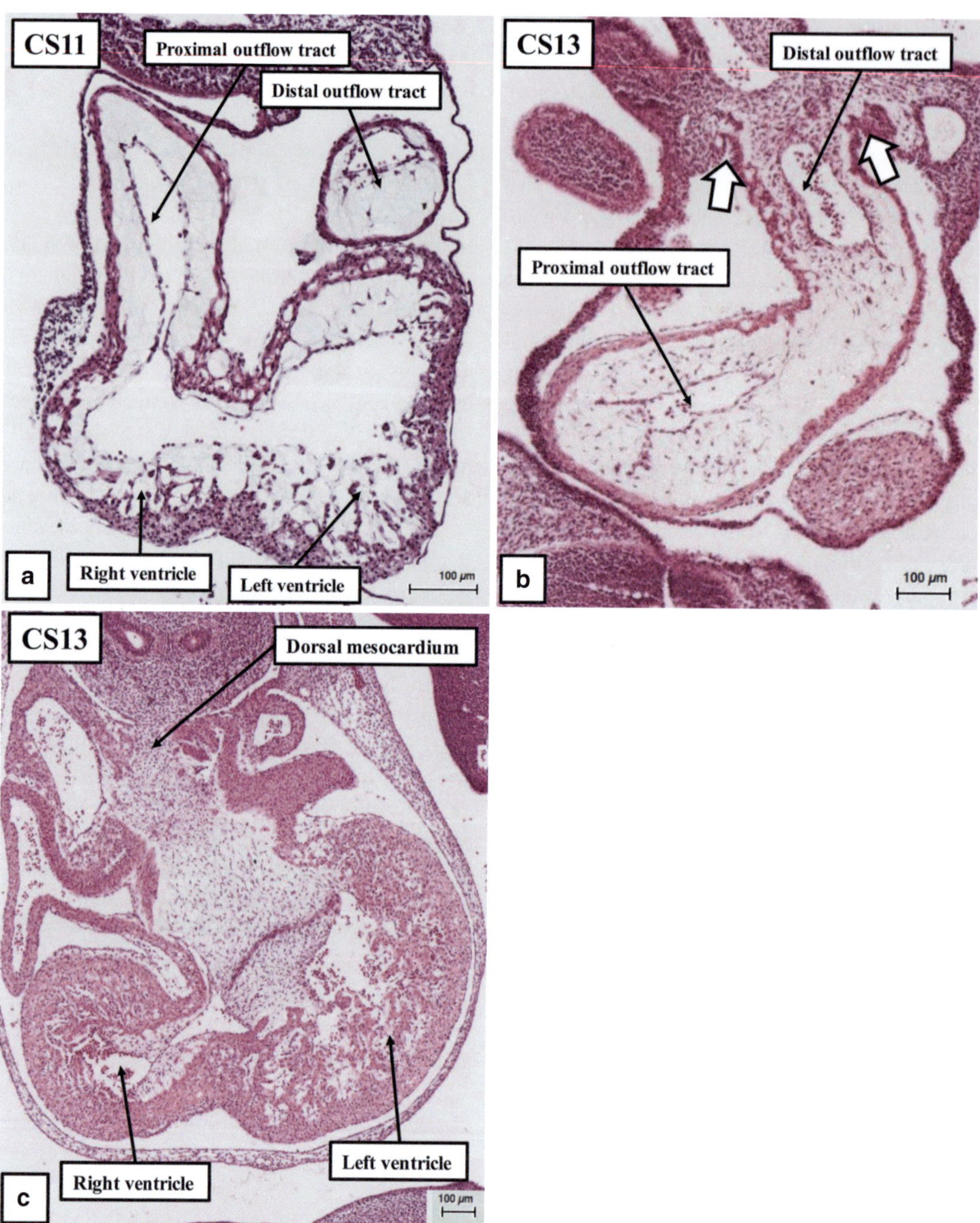

Fig. 1.1 The panels show frontal sections taken from three different human embryos at CS 13, which represents around 32 days of development subsequent to fertilisation. Panel A shows the ventricular loop, with the developing right ventricle supporting the outflow tract. Panel B is a section through the outflow tract, showing that its walls are myocardial to the margins of the pericardial cavity (white arrows with black borders). Panel C is a section through the atrioventricular canal, which is supported exclusively at this stage by the developing left ventricle. Note that the ventricular walls are made up mostly of trabeculations, with a very thin compact layer

flow tract, nonetheless, remains supported exclusively by the developing right ventricle. A significant change has taken place, however, with regard to the extent of its myocardial walls. The entirety of the developing right ventricle, including the outflow tract, is known to be formed by migration of cells into the heart tube from the so-called second heart field. Additional cells continue to populate the arterial pole of the tube between CSs 13 and 15. Unlike the initial migrations, the new cells are non-myocardial. They form the intrapericardial components of the arterial trunks [23]. At the same time, a protrusion extends from the dorsal wall of the aortic sac into the cavity of the distal outflow tract. This separates the newly formed non-myocardial component into the intrapericardial aorta and pulmonary trunk. By CS 15, the protrusion has fused with the distal margins of the mesenchymal cushions that themselves fuse to separate the remainder of the outflow tract (Fig. 1.2).

The cushions themselves are derived by a process of epithelial-to-mesenchymal transformation within the cardiac jelly that extends throughout the outflow tract. Concomitant with the appearance of the non-myocardial walls to form the distal part of the outflow tract, the distal margins of the cushions regress towards the base of the developing right ventricle in parallel with proximal regression of the distal myocardial border. At the same time, swellings are formed at the proximal ends of the tongues of the non-myocardial tissues that are forming the parietal walls of the intrapericardial arterial trunks. These swellings, identified by Kramer as the intercalated valvar swelling [24], interpose between the parietal distal margins of the major cushions. In this way, they permit the recognition of the primordiums of the developing arterial root within the area that can now be nominated as the middle part of the outflow tract [23]. It is within this middle part that the distal outflow cushions, along

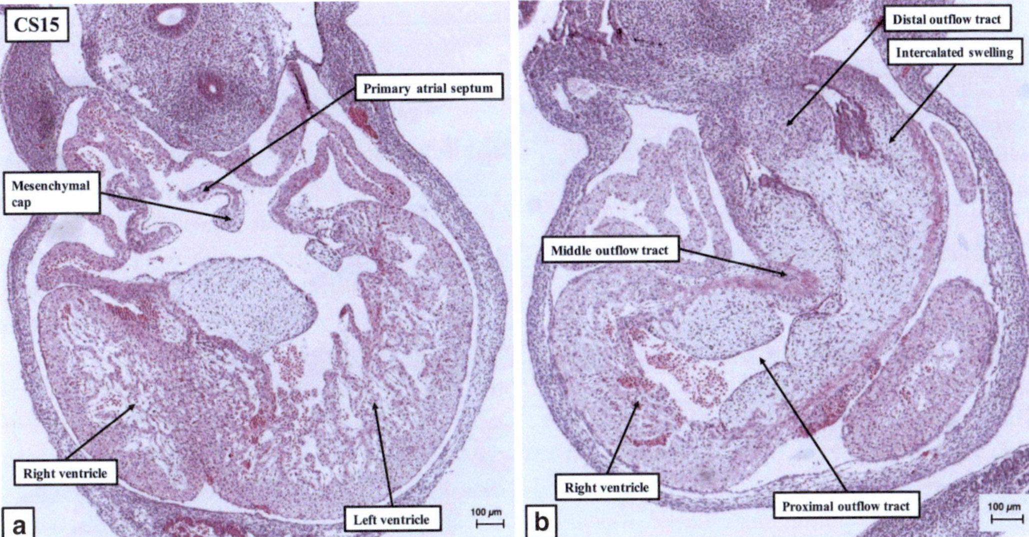

Fig. 1.2 The images show sections from the same human embryo at Carnegie stage (CS) 15, when the embryo is around 36 days old. Panel A is a section through the atrioventricular canal, which has expanded to provide the right ventricle with its inlet component. The primary atrial septum is growing towards the canal, and will separate the right and left atrial chambers. Note that the ventricular walls continue to be formed primarily by a meshwork of trabeculations, with a thin compact component. Panel B shows the developing outflow tract, which is being separated into the aortic and pulmonary channels. It now possesses three parts, with the middle part delineated by the extent of the so-called intercalated valvar swellings, which will form the non-adjacent leaflets of the aortic and pulmonary valves. In this image, only the pulmonary swelling is shown. The distal myocardial border has now regressed to the level of the junction between the distal and middle parts of the outflow tract

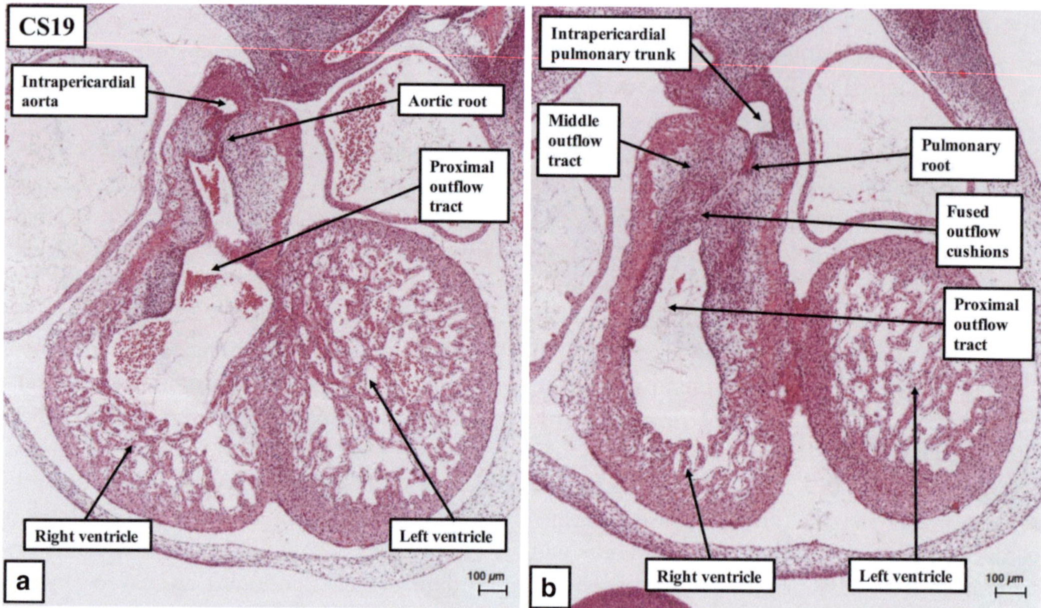

Fig. 1.3 The images show frontal sections from the same human embryo at Carnegie stage (CS) 17, when around 40 days have passed subsequent to fertilisation. Panel A shows the developing aortic root, which has been separated from the developing pulmonary root, which is shown in Panel B. Both roots remain supported by the developing right ventricle, and both are enclosed within the collar of the middle myocardium. The protrusion from the dorsal wall of the aortic sac has fused with the distal margins of the outflow cushions, which themselves have fused in the middle part of the outflow tract. The cushions, however, remain to fuse in the proximal outflow tract. The ventricular walls remain formed predominantly by trabeculations, with each trabeculation surrounded by its own endothelial sleeve. As yet, it is not possible to recognise any epicardial vascular channels

with the intercalated valvar swellings, remodel to produce the leaflets of the arterial valves. It is within this middle myocardial collar, furthermore, that we see the initial formation of vascular endothelial channels. Additional channels, nonetheless, form within the walls of the distal nonmyocardial outflow tract. These distal vessels have been dubbed the "peritruncal plexus" [7]. The crown-like plexus formed with the myocardial walls of the middle part of the outflow tract is discrete from the peritruncal plexus found within the distal outflow tract. Indeed, it is arguable that, so as to understand the relationships to congenital malformations, it is the fate of this middle part of the outflow tract that is the key to understanding.

The fusion of the protrusion formed from the dorsal wall of the aortic sac with the distal margins of the outflow cushions is the prelude to separation of the middle part of the outflow tract into the future aortic and pulmonary roots. This separation can be seen by CS 17, when the embryo has passed through around 40 days subsequent to fertilisation (Fig. 1.3). Subsequent to the fusion of the protrusion from the dorsal wall of the aortic sac with the distal margins of the outflow cushions, the arterial roots are separated one from the other, but as yet there has been no remodelling of the distal margins of the cushions and the intercalated valvar swellings, which remain flush with the distal myocardial border. And it is the myocardial border that marks the boundary between the middle part of the outflow tract and its distal nonmyocardial components. The ventricular walls at this stage, furthermore, remain formed predominantly by the meshwork of trabeculations. As yet, it is not possible to recognise any formation of vascular channels within the epicardial covering of the chambers, nor within the thin compact components of the ventricular walls. It first becomes possible to recognise the beginning of remodelling to produce arterial valvar leaflets at

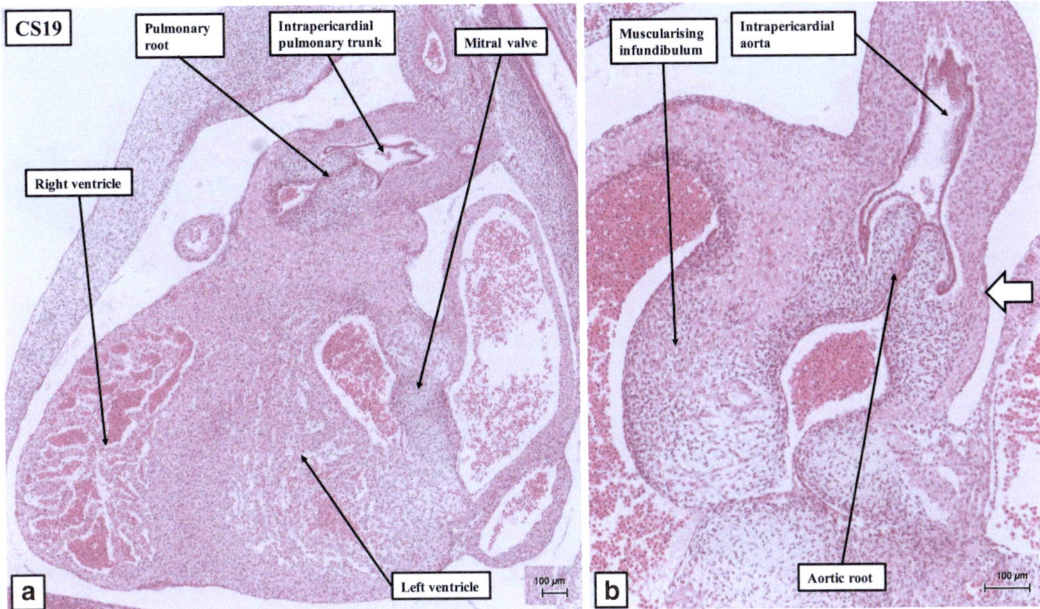

Fig. 1.4 The images are sagittal sections through a human embryo at Carnegie stage (CS) 19, when the embryo is almost 7 weeks old. Panel A shows a cut through the left side, showing the developing pulmonary root. Panel B is a higher-powered image through the dorsally located aortic root. The root remains aligned with the cavity of the right ventricle, but the proximal cushions by now have fused with each other to build a shelf, which connects the root with the cavity of the left ventricle. The fused proximal cushions are now myocardialising, and will eventually largely form the infundibulum of the right ventricle. The cushion shown in the image will fuse with the tubercles of the atrioventricular cushions to close the tertiary interventricular communication. The distal margins of the cushions are beginning to remodel to form the leaflets of the arterial valves, but remain encased in a collar of the middle outflow tract myocardium. The ventricular walls, however, remain formed mostly by trabeculations. There is still no evidence of the formation of epicardial vascular channels

CS 19, when the embryo is almost 7 weeks old. Even at this stage, nonetheless, the middle part of the outflow tract remains encased almost exclusively within its myocardial collar (Fig. 1.4). By this stage, the proximal outflow cushions have themselves fused, thus building a shelf in the roof of the right ventricle. This process creates a channel between the aortic root, which is still supported by the right ventricle, and the interventricular communication. A channel still persists, however, between the aortic root and the cavity of the right ventricle. The closure of this aorto-right ventricular channel, by tubercles derived from the atrioventricular cushions, serves to convert the interventricular foramen into the outflow tract for the left ventricle. The tubercles then become the membranous part of the septum. By this stage, the remodelling of the cushions and the intercalated valvar swellings, producing the

leaflets of both arterial valves, is obvious (Fig. 1.4). Both arterial roots, nonetheless, remain largely encased within the turret of the middle outflow tract myocardium. And the ventricular walls remain largely trabeculated. Still there has been no formation of any epicardial vascular channels, nor arterial channels within the thin compact ventricular walls.

Only during CSs 21 and 22, when the embryo is at the beginning of the eighth week of development, does it become possible to recognise the appearance of vascular channels. These are formed initially in the developing atrioventricular and interventricular grooves, but also in abundance within the myocardial walls that continue to surround the middle part of the outflow tract (Fig. 1.5). The channels in the atrioventricular and interventricular grooves will form the major epicardial arteries. In addition to these endothe-

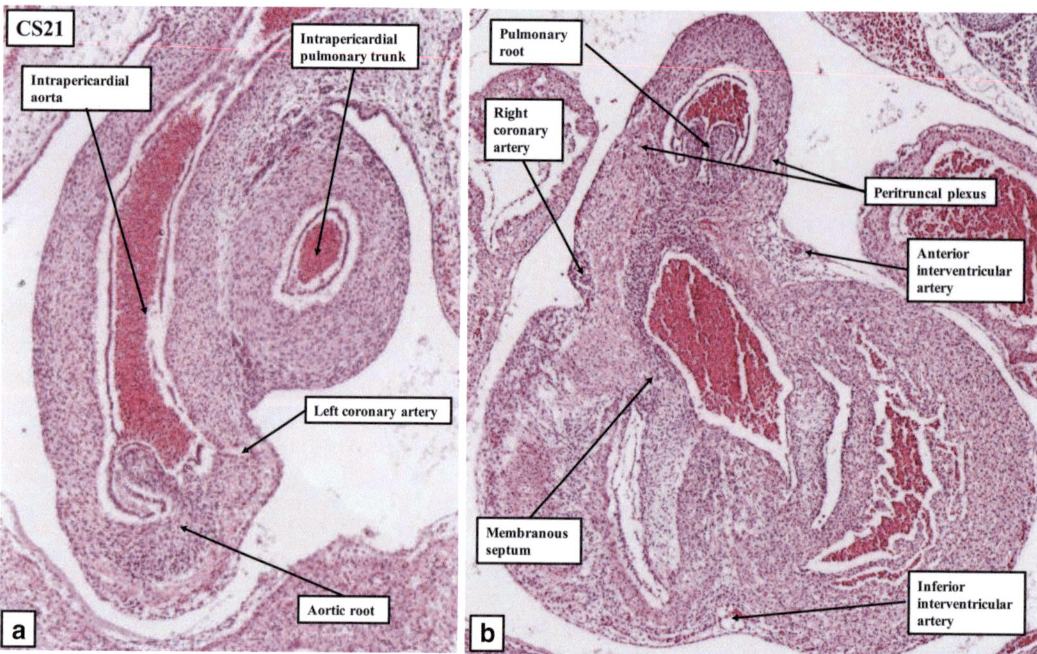

Fig. 1.5 The frontal sections are taken from a human embryo at Carnegie stage (CS) 21, when the embryo is at the beginning of the eighth week of development. It is at this stage that it first becomes possible to recognise the endothelial channels that will become the coronary arteries. As shown in Panel A, the stem of the left coronary artery is emerging from the intrapericardial aorta. It is distal to the boundary with the developing aortic root. As shown in panel B, the tubercles of the atrioventricular cushions have fused to close the persisting communication between the aortic root and the right ventricle, even though the aortic root itself remains aligned with the cavity of the right ventricle. It is now possible to recognise the endothelial channels that will become the major coronary arteries, along with an extensive plexus within the myocardial walls that still enclose the middle part of the outflow tract. As yet, however, there has been minimal formation of the arterial walls of the valvar sinuses. The compact component of the ventricular walls, however, is now beginning the thicken

lial channels, an extensive circumferential plexus can now be recognised within the myocardial walls that continue to surround the middle part of the outflow tract. Although the distal cushions and swellings have undergone additional remodelling as they form the valvar leaflets, they still remain supported, in their larger part, by the myocardium of the middle part of the outflow tract. Significantly, however, endothelial channels can now be seen growing out of the aortic trunk just distal to the myocardial border. These channels form the main stems of the coronary arteries. The stem of the left coronary artery is recognisable in the embryo shown in Fig. 1.5. In another embryo in the Human Developmental Biology Resource (HDBR) archive, considered to represent CS 22, it is possible to recognise the stem of the right coronary artery. As with the stem of the left coronary artery shown in Fig. 1.5b, it arises from the intrapericardial aorta distal to the border of the myocardium surrounding the middle part of the outflow tract (Fig. 1.6).

CS 23 marks the end of the embryonic period of development, by which time the embryo is 8 weeks old. By this stage, ongoing growth of the non-myocardial tissues permits recognition of the beginning of the formation of the arterial valvar sinuses. At CS 23, however, the stems of the right and left coronary arteries remain at the level of the sinutubular junction. They take a transmural course within the adventitial lining of the developing sinuses merge before they merge with the major coronary arteries, which by this stage have developed from the circumferential plexus initially formed within the myocardial walls of the middle part of the outflow tract. Although the compact layer of the ventricular walls has begun to thicken, the trabecular meshwork remains

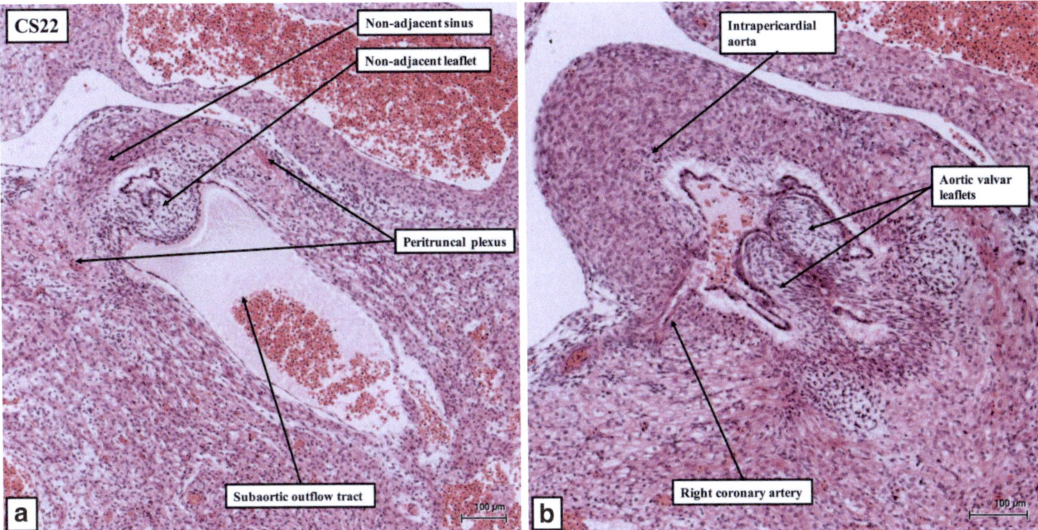

Fig. 1.6 The sections are taken through the developing left ventricular outflow tract of a human embryo at Carnegie stage (CS) 22, in the eighth week of development. Panel A shows the vascular channels that form the peritruncal plexus within the myocardial walls of the middle part of the outflow tract. Note the ongoing remodelling of the intercalated valvar swelling to form the non-adjacent leaflet of the aortic valve. Panel B shows how the stem of the right coronary artery is growing out of the intrapericardial aorta just distal to the myocardial border. It is extending to join with the endothelial channels of the peritruncal plexus

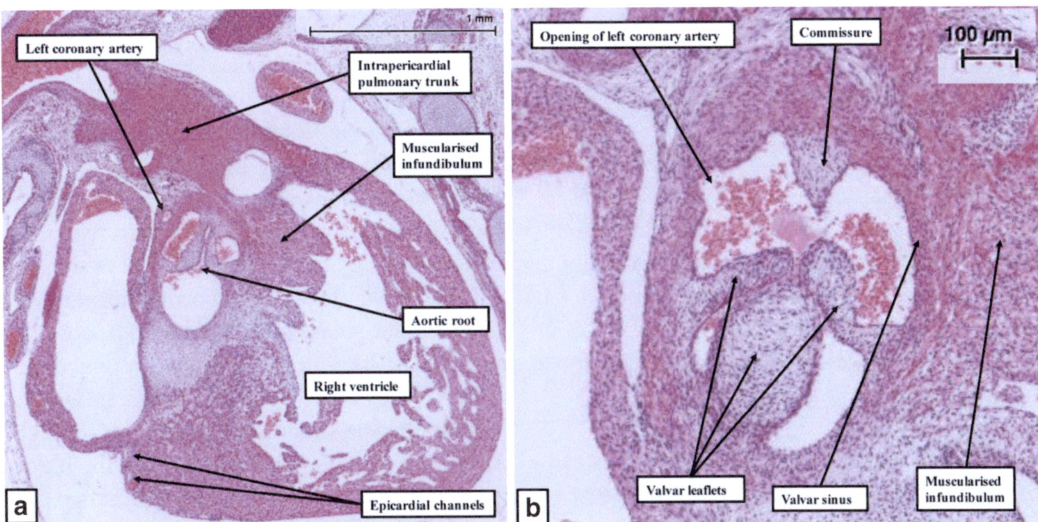

Fig. 1.7 The sections are taken from a human embryo at Carnegie stage 23, which is at the end of the eighth week of development. Panel A shows an oblique cut through the right ventricle, the aortic root, and the pulmonary trunk. The stem of the left coronary artery can be seen taking an intramural course through the adventitial lining of the developing left coronary arterial sinus. Panel B is a magnified view taken from the next serial section to the right. It shows that the opening of the artery, at this stage, is at the level of the developing sinutubular junction

prominent. Although the major epicardial coronary arteries are recognisable within the atrioventricular and interventricular grooves in the particular embryo representing CS 23 in the HDBR archive, there is still no evidence of the formation of arterial channels within the developing compact ventricular walls (Fig. 1.7). Although it was not possible to identify endothelial chan-

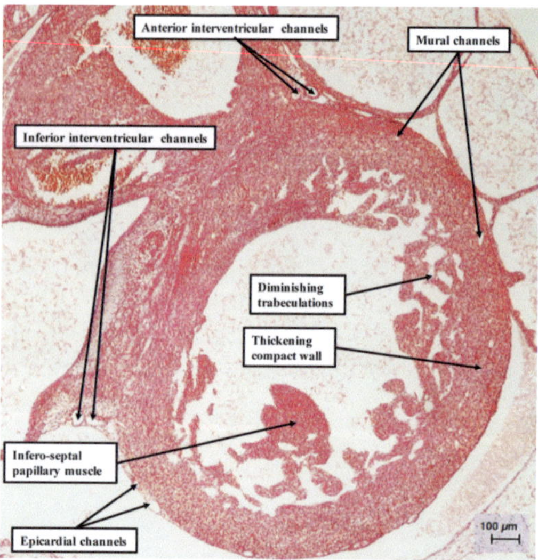

Fig. 1.8 The image shows the short axis of the left ventricle in a human embryo graded at Carnegie stage 22, which is in the eighth week of development. In this embryo, it is possible to recognise developing endothelial channels in both the interventricular grooves and the compact walls. The trabeculations are diminishing in their thickness, while the compact wall is thickening

nels within the walls of the embryo shown in Fig. 1.7, which had been graded as CS 23, it was possible to identify the channels in another human embryo retained in the Hamilton archive. This embryo had been considered to represent stage 22 (Fig. 1.8). The mural channels had only an endothelial wall. The vessels developing within the interventricular grooves, in contrast, were duplicated. One of the channels in both grooves, furthermore, was developing a smooth muscular component as part of its walls.

Evidence from Murine Development

At the moment, our access to human embryos is limited by the number of datasets available in the Human Developmental Biology Resource. Other datasets are in the process of preparation, and we anticipate being able to generate further information regarding the fate of the vascular channels seen already at CS 22. In this regard, we will further be able to assess the formation of the valvar

sinuses as we prepare material from the early weeks of the foetal period of development. We are able, nonetheless, already to support our concept of development on the basis of the availability of a large number of murine embryos and foetuses prepared using the technique of episcopic microscopy. In the mouse heart, the intrapericardial aorta becomes separated from the pulmonary trunk within the distal outflow tract at embryonic day 12.5. Embryonic day 13.5 in the mouse is the stage of beginning of closure of the embryonic interventricular communication, and hence comparable to CS 21 in humans. It is at this stage in the mouse that it becomes possible to identify the outgrowth of buds from the intrapericardial aortic trunk. As in humans, the buds originate distal to the boundary between the distal and middle parts of the outflow tract (Fig. 1.9).

By embryonic day 14.5, which is the day on which the interventricular communication is closed in the mouse, the orifices of the coronary arteries are evident in all embryos. The orifice of the right coronary artery, however, remains distal to the developing sinutubular junction, while the orifice of the left coronary artery is typically found at the level of the junction (Fig. 1.10).

With ongoing development during the foetal period, there is further regression of the distal border of the myocardium covering the middle part of the outflow tract, with this regression accompanied by further development of the arterial valvar sinuses. And, concomitant with the growth of the sinuses, the orifices of the coronary arteries are translocated so that, by embryonic day 15.5, they take their origin within the sinuses, proximal to the sinutubular junction (Fig. 1.11). At the same time, as was the case in the human heart, there is thickening of the compact components of the ventricular walls, accompanied by reciprocal diminution in thickness of the trabeculations. The trabeculations do coalesce to form the papillary muscles of the developing atrioventricular valves (Fig. 1.12). In the right ventricle, the trabeculations also coalesce to form the septomarginal and septoparietal trabeculations, with one trabeculation becoming prominent as the moderator band.

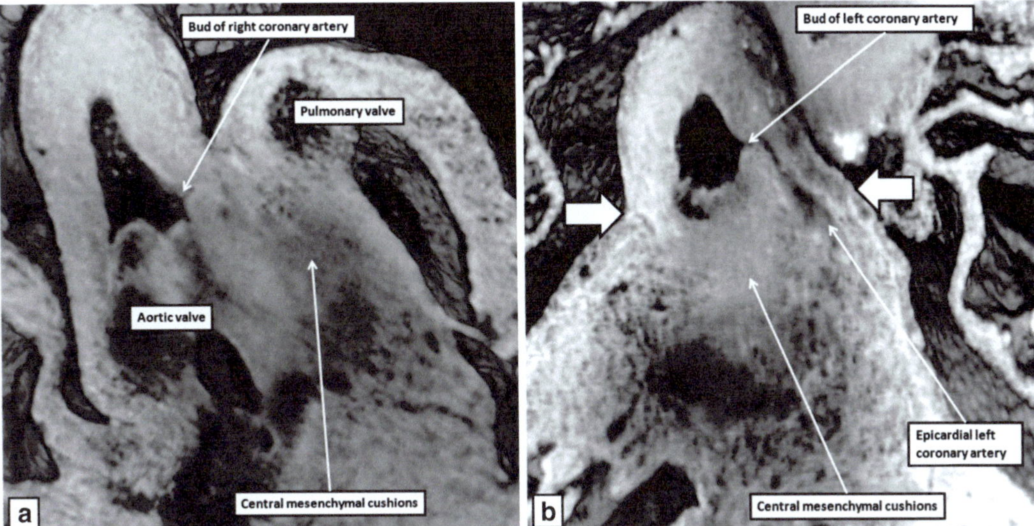

Fig. 1.9 The images are taken from the same three-dimensional dataset prepared from a mouse embryo at embryonic day 13.5. Panel A shows the origin of the bud of the right coronary artery distal to the boundary between the distal and middle parts of the outflow tract. Panel B shows the bud of the left coronary artery, again originating distal to the myocardial border, which is shown by the white arrows with black borders. The section showing the left coronary artery, however, has been taken to show its connection with the arteries developing from the peritruncal plexus within the myocardial wall of the middle part of the outflow tract

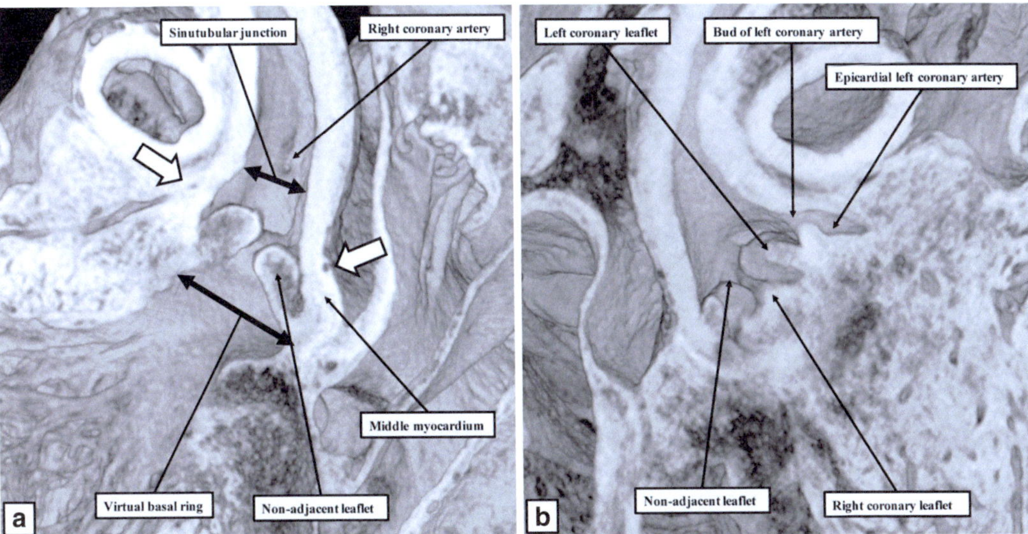

Fig. 1.10 The images are taken from a three-dimensional dataset prepared from a mouse embryo at embryonic day 14.5. Panel A shows how, at this stage, the orifice of the right coronary artery remains distal to the developing sinutubular junction. The left coronary artery, as shown in panel B, connects with the aortic root at the level of the sinutubular junction, with the epicardial component of the artery within the myocardial wall of the middle part of the outflow tract

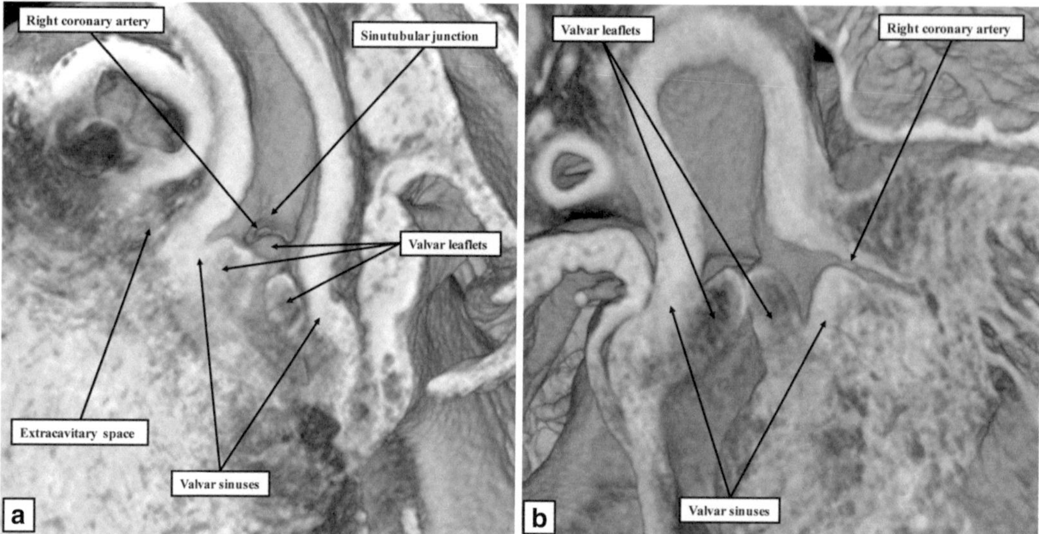

Fig. 1.11 The images are from a dataset prepared from a mouse foetus at embryonic day 15.5. Both coronary arteries have now been remodelled so as to arise within the valvar sinuses proximal to the sinutubular junction. These images show the origin of the right coronary artery, seen from the aspect of the right coronary aortic sinus in panel (**a**), and in cross-section in panel (**b**)

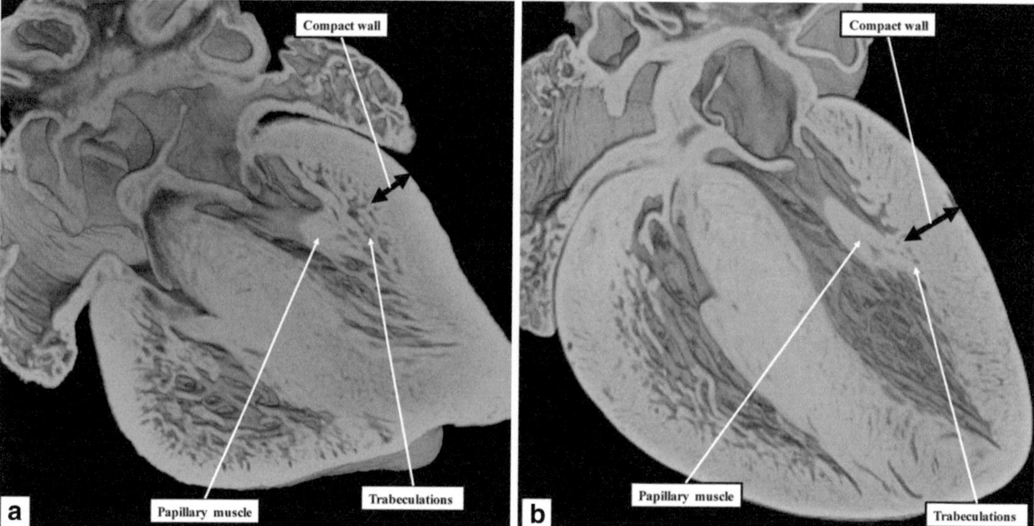

Fig. 1.12 The images are four chamber sections through the ventricular mass of mouse foetuses at embryonic day 15.5 (panel A) and 18.5 (panel B). They show how, subsequent to closure of the embryonic interventricular communication at embryonic day 14.5, there is ongoing thickening of the compact layer of the ventricular walls, with diminution in the part made of trabeculations. The trabeculations themselves, whilst not coalescing to form the compact wall, do come together to form the papillary muscles of the atrioventricular valves

Comment

The evidence from both developing human and murine embryos shows that the key stages of development of the coronary arteries take place during the transition from the embryonic to the foetal stages. It is at these stages, representing CSs 19 through 23 in human development, and then continuing through the initial weeks of foetal development subsequent to 8 weeks after fertilisation, that there is closure of the embryonic interventricular communication. This is combined with the transition during which the ventricular walls change to have predominantly compact rather trabeculated walls. The comparable changes in murine development take place during embryonic days 13.5 through 15.5. It is during these stages, furthermore, that the epicardial coronary arteries achieve their connection with the aortic root. Over the same period, the arterial circulation is developed with compact ventricular walls.

The manner of connection of the epicardial coronary arteries with the aortic root has long been controversial. The process was initially suggested to depend on the outgrowth of stems from the arterial roots. The stems, however, were alleged to sprout not only from the aortic sinuses, but also from the sinuses of the pulmonary root [25]. This notion was supplanted by the belief that the stems grew into the aortic root from the crown-like plexus formed within the middle part of the outflow tract [6]. The evidence is now overwhelming that the stems do, indeed, bud out from the aortic component of the outflow tract [7, 8, 19]. Our morphological evidence, however, reveals that the stems grow out from walls of the intrapericardial aorta distal to the developing sinutubular junction. They can first be recognised prior to any formation of the arterial valvar sinuses. Only with the ongoing formation of the sinuses are the arterial orifices translocated to achieve their anticipated definitive positions proximal to the sinutubular junctions. Lack of such translocation provides an obvious explanation for the frequent finding of distal origin of the coronary arteries relative to the sinutubular junction in otherwise normal hearts [26]. It is unlikely

to be coincidental, furthermore, that the high origin of the left coronary artery is a frequent finding in the setting of the aortic valve with two leaflets [27]. These findings point to an obvious relationship between maldevelopment of the arterial roots and abnormal origin of the coronary arteries. Further evidence in this regard is provided by the association of origin of the left coronary artery from the pulmonary trunk with the persistence of the aortopulmonary foramen as an aortopulmonary window [28]. The latter finding then points to completion of separation of the intrapericardial trunks and arterial roots one from the other as underscoring appropriate budding of the coronary arterial stems. It has been suggested that this process might be guided by "aortic cardiomyocytes" [7]. This term, however, is a contradiction in itself. The walls of the arterial valvar sinuses contain smooth muscle cells, rather than cardiomyocytes. The aortic root does have myocardium incorporated at the bases of the two sinuses that give rise to the coronary arteries. This myocardium is formed by the so-called "myocardialisation" of the outflow cushions. Its location at the bases of the aortic sinuses that usually give rise to the coronary arteries, nonetheless, could, be influential in determining the appropriate origin of the developing arterial stems. All three sinuses of the pulmonary root, however, are supported by comparable crescents of myocardium. Those arguing in favour of the role of "aortic cardiomyocytes" suggest that such cells are lacking in the pulmonary root [7]. This is manifestly not the case. The arterial stems, furthermore, originate distal to the myocardial border. And, when first formed, they take an intramural course through the adventitial linings of the developing sinusal walls. Abnormal development of the sinuses themselves, therefore, is more likely to be responsible for origin of one or other of the major coronary arteries from an inappropriate valvar sinus. Further studies on the mechanism of formation of the sinusal walls, and the incorporation of the coronary arterial orifices within the sinuses, will be required to resolve these issues.

The same goes for clarifying the morphogenesis of fistulous communications between the ventricular cavities and the epicardial coronary arteries. Such fistulous communications can be found as isolated lesions [3]. Much more frequently they are found as complicating malformations in the setting of hypoplasia of either the right or left ventricle when there is atresia of the arterial valve and an intact ventricular septum. When found in the setting of pulmonary atresia with an intact ventricular septum, the fistulous communications are most frequent when there is a so-called "unipartite" arrangement of the cavity. This occurs when mural hypertrophy has overgrown the apical trabecular and outlet ventricular components [29]. The finding implies that the insult responsible for the pulmonary atresia occurred early in foetal development, but subsequent to closure of the embryonic interventricular communication. When found in the setting of hypoplastic left heart syndrome, in contrast, the fistulous communications are found only in those phenotypes that include mitral stenosis rather than mitral atresia [30]. In both instances, nonetheless, the arrangements are suggestive that increased ventricular pressure is involved in creating the communications from the ventricular cavity, via the mural arterial circulation, to the epicardial coronary arteries, with the latter vessels then frequently becoming ectatic. Further investigations on the timing and mechanisms of formation of the mural arterial channels will be required to resolve these issues.

Acknowledgements Our study would not have been possible without access to the Human Developmental Biology Resource, housed at Newcastle University. We express our thanks to all those who prepared the datasets and made them available for online evaluation. We are also indebted to the archivists of the Hamilton collection of human embryos, initially housed at Charing Cross Hospital Medical School, transferred to St George's Medical University, but now maintained, along with the Boyd archive, at Cambridge University. Selected murine datasets are available for study in the website of the Crick Institute, London.

References

1. Rhee S, Chung JI, King DA, D'amato G, Paik DT, Duan A, Chang A, Nagelberg D, Sharma B, Jeong Y, Diehn M, Wu JC, Morrison AJ, Red-Horse K. Endothelial deletion of Ino80 disrupts coronary angiogenesis and causes congenital heart disease. Nat Commun. 2018;9:368–84.
2. Anderson RH, Jensen B, Mohun TJ, Petersen SE, Aung N, Zemrak F, Planken RN, MacIver DH. Key questions relating to left ventricular noncompaction cardiomyopathy-is the emperor still wearing any clothes? Can J Cardiol. 2017;33:747–57.
3. Perez-Pomares JM, de la Pompa JL, Franco D, et al. Congenital coronary artery anomalies: a bridge from embryology to anatomy and pathophysiology—a position statement of the development, anatomy, and pathology ESC working group. Cardiovasc Res. 2016;109:204–16.
4. Ogden JA. The origin of coronary arteries [Abstr]. Circulation. 1988;38:150.
5. Folkman J, Haudenschild C. Angiogenesis in vitro. Nature. 1980;288:551–6.
6. Bogers AJJC, Gittenberger-de Groot A, Poelmann R, et al. Development of the origin of the coronary arteries, a matter of ingrowth or outgrowth? Anat Embryol (Berl). 1989;180:437–41.
7. Chen HI, Poduri A, Numi H, et al. VEGF-C and aortic cardiomyocytes guide coronary artery stem development. J Clin Invest. 2014;124:4899–914.
8. Spicer DE, Henderson DJ, Chaudhry B, Mohun TJ, Anderson RH. The anatomy and development of normal and abnormal coronary arteries. Cardiol Young. 2015;25:1493–503.
9. Risau W, Flamme I. Vasculogenesis. Annu Rev Cell Biol Dev Biol. 1995;11:73–91.
10. Viragh S, Challice C. The origin of the epicardium and the embryonic myocardial circulation in the mouse. Anat Rec. 1981;201:157–68.
11. Poelmann R, Gittenberger-de Groot A, Mentink M, et al. Development of the cardiac coronary vascular endothelium, studied with antiendothelial antibodies, in chicken-quail chimeras. Circ Res. 1993;73:559–68.
12. Perez-Pomares JM, Macias D, Garcia-Garrido L, et al. The origin of the subepicardial mesenchyme in the avian embryo: an immunohistochemical and quailchick chimera study. Dev Biol. 1998;200:57–68.
13. Red-Horse K, Ueno H, Weissman IL, Krasnow M. Coronary arteries form by developmental reprogramming of venous cells. Nature. 2010;464:549–53.
14. Katz TC, Singh MK, Degenhardt K, et al. Distinct compartments of the proepicardial organ give rise to coronary vascular endothelial cells. Dev Cell. 2012;22:639–50.
15. Wu B, Zhang Z, Lui W, et al. Endocardial cells form the coronary arteries by angiogenesis through myocardial-endocardial VEGF signaling. Cell. 2012;151:1083–96.
16. Tian X, Hu T, Zhang H, et al. De novo formation of a distinct coronary vascular population in neonatal heart. Science. 2014;345:90–4.
17. Arima Y, Miyagawa-Tomita S, Maeda K, et al. Preotic neural crest cells contribute to coronary artery smooth muscle involving endothelin signalling. Nat Commun. 2012;3:1267.
18. Mellgren AM, Smith CL, Olsen GS, et al. Platelet-derived growth factor receptor beta sig-

naling is required for efficient epicardial cell migration and development of two distinct coronary vascular smooth muscle cell populations. Circ Res. 2008;103:1393–401.

19. Theveniau-Ruissy M, Perez-Pomares JM, Parisot P, Baldini A, Miquerol L, Kelly RG. Coronary stem development in wild-type and Tbx1 null mouse hearts. Dev Dyn. 2016;245:445–59.

20. Ruiz-Villalba A, Ziogas A, Ehrbar M, Perez-Pomares JM. Characterization of epicardial derived cardiac interstitial cells: differentiation and mobilization of heart fibroblast progenitors. PLoS One. 2013;8:e53694.

21. Ruiz-Villalba A, Simon AM, Pogontke C, et al. Interacting resident epicardium-derived fibroblasts and recruited bone marrow cells form myocardial infarction scar. J Am Coll Cardiol. 2015;65:2057–66.

22. O'Rahilly R, Muller F. Developmental stages in human embryos: revised and new measurements. Cells Tissues Organs. 2010;192:73–84.

23. Anderson RH, Chaudhry B, Mohun TJ, Bamforth SD, Hoyland D, Phillips HM, Webb S, Moorman AF, Brown NA, Henderson DJ. Normal and abnormal development of the intrapericardial arterial trunks in humans and mice. Cardiovasc Res. 2012;95:108–15.

24. Kramer TC. The partitioning of the truncus and conus and the formation of the membranous portion of the interventricular septum in the human heart. Am J Anat. 1942;71:343–70.

25. Hackensellner HA. Aksessorische Kransgeffäsanlagen der Arteria pulmonalis unter 63 meschlichen Embyonenserien mit einer grössten Lange von 12 bis 36 mm. Mikroscop Forschung. 1956;62:153–63.

26. Muriago M, Sheppard M, Ho S, Anderson R. The location of the coronary arterial orifices in the normal heart. Clin Anat. 1997;10:1–6.

27. Lerer PK, Edwards WD. Coronary arterial anatomy in bicuspid aortic valve. Necropsy study of 100 hearts. Br Heart J. 1981;45:142–7.

28. Hlavacek A, Loukas M, Spicer D. Anderson RH anomalous origin and course of the coronary arteries. Cardiol Young. 2010;20(Suppl 3):20–5.

29. Bull C, de Leval M, Mercanti C, Macartney FJ, Anderson RH. Pulmonary atresia with intact ventricular septum: a revised classification. Circulation. 1982;66:266–71.

30. Stephens EH, Gupta D, Bleiweis M, Backer CL, Anderson RH, Spicer DE. Coronary arterial abnormalities in Hypoplastic left heart syndrome: pathologic characteristics of archived specimens. Semin Thorac Cardiovasc Surg. 2020;32:531–8.

Congenital Anomalies of Coronary Arteries: Anatomy, Embryology and Risk of Sudden Death

Stefania Rizzo, Cristina Basso, Michela Muriago, and Gaetano Thiene

Anatomy of Coronary Arteries with Historical Notes

Arturo Banchi, assistant in anatomy to Prof. Chiarugi in Florence, published in 1903 the paper entitled "Morfologia delle arteriae coronariae cordis" (Fig. 2.1), first introducing the concept of coronary arterial patterns [1] (Fig. 2.2).

(a) Right dominant when the right coronary artery gives origin to the posterior descending artery ("branch of the posterior longitudinal groove") and branches to the posterior wall of the left ventricle.

(b) Left dominant when the posterior descending coronary artery and branches to the posterior left ventricular wall take origin from the left circumflex artery ("circumflex branch").

(c) Balanced when the posterior descending coronary artery takes origin from the right coronary artery whereas branches to the posterior left ventricular wall originate from the left circumflex artery.

At that time, the cause of myocardial infarction, by sudden coronary thrombotic occlusion, was not yet established. Nowadays, we are well aware of how much important is the coronary arterial pattern for the site and extension of myocardial infarction ("infarct related artery"). Moreover, among Bianchi's drawings, a coronary arterial branch called "right atrial branch" is well evident, arising from the right coronary artery in right dominant pattern and from the left circumflex artery in the left dominant pattern. We know that it is the artery for the sino-atrial node, which at that time had not been yet discovered as the cardiac pacemaker.

The variability of coronary artery network was confirmed with post-mortem casts by Giorgio Baroldi. His book, published in 1967, is known as the "Bible" of the anatomy and pathology of coronary arteries [2] (Fig. 2.3).

Overall, these information, deriving from research of anatomists and pathologists, would have become fundamental for the development of in vivo diagnosis, invented by Mason Sones at the Cleveland Clinic (Fig. 2.4) in 1962 by coronary angiography [3] and followed by surgical therapy of coronary artery disease, with aorto-coronary by-pass with saphenous vein by Renè Favaloro in 1967 [4] (Fig. 2.5).

S. Rizzo · C. Basso · G. Thiene (✉)
Department of Cardio-Thoraco-Vascular Sciences and Public Health, University of Padua, Medical School, Padua, Italy
e-mail: s.rizzo@unipd.it; cristina.basso@unipd.it; gaetano.thiene@unipd.it

M. Muriago
Internal Medicine, Pietro Milani Ospital, Noventa Vicentina, Vicenza, Italy

© Springer Nature Switzerland AG 2023
G. Butera, A. Frigiola (eds.), *Congenital Anomalies of Coronary Arteries*,
https://doi.org/10.1007/978-3-031-36966-7_2

Fig. 2.1 Title page of
Dott. Banchi paper

Istituto Anatomico di Firenze, diretto dal Prof. G. Chiarugi.

Banchi Dott. Arturo

Aiuto e Libero docente.

Morfologia delle *arteriae coronariae cordis*.

(Con 38 figure)

Ricevuta il 15 giugno 1903

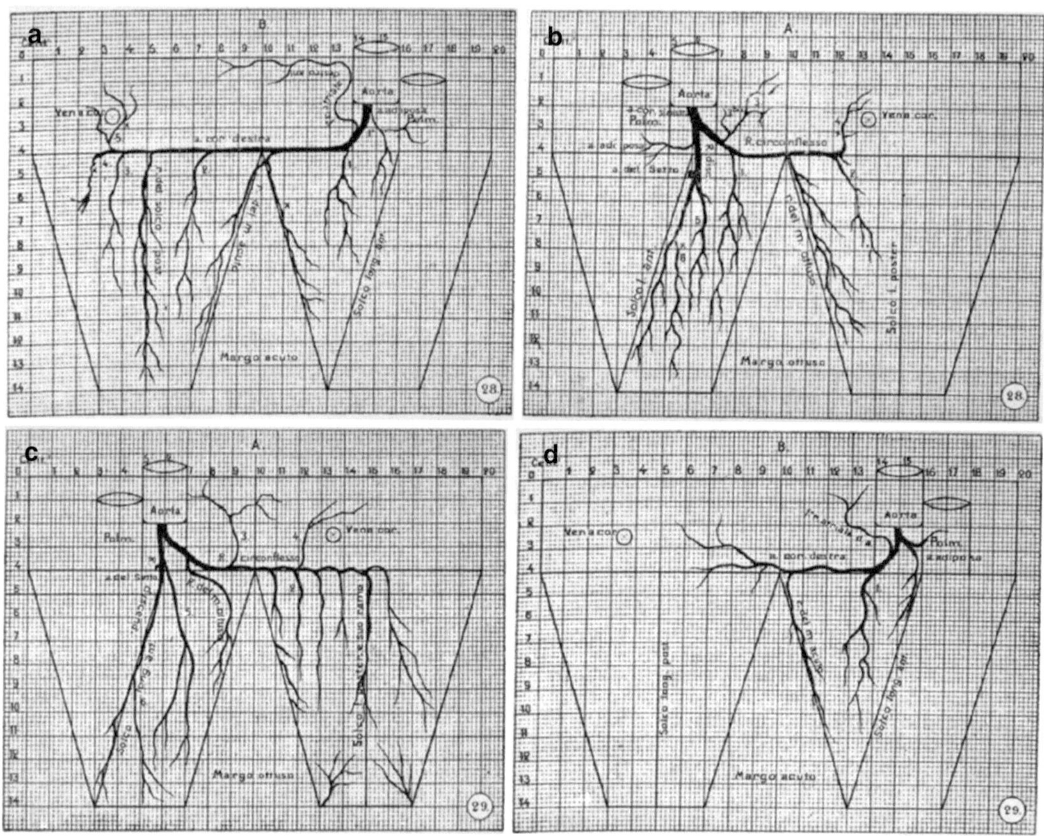

Fig. 2.2 The original drawings of coronary artery patterns. (**a**, **b**) Right dominance and (**c**, **d**) left dominance. From
Banchi A [1]

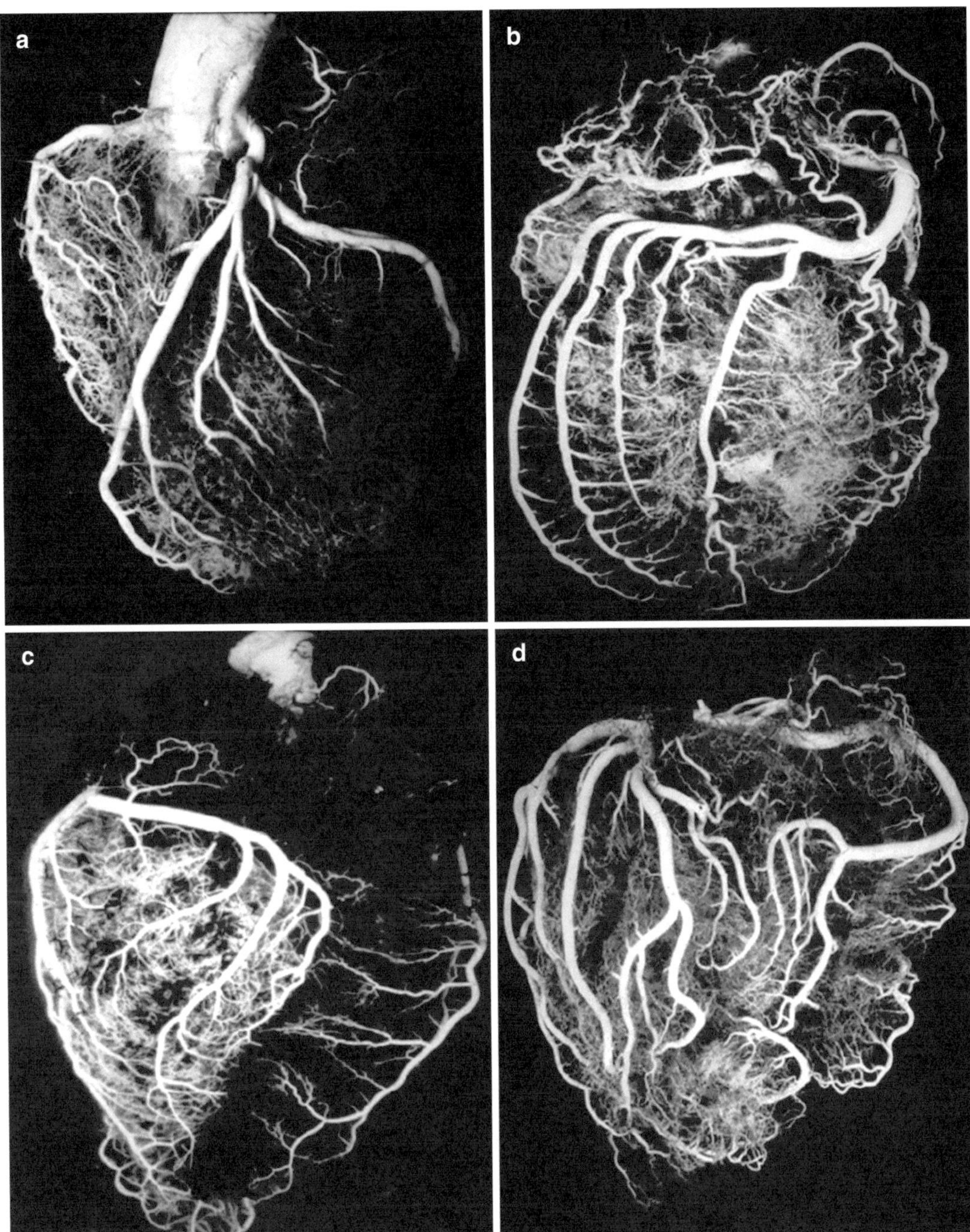

Fig. 2.3 Postmortem casts of coronary arteries. (**a**) Left coronary artery anatomy, (**b**) dominant right pattern, (**c**) dominant left pattern, and (**d**) balanced pattern. From Baroldi G et al. [2]

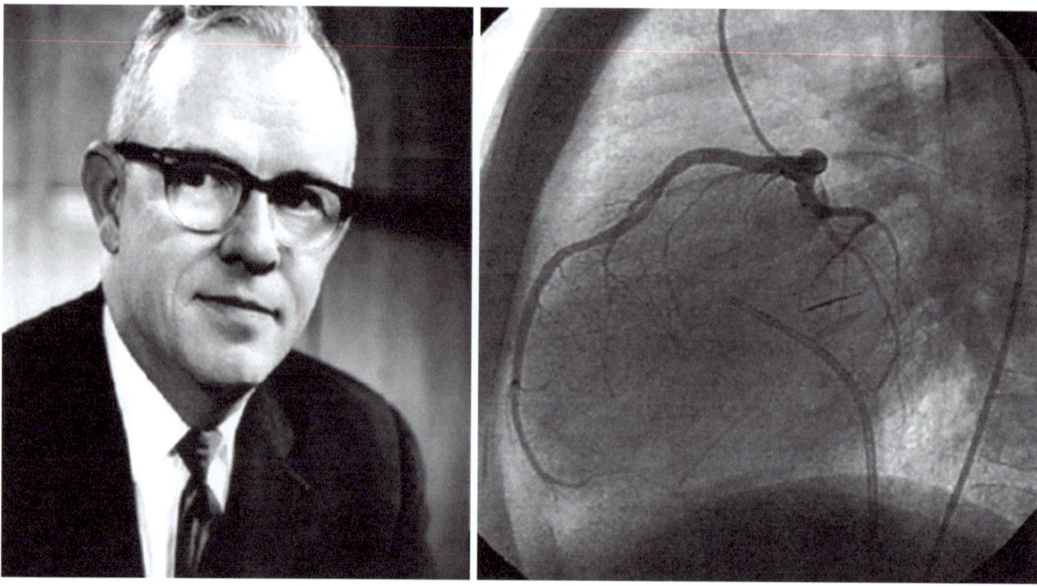

Fig. 2.4 Mason Sones (1918–1985), the inventor of selective coronary angiography (1962)

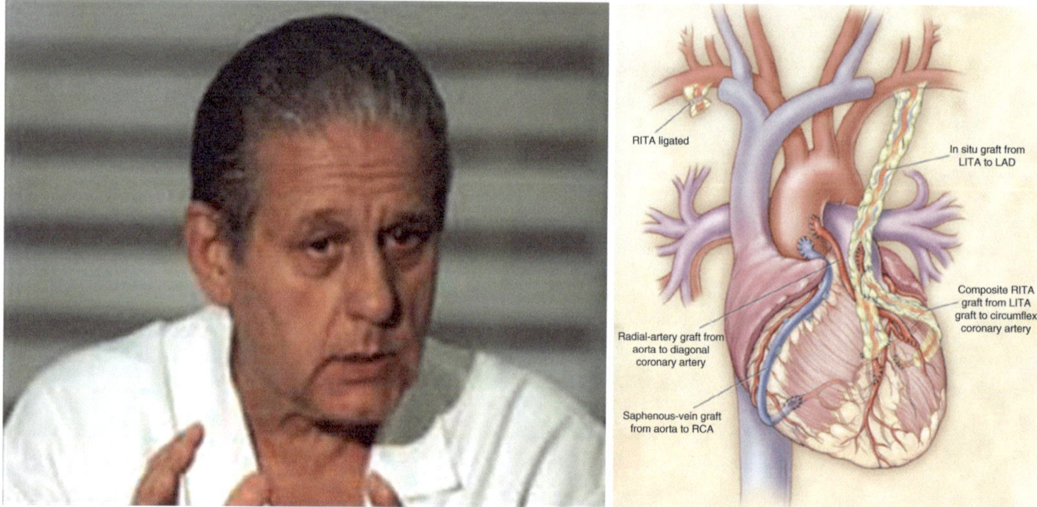

Fig. 2.5 René Favaloro (1923–2000). The inventor of aorto-coronary bypass with autologous saphenous vein (1967)

Embryology of Coronary Arteries

Both subepicardial coronary arteries (CAs) and veins derive from epicardial cells [5, 6].

Their development begins with the formation of a plexus-like vasculature, located in the subepicardium, which invades the myocardium and develops small vessels and capillaries.

Earlier, the myocardial blood supply originated directly from the ventricular cavities through the intertrabecular spaces lined by endocardium (Fig. 2.6a). This source of blood to the primitive spongy myocardium disappears with the myocardial compaction (Fig. 2.6b). At this point, the whole intramyocardial vascularization consists of vessels with endothelium derived from the subepicardium [6–8].

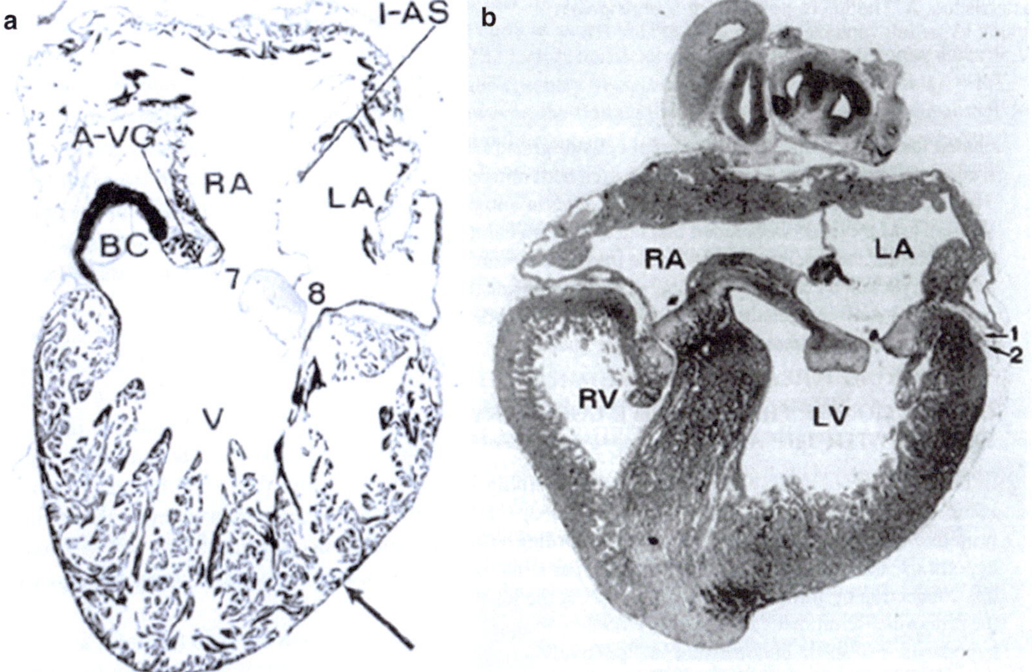

Fig. 2.6 Embryology of the myocardium. (**a**) Spongy myocardium with blood supply deriving directly from the endocardium of the ventricular cavities. (**b**) The myocardium becomes compact, with blood supply deriving from the subepicardial vasculature

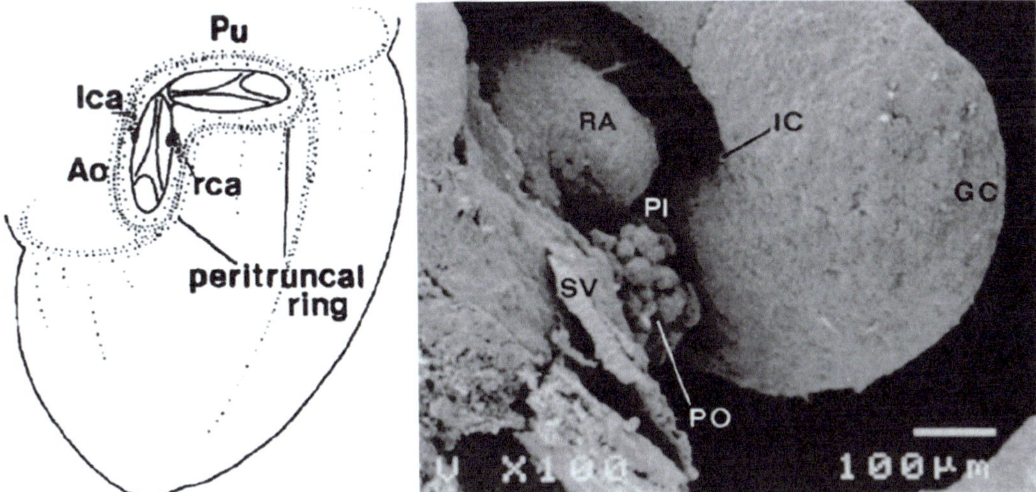

Fig. 2.7 Origin of coronary arterial stems from the peritruncal epicardial ring

The origin of both CAs and veins, whether intra- or extramural, is similar. Their definitive identity and function depend upon the connection, arteries with the aorta, and veins with the sinus venosus.

A subepicardial network of cells surrounds the orifices of the great arteries (peritruncal ring) and eventually connects with the facing aortic sinuses [5, 9] (Fig. 2.7). The question is whether the development of CAs origin is a matter of ingrowth or outgrowth [10]. There are two hypotheses to explain the connection.

The first is the outgrowth hypothesis, namely, the development of sprouts or buds from the aortic wall of facing sinuses, capturing the peritruncal ring of coronary subepicardial arterial vasculature [5, 11] (Fig. 2.8).

The second developmental hypothesis is supported by the observation that the prongs of the peritruncal ring penetrate the aortic wall and make contact with the endothelial lining of the aorta [9, 10] (Fig. 2.9).

Until the late 1980s, it was thought that CAs entirely derived from an aortic endothelial outgrowth that would expand to form the complete coronary system, including coronary veins. Further research in avian models partially argued against this, demonstrating that CA endothelial cells do not bud from the aortic root, but instead grow into the aortic wall from the aortic peritruncal plexus to connect to the systemic circulation, most likely under the guidance of vascular endothelial growth factor (VEGF) and periaortic cardiomyocytes. At least part of the early arterial coronary vascular system forms through a process of vasculogenesis with subsequent fusion of endothelial cell clusters to form new blood vessels [12, 13].

Recent investigations confirmed that the proximal CAs do not grow from the aorta. In the contrary, they develop from the peritruncal ring of the subepicardial vascular plexus [14, 15] penetrating into the aorta.

Septation of the arterial pole of the heart (42 days in the human embryo) precedes the appearance of coronary ostia when cells from the peritruncal ring migrate into the aortic root. Septation therefore cannot be responsible for the final position of coronary orifices.

Formation of the left CA precedes the right CA.

Moreover, unlike from the tunica media of the ascending aorta, the tunica media of the CAs does not derive from the neural crest.

Cellular cross-talks and signaling pathways take place (notch and hippo signals, transcription factors, angiogenic molecules, and apoptosis) [16–20]. VEGF plays a crucial role in the development of coronary ostia and main stem formation [14]. Absence of VEGF was shown to inhibit ostia formation. Epicardial inhibition, reducing apoptotic remodelling at the ventricular-arterial junction, alters vascular connection with the aorta and may produce CA anomalies equal to those observed in humans [21].

Why the primitive subepicardial coronary arterial vasculature tends to connect with the facing aortic sinuses, instead of facing pulmonary sinuses, is still a mystery. The explanation cannot be the posterior position of the aorta since in

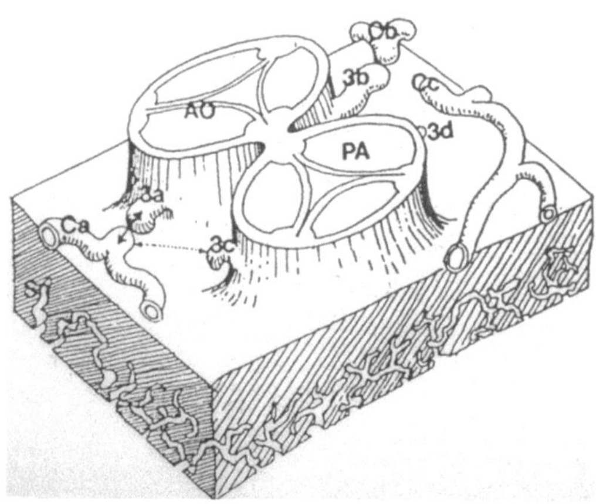

Fig. 2.8 The hypothesis according to which sprouts or buds arise from the facing aortic sinuses and make contact with the subepicardial coronary vasculature

Fig. 2.9 Ingrowth Developmental Hypothesis with cells of the peritruncal ring penetrating the aortic wall. (**a–e**) show the progression of the ingrowth of epicardial cells trouth thye aortic wall until the endocardium

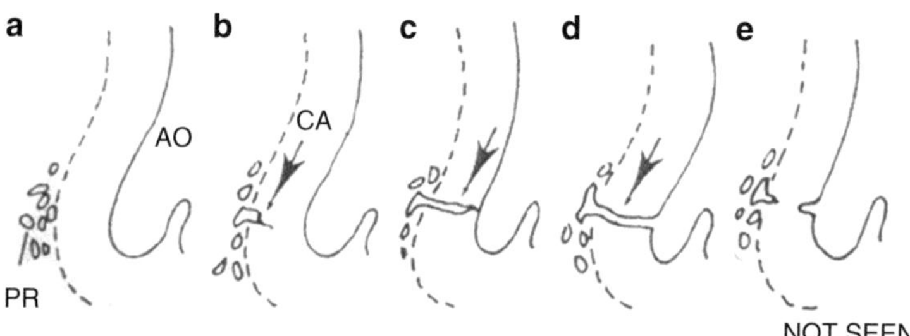

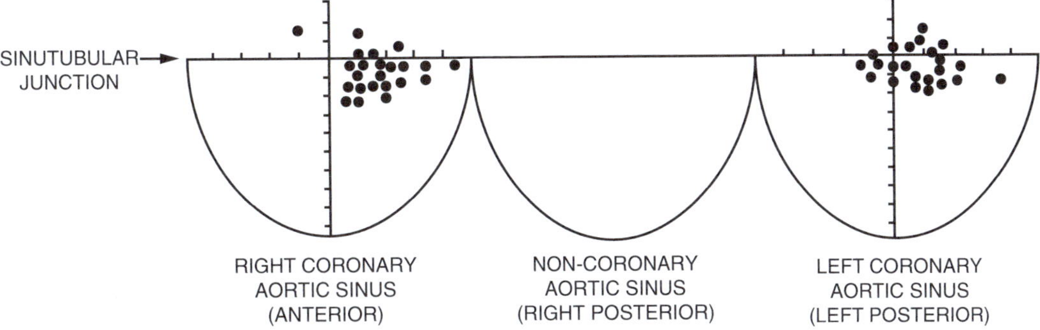

Fig. 2.10 The topographical variability of coronary artery orifices in normal hearts. From Muriago M. et al. [32]

transposition of the great arteries (TGA), where the aorta is anterior, the CAs regularly arise from the facing sinuses of the aorta. Indeed, an anomalous origin of a coronary artery from the posterior pulmonary artery in TGA is quite rare [22, 23].

Coronary Artery Anomalies

The incidence of reported coronary artery anomalies is [15, 24–29]

- 0.17% in autopsy,
- 1.2% in coronary angiography, and
- 0.17% in echo series.

Ogden [30] distinguished major anomalies, like coronary artery origin from the pulmonary artery, and minor anomalies, such as high take off, single coronary artery, and origin from a wrong coronary sinus. However, this classification turned out to be untenable, since even some Ogden "minor" anomalies were proven to be life-threatening as well.

Familial clustering of coronary artery anomalies has been sporadically reported [31]. It does not exceed the rate of recurrence in siblings and off-springs of other congenital heart diseases and, as such, they cannot be considered a Mendelian disorder.

There is a large spectrum of coronary artery anomalies, from variants of normal without functional significance to real morbid entities at risk of myocardial infarction and sudden death.

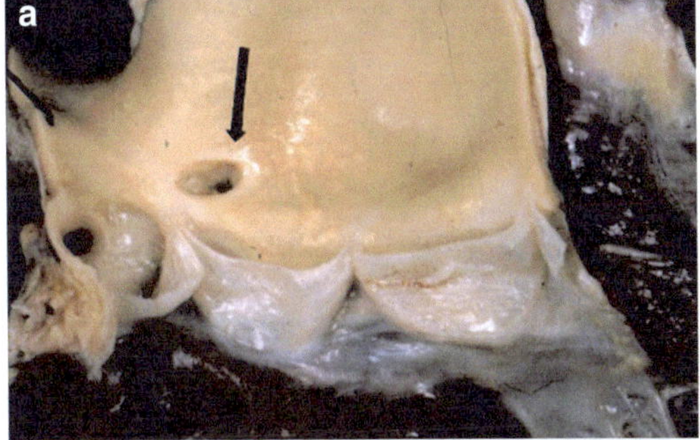

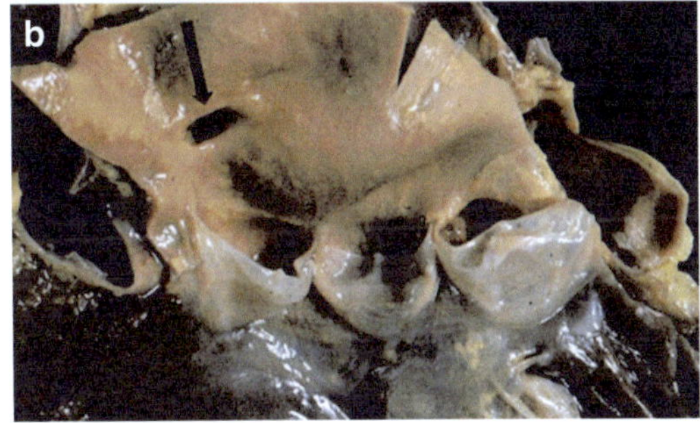

Fig. 2.11 (a) The right coronary artery orifice (arrow) is just above (2 mm) the sino-tubular junction, within normal limits. (b) The right coronary orifice (arrow) is well above the sino-tubular junction (10 mm), over the threshold of normal limits. From Thiene, G., Corrado, D., Basso, C. (2016). Coronary Artery Disease. In: Sudden Cardiac Death in the Young and Athletes. Springer, Milano. https://doi.org/10.1007/978-88-470-5776-0_3

(a) *Variants of normal*

- High take off from the aortic root with coronary ostium located less than 2.5 mm above the sino-tubular junction [32, 33] (Figs. 2.10 and 2.11).

Fig. 2.12 The first historical description of myocardial bridge made in 1834 by Leopoldo and Floriano Caldani, Professors of Anatomy at the University of Padua

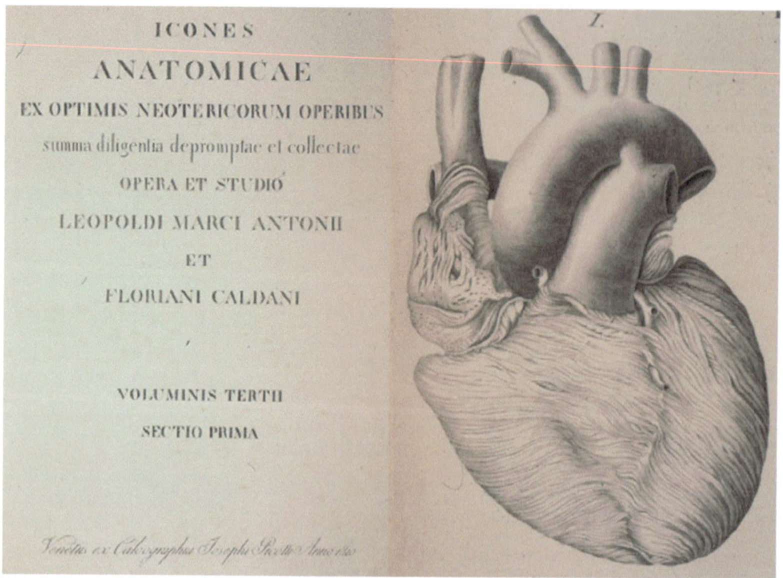

- Myocardial bridge with a short, not deep intramural course of a coronary artery branch (mostly descending coronary artery), observed in 30% of individuals [33–38] (Fig. 2.12).
- Separate origin of the left anterior descending and left circumflex arteries, in the absence of left coronary trunk [33, 39].
- Double left anterior descending coronary artery [2, 33] (Fig. 2.13).
- Left anterior descending coronary artery taking origin from the right coronary artery and crossing the pulmonary infundibular, at risk during surgical infundibulotomy [39].

(b) *Uncertain morbid significance*

- High take off-ostium located >2.5 mm from the sino-tubular junction [40, 41] (Fig. 2.14)
- Origin of the right coronary artery from the left sinus
- Single coronary artery (Fig. 2.15)
- Valve-like ridge in front of a coronary ostium [42] (Fig. 2.16)

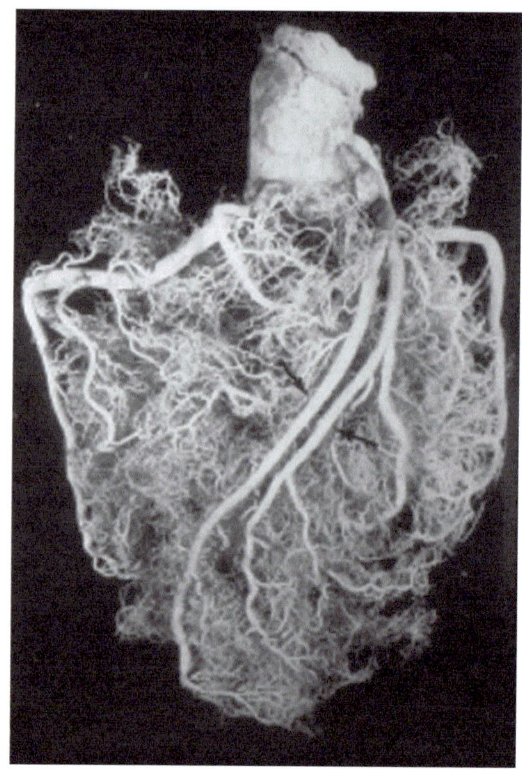

Fig. 2.13 Double left anterior descending coronary artery

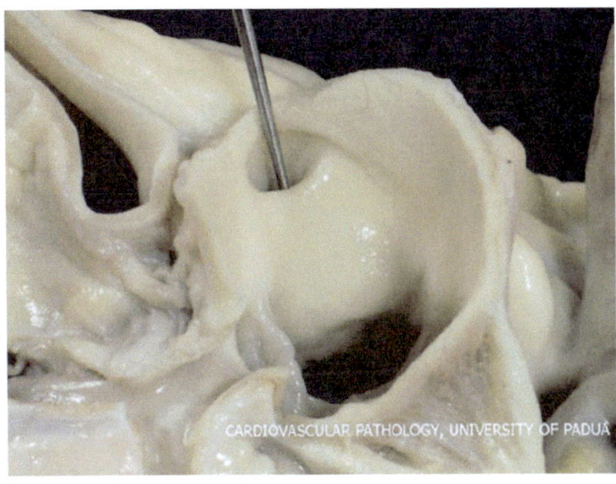

Fig. 2.14 High take off

- Short and superficial myocardial bridge in HCM [43–47] (Fig. 2.17)
- Congenital coronary aneurysm

(c) *Anomalies at risk of sudden death (as sole explanation of fatal outcome)*

- Origin from the pulmonary artery [48, 49] (Fig. 2.18)
- Origin of the left coronary artery from wrong right aortic sinus [50–55] (Fig. 2.19)

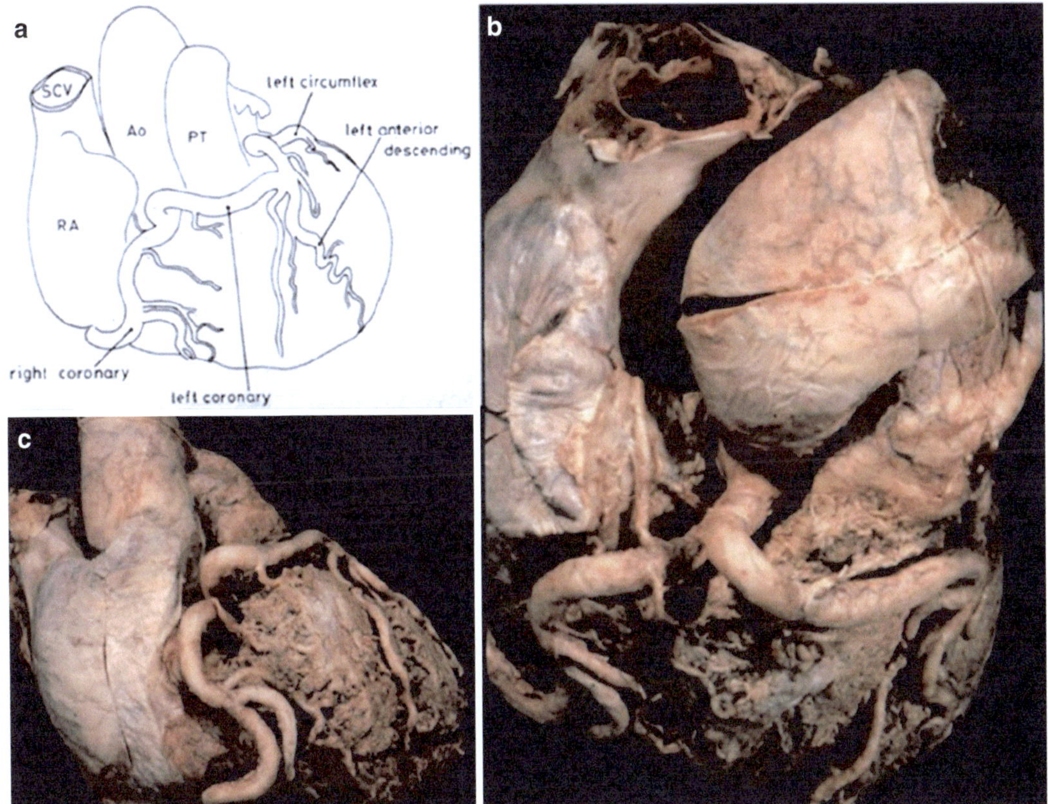

Fig. 2.15 Single right coronary artery. (**a**) Drawing of gross picture (**b**) and (**c**). *AO* aorta, *PA* pulmonary trunc, *RA* right atrium, *SCV* superior caval vein

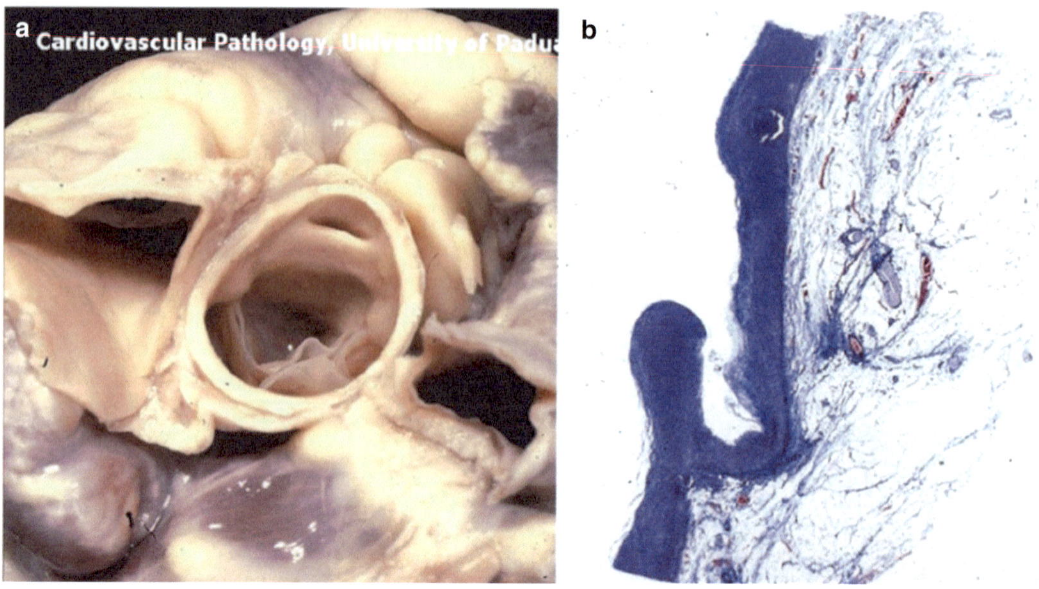

Fig. 2.16 Valve-like ridge obstructing the left coronary ostium. (**a**) gross view; (**b**) histology, Azan-Mallory stain

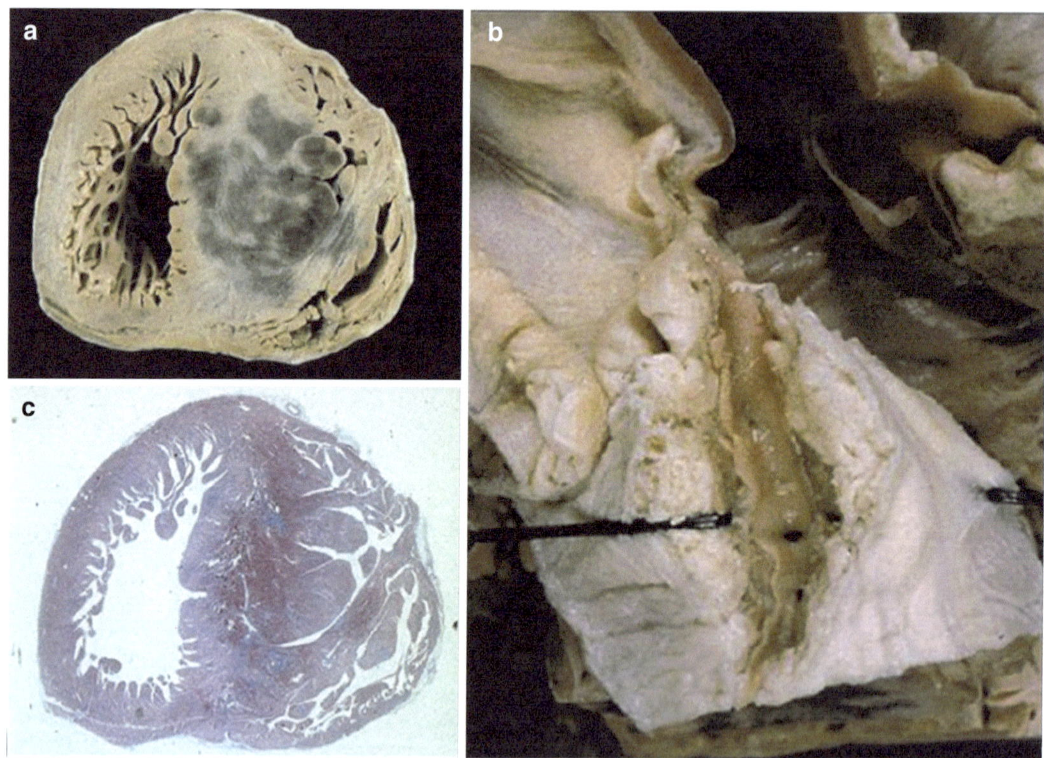

Fig. 2.17 The heart of a boy with Hypertrophic Cardiomyopathy. A cross-section of the heart (**a**) remarkable asymmetric septal hypertrophy (25-mm septal thickness vs 7-mm thickness of the left ventricular free wall); in the center is a dark red area. (**b**) the anterior view of the heart. The proximal middle tract of the left anterior descending coronary artery show a deep and long intramural course. The region of the first and second septal perforators corresponds to the location of the myocardial bridging. A panoramic histologic view (**c**) shows coagulation and reperfusion necrosis of the septal myocardium (trichrome–Heidenhain stain). From Gori F et al. [47]

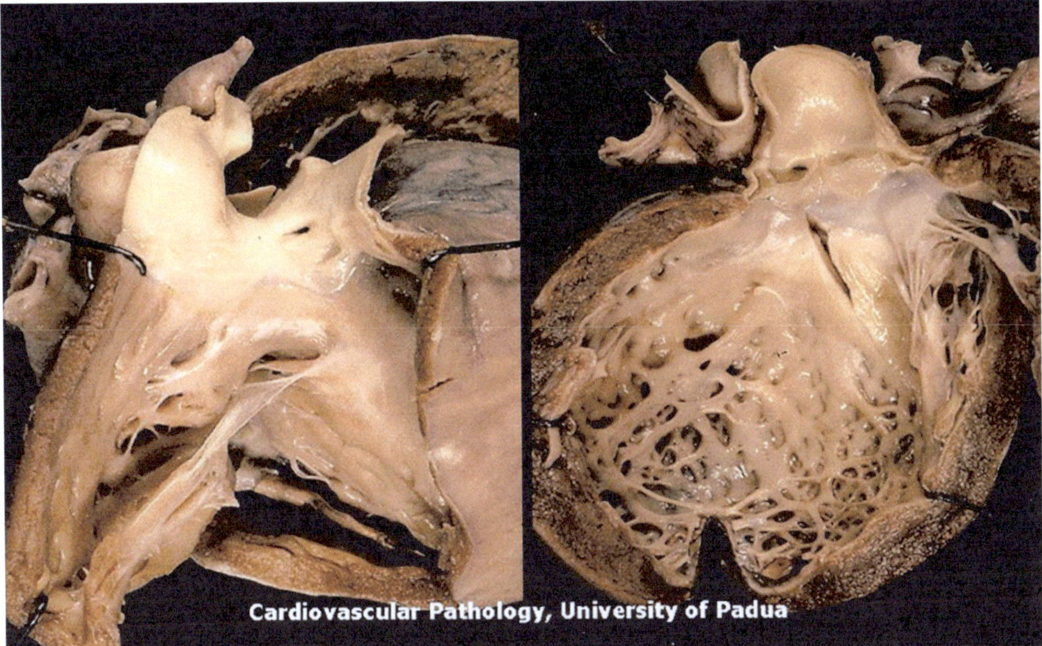

Fig. 2.18 Origin of the left coronary artery from the pulmonary artery. From Thiene, G., Corrado, D., Basso, C. (2016). Coronary Artery Disease. In: Sudden Cardiac Death in the Young and Athletes. Springer, Milano. https://doi.org/10.1007/978-88-470-5776-0_3

- Myocardial bridge, deep >5 mm, long >2.5 cm with a myocardial circular sleeve with disarray [56, 57] (Fig. 2.20)
- Left circumflex from right sinus coronary artery, with retro-aortic course [56, 58, 59] (Fig. 2.21)

- Coronary ostia sequestration [60] (Fig. 2.22).
- Coronary fistula

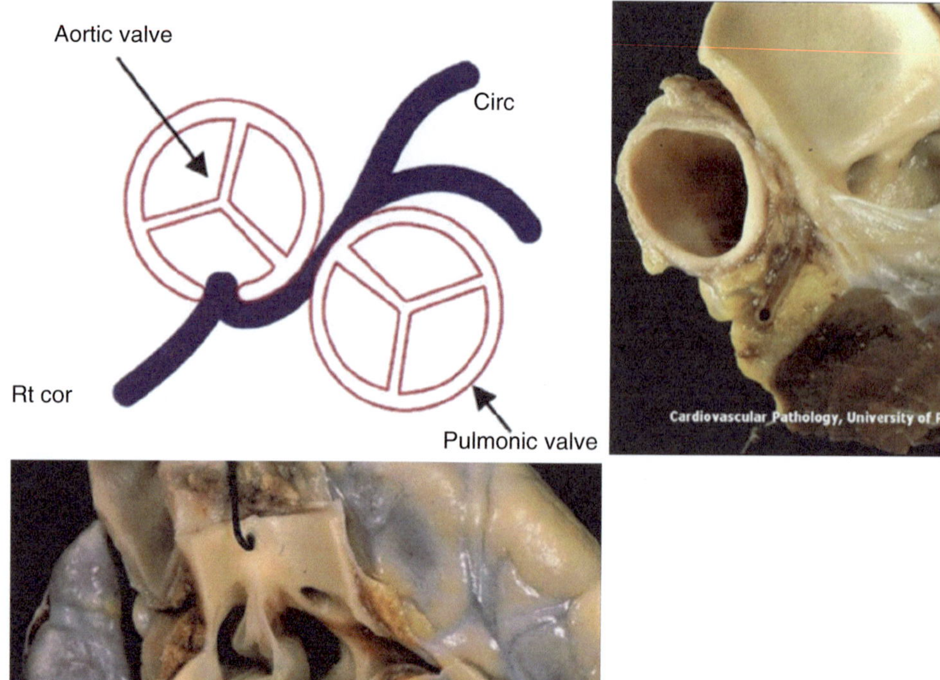

Fig. 2.19 Origin of the left coronary artery from the wrong right aortic sinus. From Thiene, G., Corrado, D., Basso, C. (2016). Coronary Artery Disease. In: Sudden Cardiac Death in the Young and Athletes. Springer, Milano. https://doi.org/10.1007/978-88-470-5776-0_3

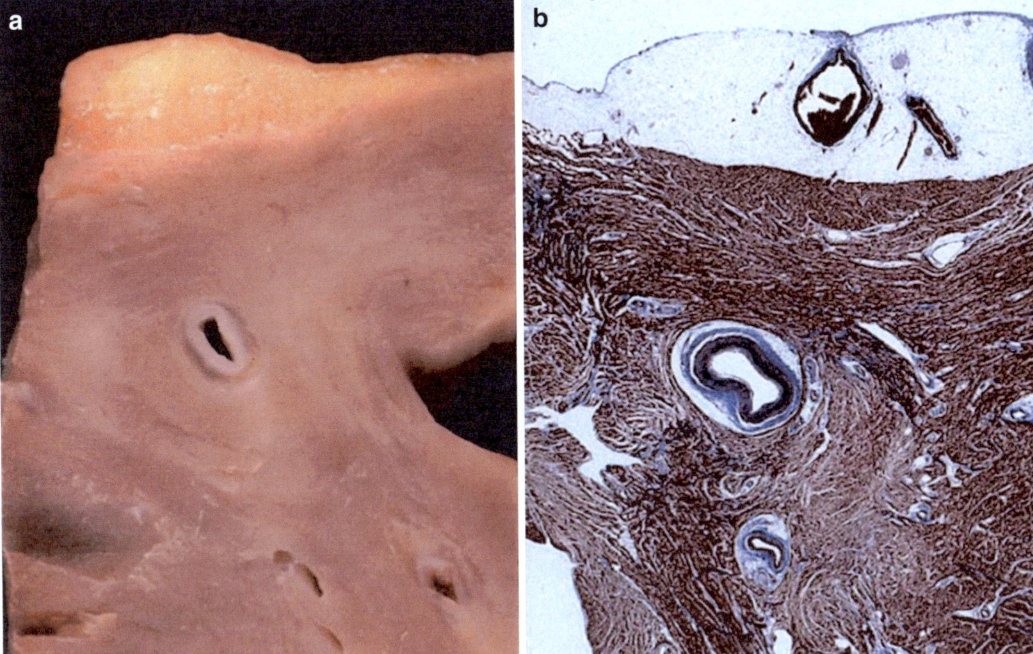

Fig. 2.20 Myocardial bridge with deep intramural course: the coronary segment is completely surrounded by a myocardial sleeve. Gross (**a**) and histological views (**b**). Azan Mallory stain. From Thiene, G., Corrado, D., Basso, C. (2016). Coronary Artery Disease. In: Sudden Cardiac Death in the Young and Athletes. Springer, Milano. https://doi.org/10.1007/978-88-470-5776-0_3

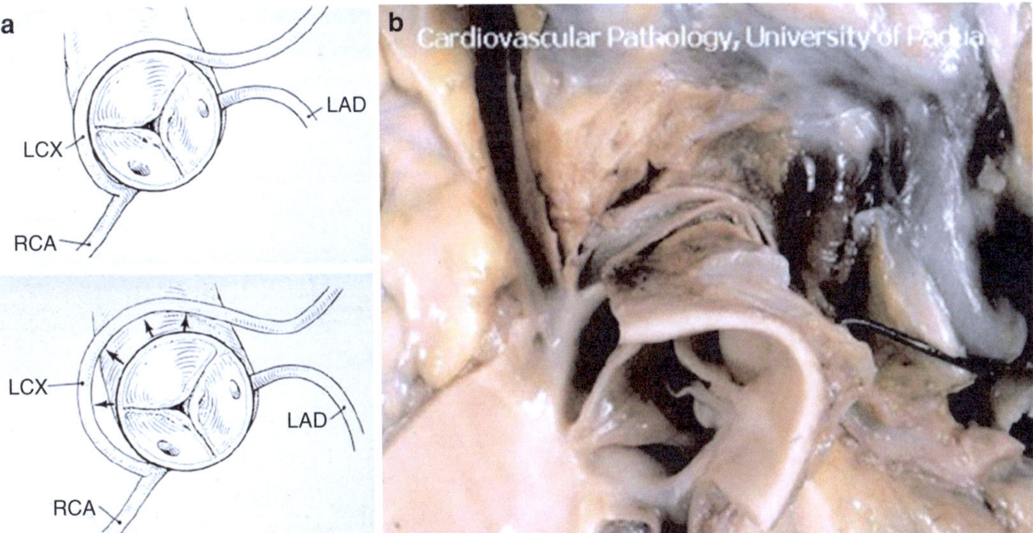

Fig. 2.21 LCx from RCA (**a**) Diagram with origin of the left circumflex artery from the right coronary artery and retro-aortic course. From Roberts [39]. (**b**) Gross view of the aortic root. Arrow indicates the retro-aortic course of the anomalous left circumflex artery. From Thiene, G., Corrado, D., Basso, C. (2016). Coronary Artery Disease. In: Sudden Cardiac Death in the Young and Athletes. Springer, Milano. https://doi.org/10.1007/978-88-470-5776-0_3

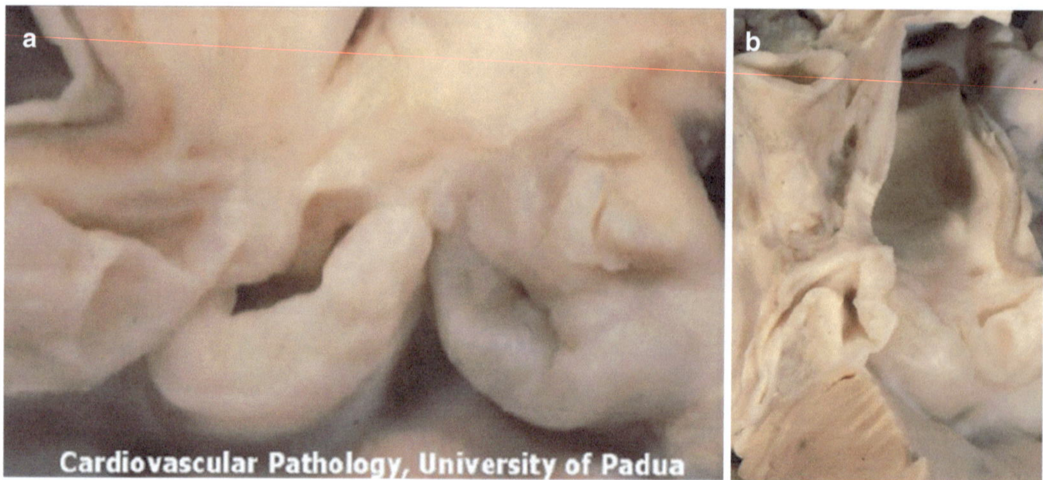

Fig. 2.22 Coronary ostia sequestration in Williams syndrome

Coronary Artery Anomalies and Sudden Cardiac Death

Coronary artery anomalies account for a significant burden of sudden cardiac deaths in the young and particularly in athletes [61–70]. Of 75 consecutive cases of sudden death in athletes, studied pathologically in the time interval 1981–2014 in the Veneto Region, Italy, 12 (16%) (Fig. 2.23) were ascribed to congenital malformations of coronary arteries, either of origin or course [71]. They represent the third morbid entity as the sole explanation of the fatal outcome, following arrhythmogenic cardiomyopathy (27%) and coronary atherosclerosis (24%). Clearly, their detection at pre-participation screening for competitive sports eligibility plays a fundamental role in sudden death prevention [72]. It represents a great challenge, since it requires clinical imaging, ECG (both 12 leads basal and stress test) having a scarce sensibility to raise the suspicion.

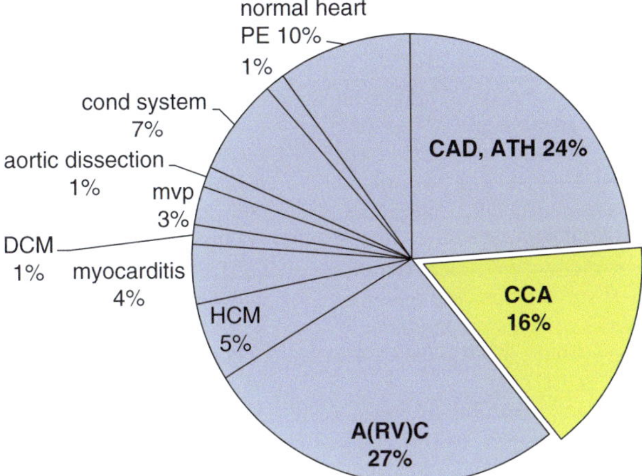

Fig. 2.23 Causes of Sudden Cardiac Death in 75 athletes, Veneto Region Registry, Italy (1981–2014). Coronary artery anomalies accounted for 16% of cases. *A(RV)C* arrhythmogenic right ventricular cardiomyopathy, *CAD* coronary artery disease, *ATH* atherosclerosis, *CCA* congenital coronary anomalies, *DCM* dilated cardiomyopathy, *HCM* hypertrophic cardiomyopathy, *mpv* mitral valve prolapse, *PE* pulmonary embolism

Causal Relationship Between Coronary Artery Anomalies and SCD

According to the autopsy guidelines for the study of SCD cases of the Association for European Cardiovascular Pathology [73, 74]:

1. Only the origin from the pulmonary trunk should be considered as a *certain* cause of SCD.
2. The origin of left coronary artery from the opposite wrong right sinus of Valsalva has been classified as a *highly probable* cause of SCD.
3. Other forms (right from left sinus, left circumflex from right sinus and retro-aortic course, high take off, and myocardial bridging) are classified as *uncertain* cause.
4. If uncertain, in the absence of other structural abnormalities, molecular investigation together with family genetic study cascade should be carried to rule out pathogen mutations for channelopathies.

References

1. Banchi A. Le. variazioni delle arteriae coronariae cordis e la morfologia di questi vasi. Sperimentale. 1903;57:367–9.
2. Baroldi G, Scomazzoni G. Coronary circulation in the Normal and pathologic heart. Washington DC: Office of the Surgeon General, Department of the Army; 1967. p. 1–37.
3. Sones FM, Shirey EK. Cine coronary arteriography. Mod Concepts Cardiovasc Dis. 1962;31:735–8.
4. Effler DB, Groves LK, Suarez EL, Favaloro RG. Direct coronary artery surgery with endarterotomy and patch-graft reconstruction. Clinical application and technical considerations. J Thorac Cardiovasc Surg. 1967;53(1):93–101.
5. de la Cruz MV, Moreno-Rodriguez R, Angelini P. ontogeny of the coronary vessels. In: Angelini P, Fairchild VD, editors. Coronary artery anomalies: a comprehensive approach. Philadelphia, PA: Lippincott; 1999. p. 11–6.
6. Winter EM, Gittenberger-de Groot AC. Epicardium-derived cells in cardiogenesis and cardiac regeneration. Cell Mol Life Sci. 2007;64:692–703. https://doi.org/10.1007/s00018-007-6522-3.
7. Waldo KL, Willner W, Kirby ML. Origin of the proximal coronary artery stems and a review of ventricular vascularization in the chick embryo. Am J Anat. 1990;188:109–20. https://doi.org/10.1002/aja.1001880202.

8. Poelmann RE, Gittenberger-de Groot AC, Mentink MM, Bökenkamp R, Hogers B. Development of the cardiac coronary vascular endothelium, studied with antiendothelial antibodies, in chicken-quail chimeras. Circ Res. 1993;73:559–68. https://doi.org/10.1161/01.RES.73.3.559.

9. Bogers AJ, Gittenberger-de Groot AC, Dubbeldam JA, Huysmans HA. The inadequacy of existing theories on development of the proximal coronary arteries and their connexions with the arterial trunks. Int J Cardiol. 1988;20:117–23. https://doi.org/10.1016/0167-5273(88)90321-X.

10. Bogers AJ, Gittenberger-de Groot AC, Poelmann RE, Péault BM, Huysmans HA. Development of the origin of the coronary arteries, a matter of ingrowth or outgrowth? Anat Embryol (Berl). 1989;180:437–41. https://doi.org/10.1007/BF00305118.

11. Angelini P. Normal and anomalous coronary arteries: definitions and classification. Am Heart J. 1989;117:418–34. https://doi.org/10.1016/0002-8703(89)90789-8.

12. Pérez-Pomares JM, Macías D, García-Garrido L, Muñoz-Chápuli R. The origin of the subepicardial mesenchyme in the avian embryo: an immunohistochemical and quail-chick chimera study. Dev Biol. 1998;200:57–68. https://doi.org/10.1006/dbio.1998.8949.

13. Mikawa T, Fischman DA. Retroviral analysis of cardiac morphogenesis: discontinuous formation of coronary vessels. Proc Natl Acad Sci U S A. 1992;89:9504–8. https://doi.org/10.1073/pnas.89.20.9504.

14. Tomanek R, Angelini P. Embryology of coronary arteries and anatomy/pathophysiology of coronary anomalies. A comprehensive update. Int J Cardiol. 2019;281:28–34. https://doi.org/10.1016/j.ijcard.2018.11.135.

15. Pérez-Pomares JM, de la Pompa JL, Franco D, Henderson D, Ho SY, Houyel L, et al. Congenital coronary artery anomalies: a bridge from embryology to anatomy and pathophysiology–a position statement of the development, anatomy, and pathology ESC working group. Cardiovasc Res. 2016;109:204–16. https://doi.org/10.1093/cvr/cvv251.

16. Eralp I, Lie-Venema H, DeRuiter MC, van den Akker NMS, Bogers AJJC, Mentink MMT, et al. Coronary artery and orifice development is associated with proper timing of epicardial outgrowth and correlated Fas-ligand-associated apoptosis patterns. Circ Res. 2005;96:526–34. https://doi.org/10.1161/01.RES.0000158965.34647.4e.

17. Mu H, Ohashi R, Lin P, Yao Q, Chen C. Cellular and molecular mechanisms of coronary vessel development. Vasc Med. 2005;10:37–44. https://doi.org/10.1191/1358863x05vm584ra.

18. Lie-Venema H, Gittenberger-de Groot AC, van Empel LJ, Boot MJ, Kerkdijk H, de Kant E, et al. Ets-1 and Ets-2 transcription factors are essential for normal coronary and myocardial development in chicken embryos. Circ Res. 2003;92:749–56. https://doi.org/10.1161/01.RES.0000066662.70010.DB.

19. van den Akker NM, Caolo V, Wisse LJ, Peters PP, Poelmann RE, Carmeliet P, et al. Developmental coronary maturation is disturbed by aberrant cardiac vascular endothelial growth factor expression and notch signalling. Cardiovasc Res. 2008;78:366–75. https://doi.org/10.1093/cvr/cvm108.

20. Lavine KJ, Ornitz DM. Shared circuitry: developmental signaling cascades regulate both embryonic and adult coronary vasculature. Circ Res. 2009;104:159–69. https://doi.org/10.1161/CIRCRESAHA.108.191239.

21. Gittenberger-de Groot AC, Vrancken Peeters MP, Bergwerff M, Mentink MM, Poelmann RE. Epicardial outgrowth inhibition leads to compensatory mesothelial outflow tract collar and abnormal cardiac septation and coronary formation. Circ Res. 2000;87:969–71. https://doi.org/10.1161/01.RES.87.11.969.

22. Chandrasekhar S, Caldwell RL, Brown JW. Anomalous origin of the left coronary artery from the pulmonary artery in D-transposition of great vessels. Am Heart J. 1994;127:722–3. https://doi.org/10.1016/0002-8703(94)90694-7.

23. Yamagishi M, Emmoto T, Wada Y, Oka T. Transposition of the great arteries with anomalous origin of the left coronary artery from the pulmonary artery. Ann Thorac Surg. 1998;66:1416–8. https://doi.org/10.1016/S0003-4975(98)00788-7.

24. Yildiz A, Okcun B, Peker T, Arslan C, Olcay A, Bulent VM. Prevalence of coronary artery anomalies in 12,457 adult patients who underwent coronary angiography. Clin Cardiol. 2010;33(12):E60–4.

25. Yamanaka O, Hobbs RE. Coronary artery anomalies in 126,595 patients undergoing coronary arteriography. Catheter Cardiovasc Diagn. 1990;21(1):28–40.

26. Pelliccia A, Spataro A, Maron BJ. Prospective echocardiographic screening for coronary artery anomalies in 1,360 elite competitive athletes. Am J Cardiol. 1993;72(12):978–9.

27. Harikrishnan S, Jacob SP, Tharakan J, Titus T, Kumar VK, Bhat A, et al. Congenital coronary anomalies of origin and distribution in adults: a coronary arteriographic study. Indian Heart J. 2002;54(3):271–5.

28. Kardos A, Babai L, Rudas L, Gaal T, Horvath T, Talosi L, et al. Epidemiology of congenital coronary artery anomalies: a coronary arteriography study on a central European population. Catheter Cardiovasc Diagn. 1997;42(3):270–5.

29. Labombarda F, Coutance G, Pellissier A, Mery-Alexandre C, Roule V, Maragnes P, et al. Major congenital coronary artery anomalies in a paediatric and adult population: a prospective echocardiographic study. Eur Heart J Cardiovasc Imaging. 2014;15(7):761–8.

30. Ogden JA. Congenital anomalies of the coronary arteries. Am J Cardiol. 1970;25(4):474–9.

31. Youniss MA, Ghoshhajra B, Bernard S, Bhatt AB, Aranki SF, MacGillivray TE, et al. Familial anomalous origin of right coronary artery from the left coronary sinus. Am J Cardiol. 2018;122(10):1800–2.

32. Muriago M, Sheppard MN, Ho SY, Anderson RH. Location of the coronary arterial orifices in the normal heart. Clin Anat. 1997;10:297–302. https://doi.org/10.1002/(SICI)1098-2353(1997)10:5<297::AID-CA1>3.0.CO;2-O.

33. Thiene G, Frescura C, Padalino M, Basso C, Rizzo S. Coronary arteries: Normal anatomy with historical notes and embryology of Main stems. Front Cardiovasc Med. 2021;8:649855.

34. Caldani L, Caldani F. Icones anatomicae ex optimis neotericum operibus summa diligentia depromptae et collected. In: Picotti J, editor. Venetiis ex Calcographia; 1810.

35. Alegria JR, Herrmann J, Holmes DR Jr, Lerman A, Rihal CS. Myocardial bridging. Eur Heart J. 2005;26(12):1159–68.

36. Angelini P, Trivellato M, Donis J, Leachman RD. Myocardial bridge: a review. Prog Cardiovasc Dis. 1983;26:75–88. https://doi.org/10.1016/0033-0620(83)90019-1.

37. Corban MT, Hung OY, Eshtehardi P, Rasoul-Arzrumly E, McDaniel M, Mekonnen G, et al. Myocardial bridging: contemporary understanding of pathophysiology with implications for diagnostic and therapeutic strategies. J Am Coll Cardiol. 2014;63(22):2346–55.

38. Mohlenkamp S, Hort W, Ge J, Erbel R. Update on myocardial bridging. Circulation. 2002;106(20):2616–22.

39. Roberts WC. Major anomalies of coronary arterial origin seen in adulthood. Am Heart J. 1986;111:941–63. https://doi.org/10.1016/0002-8703(86)90646-0.

40. Purvis J, Howe A, Morgan D. Aortic step: a clue to unusually high origin of right coronary artery. Heart. 2010;96(16):1334.

41. Loukas M, Andall RG, Khan AZ, Patel K, Muresian H, Spicer DE, et al. The clinical anatomy of high take-off coronary arteries. Clin Anat. 2016;29(3):408–19.

42. Virmani R, Chun PK, Goldstein RE, Robinowitz M, McAllister HA. Acute takeoffs of the coronary arteries along the aortic wall and congenital coronary ostial valve-like ridges: association with sudden death. J Am Coll Cardiol. 1984;3(3):766–71.

43. Thiene G, Rizzo S, Frescura C, Basso C. Chapter 21: specific cardiovascular diseases and competitive sports participation: coronary anomalies and myocardial bridging at risk of sudden death. In: Pressler A, Niebauer J, editors. Textbook of sports and exercise cardiology. Cham: Springer; 2020. p. 403–21. https://doi.org/10.1007/978-3-030-35374-2_21.

44. Basso C, Thiene G, Mackey-Bojack S, Frigo AC, Corrado D, Maron BJ. Myocardial bridging, a frequent component of the hypertrophic cardiomyopathy phenotype, lacks systematic association with sudden cardiac death. Eur Heart J. 2009;30(13):1627–34.

45. Bourassa MG, Butnaru A, Lesperance J, Tardif JC. Symptomatic myocardial bridges: overview of ischemic mechanisms and current diagnostic and treatment strategies. J Am Coll Cardiol. 2003;41(3):351–9.

46. Schwarz ER, Gupta R, Haager PK, vom Dahl J, Klues HG, Minartz J, et al. Myocardial bridging in absence of coronary artery disease: proposal of a new classification based on clinical-angiographic data and long-term follow-up. Cardiology. 2009;112(1):13–21.

47. Gori F, Basso C, Thiene G. Myocardial infarction in a patient with hypertrophic cardiomyopathy. N Engl J Med. 2000;342(8):593–4.

48. Yau JM, Singh R, Halpern EJ, Fischman D. Anomalous origin of the left coronary artery from the pulmonary artery in adults: a comprehensive review of 151 adult cases and a new diagnosis in a 53-year-old woman. Clin Cardiol. 2011;34(4):204–10.

49. Dodge-Khatami A, Mavroudis C, Backer CL. Anomalous origin of the left coronary artery from the pulmonary artery: collective review of surgical therapy. Ann Thorac Surg. 2002;74(3):946–55.

50. Basso C, Perez-Pomares J, Thiene G, Houyel L. Coronary anomalies. In: Perez-Pomares J, Kelly R, editors. The ESC textbook of cardiovascular development. 1st ed. Oxford: OUP; 2018. p. 250–60.

51. Angelini P, Uribe C. Anatomic spectrum of left coronary artery anomalies and associated mechanisms of coronary insufficiency. Catheter Cardiovasc Interv. 2018;92(2):313–21.

52. Angelini P, Villason S, Chan AJ, Diez J. Normal and anomalous coronary arteries in humans. In: Angelini P, editor. Coronary artery anomalies: a comprehensive approach. Philadelphia: Lippincott, Williams & Wilkins; 1999. p. 27–150.

53. Barth CW 3rd, Roberts WC. Left main coronary artery originating from the right sinus of Valsalva and coursing between the aorta and pulmonary trunk. J Am Coll Cardiol. 1986;7(2):366–73.

54. Lim JC, Beale A, Ramcharitar S. Medscape. Anomalous origination of a coronary artery from the opposite sinus. Nat Rev Cardiol. 2011;8(12):706–19.

55. Roberts WC, Siegel RJ, Zipes DP. Origin of the right coronary artery from the left sinus of valsalva and its functional consequences: analysis of 10 necropsy patients. Am J Cardiol. 1982;49(4):863–8.

56. Morales AR, Romanelli R, Boucek RJ. The mural left anterior descending coronary artery, strenuous exercise and sudden death. Circulation. 1980;62(2):230–7.

57. Cheitlin MD. The intramural coronary artery: another cause for sudden death with exercise? Circulation. 1980;62(2):238–9.

58. Piovesana P, Corrado D, Contessotto F, Zampiero A, Camponeschi M, Lafisca N, et al. Echocardiographic identification of anomalous origin of the left circumflex coronary artery from the right sinus of Valsalva. Am Heart J. 1990;119(1):205–7.

59. Corrado D, Pennelli T, Piovesana P, Thiene G. Anomalous origin of the left circumflex coronary artery from the right aortic sinus of Valsalva and sud-

den death. Cardiovasc Pathol. 1994;3:269–71. https://doi.org/10.1016/1054-8807(94)90013-2.

60. Thiene G, Ho SY. Aortic root pathology and sudden death in youth: review of anatomical varieties. Appl Pathol. 1986;4:237–45.

61. Basso C, Corrado D, Thiene G. Congenital coronary artery anomalies as an important cause of sudden death in the young. Cardiol Rev. 2001;9(6):312–7.

62. Basso C, Corrado D, Thiene G. Coronary artery anomalies and sudden death. Card Electrophysiol Rev. 2002;6(1–2):107–11.

63. Basso C, Maron BJ, Corrado D, Thiene G. Clinical profile of congenital coronary artery anomalies with origin from the wrong aortic sinus leading to sudden death in young competitive athletes. J Am Coll Cardiol. 2000;35(6):1493–501.

64. Frescura C, Basso C, Thiene G, Corrado D, Pennelli T, Angelini A, et al. Anomalous origin of coronary arteries and risk of sudden death: a study based on an autopsy population of congenital heart disease. Hum Pathol. 1998;29:689–95. https://doi.org/10.1016/S0046-8177(98)90277-5.

65. Burke AP, Farb A, Virmani R, Goodin J, Smialek JE. Sports-related and non-sports-related sudden cardiac death in young adults. Am Heart J. 1991;121(2 Pt 1):568–75.

66. Angelini P, Cheong BY, Lenge De Rosen VV, Lopez A, Uribe C, Masso AH, et al. High-risk cardiovascular conditions in sports-related sudden death: prevalence in 5,169 schoolchildren screened via cardiac magnetic resonance. Tex Heart Inst J. 2018;45(4):205–13.

67. Cheitlin MD, MacGregor J. Congenital anomalies of coronary arteries: role in the pathogenesis of sudden cardiac death. Herz. 2009;34(4):268–79.

68. Taylor AJ, Rogan KM, Virmani R. Sudden cardiac death associated with isolated congenital coronary artery anomalies. J Am Coll Cardiol. 1992;20(3):640–7.

69. Corrado D, Thiene G, Cocco P, Frescura C. Non-atherosclerotic coronary artery disease and sudden death in the young. Br Heart J. 1992;68(6):601–7.

70. Cheitlin MD, De Castro CM, McAllister HA. Sudden death as a complication of anomalous left coronary origin from the anterior sinus of Valsalva, A not-so-minor congenital anomaly. Circulation. 1974;50(4):780–7.

71. Thiene G, Basso C, Favretto D, Rizzo S. Sudden death in athletes: autoptic findings. In: Delise P, Zeppilli P, editors. Sport-related sudden cardiac death. Cham: Springer; 2022. p. 85–7.

72. Elias MD, Meza J, McCrindle BW, Brothers JA, Paridon S, Cohen MS. Effects of exercise restriction on patients with anomalous aortic origin of a coronary artery. World J Pediatr Congenit Heart Surg. 2017;8(1):18–24.

73. Basso C, Burke M, Fornes P, Gallagher PJ, de Gouveia RH, Sheppard M, et al. Guidelines for autopsy investigation of sudden cardiac death. Virchows Arch. 2008;452(1):11–8.

74. Basso C, Aguilera B, Banner J, Cohle S, d'Amati G, de Gouveia RH, et al. Guidelines for autopsy investigation of sudden cardiac death: 2017 update from the Association for European Cardiovascular Pathology. Virchows Arch. 2017;471(6):691–705.

Normal Coronary Flow Physiology

3

Carlo Trani, Cristina Aurigemma, and Filippo Crea

Introduction

The heart is the unique organ responsible for providing its own blood supply through the coronary circulation. Regulation of coronary blood flow is quite complex and, after over 100 years of dedicated research, is understood to depend on multiple mechanisms that include extravascular compressive forces (tissue pressure), coronary perfusion pressure, myogenic, local metabolic, endothelial as well as neural and hormonal influences [1]. Each of these determinants can have a profound influence on myocardial perfusion, largely through effects on end-effector ion channels and collectively modulate coronary vascular resistance and act to ensure an adequate refueling of oxygen and substrates. Owing to the limited anaerobic capacity of the heart, coronary vascular resistance is continuously regulated to deliver sufficient quantities of oxygen to meet any change in the demand of surrounding myocardial tissue (Fig. 3.1).

C. Trani (✉) · F. Crea
Dipartimento di Scienze Cardiovascolari, Fondazione Policlinico Universitario A. Gemelli IRCCS,
Rome, Italy

Università Cattolica del Sacro Cuore, Rome, Italy
e-mail: carlo.trani@unicatt.it; filippo.crea@unicatt.it

C. Aurigemma
Dipartimento di Scienze Cardiovascolari, Fondazione Policlinico Universitario A. Gemelli IRCCS,
Rome, Italy
e-mail: cristina.aurigemma@policlinicogemelli.it

© Springer Nature Switzerland AG 2023
G. Butera, A. Frigiola (eds.), *Congenital Anomalies of Coronary Arteries*,
https://doi.org/10.1007/978-3-031-36966-7_3

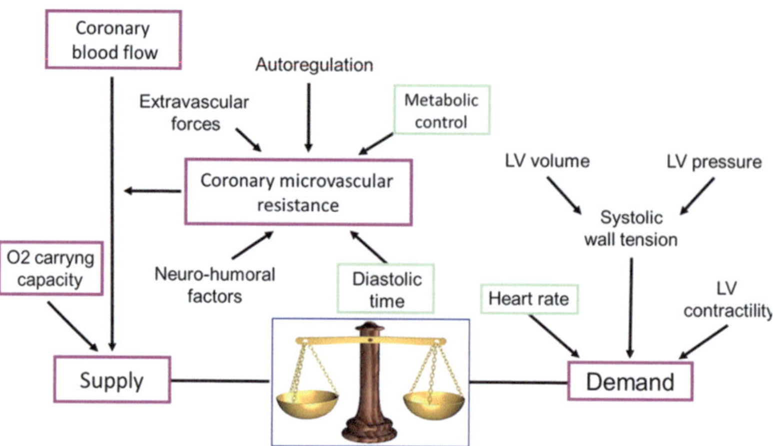

Fig. 3.1 Determinants of coronary blood flow

Physiology of Myocardial Blood Flow

The coronary circulation is divided into three compartments, the large epicardial conduit vessels (proximal compartments with vessels range from 5.0 to 0.5 mm), the prearterioles (intermediate compartments with vessels range from ≈500 to 100 μm) and the arterioles (distal compartments with vessels diameters <100 μm) (Fig. 3.2). The conduit vessels exert little resistance to flow, indeed resistance to flow progressively rises in prearterioles and arterioles. The vasomotor actions of the prearterioles are independent of diffusible myocardial metabolites, but are more responsive to changes in flow (in proximal prearterioles, 500–150 μm) and in pressure (in distal prearterioles, 150–100 μm). Instead, the tone of arterioles depends on substances produced by the surrounding cardiac myocytes, representing the place of metabolic regulation of coronary flow [2]. Flow across the myocardium largely depends on the pressure gradient between the aortic root and the right atrium (the "coronary driving pressure"). Under normal conditions, the driving pressure is fully maintained along the epicardial conduit vessels with little if any pressure loss in the distal epicardial arteries. However, intra-coronary pressures decline along the microvasculature (with most of the pressure dissipating in the 300–100 μm diameter vessels) until reaching a pressure of 20–30 mmHg, still adequate to main-

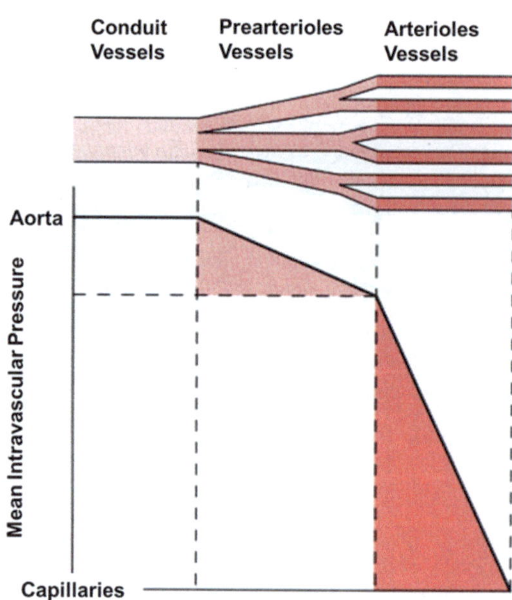

Fig. 3.2 The main anatomic features of the coronary circulation

tain a gradient across the capillaries. Extravascular resistive forces, that are directly related to the left ventricular systolic pressure, the contractile state of the myocardium, and the heart rate, represent additional determinants of the resistance to flow. The interaction between intra-coronary driving pressure and microvascular resistance is coordinated by auto-regulatory mechanisms in order to maintain adequate flow across the capillaries. The flow is mathematically described in the vascular system as a correlate to Ohm's Law

(Flow = ΔPressure/Resistance). Therefore, through this regulatory mechanism, defined "coronary autoregulation", decreases in driving pressure are compensated by decreases in resistance and conversely, increases in driving pressure by increases in resistance, so that flow remains constant for a given cardiac workload. This regulatory mechanism operates within the range of physiologic arterial pressures (60 and 200 mmHg) but fails during hypotension when flows become strongly dependent on the driving pressure [3].

The specifics of metabolism-perfusion matching are unique in the coronary circulation because of the continuous pumping and high workload of the heart. Based on a constantly functioning contractile machine, the heart demonstrates the highest per gram oxygen consumption of any organ (~50–100 µL O_2/min/g) and, as such, extracts ~70–80% of delivered oxygen even under resting conditions (coronary venous PO_2 ~ 18–20 mmHg), unlike skeletal muscle which utilizes only ~30–40% of delivered oxygen at rest (venous PO_2 ~ 40 mmHg) [4]. This high extraction percentage results in a system that is almost completely dependent on the delivery of blood to the tissue as enhancements to extraction are rather limited. Therefore, coronary vascular tone must be constantly modulated to ensure adequate myocardial perfusion. This point is evident in examination of coronary responses to a variety of physiologic perturbations including alterations in metabolism, perfusion pressure, arterial oxygen content, and/or a transient coronary artery occlusion. These well-established phenomena clearly illustrate the tight coupling between coronary blood flow and myocardial oxygen consumption (MVO_2) in response to exercise. Indeed, in non-diseased coronary vessels, whenever cardiac activity and oxygen consumption increase there is an increase in coronary blood flow that is nearly proportionate to the increase in oxygen consumption (functional hyperemia) [5]. Coronary blood flow analogously increases in response to the repayment of "oxygen-debt" occurring following the interruption of myocardial oxygen, such as a transient coronary artery occlusion (reactive hyperemia) [6]. Work-related flow increases are

initiated by a metabolically mediated decrease in microvascular resistance, involving adenosine and causing vascular smooth muscle relaxation [7]. The resulting flow is augmented by endothelium-dependent factors; higher flow velocities exert greater shear stress upon the endothelium with stimulation of the endothelial nitric oxide synthase (eNOS) and release of the smooth muscle-relaxing nitric oxide (NO). In this scenario, endothelial cells closely interact with vascular smooth muscle cells in order to adjust the vessel diameter to changes in flow velocities ("flow-mediated dilation"), both at the level of the microvessels and the epicardial conduit vessels.

In the majority of organs, the compressive tissue force is constant and therefore its contribution to the pressure gradient is only minimal yet consistent. Instead, the pattern of flow in the coronary vascular system is more complex due to the periodicity of contractions in the heart and tremendous compressive forces of the myocardium. Coronary vascular flow is described as phasic flow in that the compressive forces of systole counteract the driving force for flow in the coronary circulation and, therefore, the majority of anterograde blood flow to the left ventricle occurs during diastole (Fig. 3.3) [8]. The physiologic interaction between myocardial contraction and the phasic nature of coronary flow is further

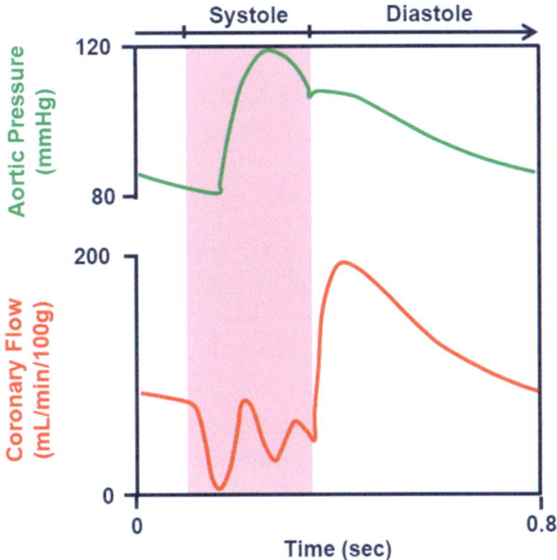

Fig. 3.3 Phasic trace of coronary blood flow

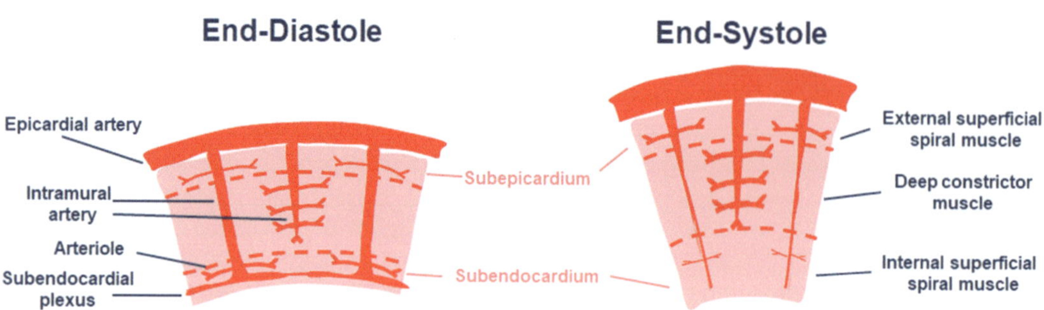

Fig. 3.4 Schematic cross-section of the myocardial wall at end-diastole and end-systole. (Figure modified from Bell JR, Fox AC. Pathogenesis of subendocardial ischemia. Am J Med Sci. 1974; 268:3–13)

complicated by the disparity in compressive forces across the wall of the left ventricle, as described in the early 1950s by Rushmer [9]. The greatest degree of vascular compression is found in endocardial layers, with little if any compressive force at the level of the epicardium (Fig. 3.4). This disparity leads to a reduced blood flow in endocardial tissue during systole as the compressive forces are of sufficient magnitude to exceed the driving force of arterial pressure. Thus, the endocardium only receives flow during diastole and is therefore extremely dependent on an adequate diastolic filling period to maintain sufficient coronary flow. By contrast, the lack of compressive forces at the epicardial layer allows for perfusion throughout the entire cardiac cycle. Therefore, there is a linear decrease in dependence on diastolic time fraction for the maintenance of coronary flow in the endocardial to epicardial direction [10]. Given the higher compressive forces and oxygen requirements of the left ventricular endocardium, there is a gradient for coronary flow across the wall of the heart. Typically, epicardial to endocardial flow ratio ranges from ~1.1–1.5 and is only partially compensated by the higher density and the lower resistance of the endocardial microcirculation. As such, the left ventricle receives ~80% of its blood supply during diastole whereas the much thinner right ventricle, which is subject to much lower myocardial tissue pressures, is primarily perfused during systole.

Coronary Flow Assessments

Maximum hyperemic flows reflect the total vasodilator capacity of the coronary circulation. Blood flow during pharmacologically stimulated vasodilation strongly depends on the driving pressure, therefore the ratio of mean arterial blood pressure over myocardial blood flow, defined as minimal coronary vascular resistance (CVR), represents an index of the coronary vasodilator capacity that is however normalized to the perfusion pressure. The coronary (or more appropriately, myocardial) flow reserve (CFR) is also been accepted as another measure of the vasodilator capacity. It reflects the ratio of hyperemic over rest myocardial blood flow, which limits its accuracy because it not only reflects the maximally achieved hyperemic blood flow, but depends also on myocardial blood flow at rest. In patients with hypertension, for example, flows at rest are elevated due to the higher myocardial work so that even when hyperemic blood flows are in the range of normal, the actual flow reserve may be diminished. Therefore, resting blood flow is adjusted to cardiac work by normalizing flows to the rate pressure product. The CFR is reported as the ratio of hyperemic to "normalized" resting blood flows [3] and it is considered an index of microvascular function with a cutoff >2.0. The index of microcirculatory resistance (IMR) is an invasive quantitative assessment of the minimum microcirculatory resistance in a target coronary artery territory. The IMR is defined as the ratio

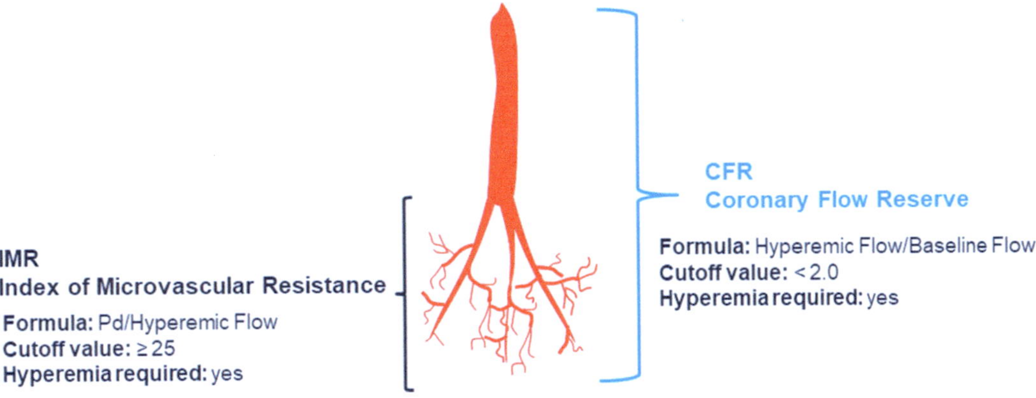

Fig. 3.5 Coronary flow assessments: coronary flow reserve (CFR) and index of microcirculatory resistance (IMR)

between the distal intracoronary pressure (Pd) and the inverse of the hyperemic mean transit time (Tmn). Because IMR incorporates only hyperemic parameters, it eliminates the variability of hemodynamics and resting vascular tone and estimates the minimum achievable microvascular resistance. Importantly, IMR is based on indirect measurements of coronary flow using Tmn, in contrast to CFR, based on direct measurements of coronary flow velocity [11]. IMR is used as a marker of microvascular dysfunction with a cutoff ≥25 (Fig. 3.5).

Vasodilator Stress Pharmacological stress with vascular smooth muscle relaxing agents (e.g. dipyridamole, adenosine, adenosine-triphosphate, and more recently, adenosine receptor subtype A2A agonists like regadenoson) reduce maximally the vascular resistance through relaxation of the vascular smooth muscle cell at the level of the microcirculation, thereby uncoupling coronary flow (supply) from myocardial work (demand). Flows during vasodilator-induced hyperemia then depend largely on the coronary driving pressure and, thus, on the arterial blood pressure, and the residual coronary resistance [12].

Sympathetic Stress Sympathetic stimulation, such as cold pressor testing, more specifically targets endothelium-related determinants of the coronary circulatory function. It increases heart rate and systolic blood pressure together with local norepinephrine release from adrenergic nerve terminals in the coronary circulation. The increase in myocardial work, as reflected by the increase in the rate pressure product, is under normal conditions associated with a proportionate increase in myocardial blood flow [13]. A metabolically induced work-related increase in flow is augmented by endothelium-related vasodilator forces. Indeed, vasoconstrictor effects on the vascular smooth muscle mediated by adrenergic stimulation are balanced by largely endothelium-related vasodilator forces affecting both the microvasculature and the epicardial conduit vessels. The endothelium-dependent modulation of flow during sympathetic stimulation corresponds to the endothelium-related flow augmentation during pharmacologically stimulated hyperemia. For example, in healthy subjects without coronary risk factors, the change in vascular resistance in response to cold pressor testing is significantly correlated with the adenosine- or dipyridamole-induced decline in CVR, suggesting proportionate contributions of endothelium-related mechanisms to both types of flow responses [3].

Positive Inotropic Stimulation Pharmacologic inotropic stimulation is an alternate to physical stress. Intravenous administration of dobutamine, a synthetic sympathomimetic amine with a dominant positive inotropic effect via stimulation of β- and α-adrenoreceptors, produces significant increases in MVO_2 and consequently commensurate increases in myocardial blood flow. The dobutamine-induced changes in MVO_2 are closely correlated to changes in myocardial work and, further, myocardial blood flow [14].

Coronary Artery Anomalies: Effect on Coronary Flow

The pathophysiology of anomalous coronary arteries originating from the opposite sinus of Valsalva (ACAOS) is not well understood. Anatomic high-risk features of slit-like ostium and proximal narrowing are not only relevant due to the reduced cross-sectional area (CSA), compared with a round vessel shape, but also due to higher resistance. Decreasing CSA increases the resistance, as a function of the height/width ratio. Furthermore, the intramural length directly increases resistance to flow (Fig. 3.6). Therefore, the increased resistance along the anomalous segment, due to the progressive deformation, results in compensatory coronary vasodilatation for the preservation of adequate perfusion at the expense of decreased CFR [15]. A two-tier concept for the pathomechanisms of ischemia in ACAOS based on the combination of a fixed

(anatomic high-risk features of slit-like ostium and proximal narrowing) and a dynamic (acute take-off angle, intramural course with the elliptic vessel shape) component is recently proposed [15]. In previous studies, none of the anatomic features correlated with ischemia, indicating a complex interaction between the different components [16]. In addition, the hemodynamic relevance depends directly on the supplied viable myocardial mass downstream of the stenosis, providing an explication for the diverging prognosis of right and left ACAOS. Moreover, ischemia is unlikely to occur every time, suggesting the presence of additional factors such as volume status and type of physical activity [17].

Fixed Component Slit-like ostium and proximal narrowing are present at rest and behave in a similar manner to classic coronary lesions. The reduction of the CSA creates flow restrictions, which can be evaluated by coronary angiography or intravascular imaging and/or the pressure gradient over the stenotic segment. Fractional flow reserve (FFR) with hyperemia induced by pharmacological vasodilatation (i.e. adenosine) was used to assess the hemodynamic relevance of ACAOS in multiple studies, but only a poor correlation with symptoms and/or anatomic features could be documented [18]. Indeed, these studies

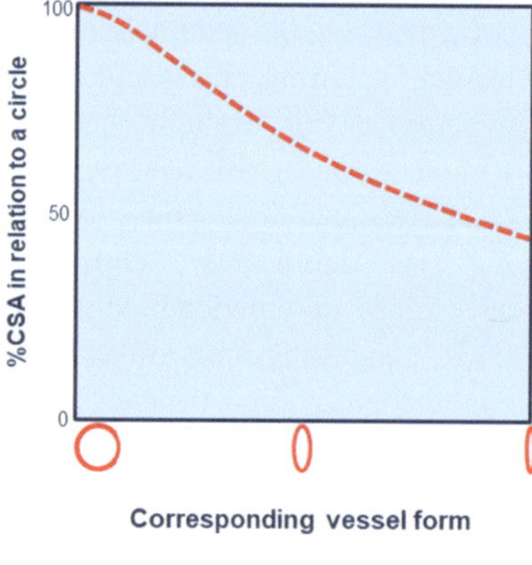

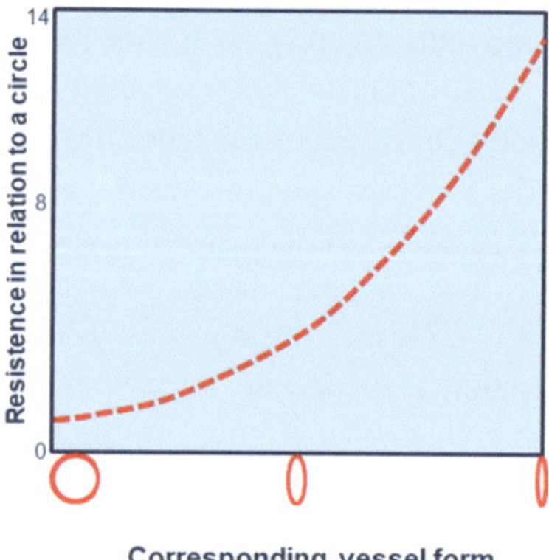

Fig. 3.6 The impact of deformed vascular shape, such as lateral compression, on coronary flow. Decreasing cross-sectional area is associate to increasing resistance as a function of the height/width ratio in a vessel with a fixed circumference is calculated (a theoretical model with the limitation that deformation will rarely result in a perfect elliptic shape). (*Figure modified from Bigler MR, Ashraf A, Seiler C, Praz F, Ueki Y, Windecker S, Kadner A, Räber L, Gräni C. Hemodynamic Relevance of Anomalous Coronary Arteries Originating From the Opposite Sinus of Valsalva-In Search of the Evidence. Front Cardiovasc Med. 2021 Jan 21;7:591326*)

assessed the fixed component alone but the dynamic component cannot be sufficiently reproduced using pharmacological stress with vasodilators.

Dynamic Component Anatomic features like acute take-off angle or lateral compression in the intramural segment have hemodynamic relevance during exercise. After the increase in heart rate, an increase of systolic blood pressure, myocardial contractility, systolic expansion, and higher wall stress of the proximal aorta can be observed because of increased dP/dt and stroke volume [19]. These modifications increase lateral compression of the intramural segment and subsequent flow resistance, affecting CFR during conditions of increased myocardial oxygen demand. This phenomenon causes myocardial ischemia that cannot be triggered by vasodilatory drugs alone. Hence, assessment of the hemodynamic component of ACAOS should be performed preferably by physical exercise or dobutamine, which increases heart rate and stroke volume. Of note, in multiple studies, FFR dobutamine was usually lower than FFR adenosine, revealing the inconstant presence of the dynamic component [20]. Increasing age, thickening, and stiffness of the aortic wall decrease distensibility, and thus, the dynamic component loses its relevance. These findings are in line with the autoptic studies that reported a decreased risk of sudden cardiac death beyond the age of 30 [16].

Stress Testing The ideal stress test for ACAOS in patients with suspected angina should be able to assess both dynamic and fixed components. Stress tests based on vasodilators (i.e. adenosine or regadenoson) fail to assess the dynamic components (i.e. dynamic lateral compression of the intramural abnormal coronary artery) and therefore may provide false negative results. Dobutamine stress test is more adequate to test both fixed and dynamic components. Unfortunately, dobutamine stress test typically achieves less than 85% of the maximal heart rate and does not result in a substantial increase in blood pressure. Therefore, a dobutamine stress test sensitized by saline infusion to prevent pre-load decrease and by atropine administration to reach 100% of the maximal heart rate, has been proposed [16]. This enhanced dobutamine stress test should be considered in patients with suspected angina and ACAOS, in particular in athletes, to predict the risk of ischemia-induced sudden death during strenuous physical exercise.

References

1. Goodwill AG, Dick GM, Kiel AM, Tune JD. Regulation of coronary blood flow. Compr Physiol. 2017;7(2):321–82.
2. Kaski JC, Crea F, Gersh BJ, Camici PG. Reappraisal of ischemic heart disease. Circulation. 2018;138(14):1463–80.
3. Schelbert HR. Anatomy and physiology of coronary blood flow. J Nucl Cardiol. 2010;17:545.
4. Duncker DJ, Bache RJ. Regulation of coronary blood flow during exercise. Physiol Rev. 2008;88:1009–86.
5. Berwick ZC, Dick GM, Moberly SP, Kohr MC, Sturek M, Tune JD. Contribution of voltage-dependent K(+) channels to metabolic control of coronary blood flow. J Mol Cell Cardiol. 2012;52:912–9.
6. Berwick ZC, Payne GA, Lynch B, Dick GM, Sturek M, Tune JD. Contribution of adenosine A(2A) and A(2B) receptors to ischemic coronary dilation: role of K(V) and K(ATP) channels. Microcirculation. 2010;17:600–7.
7. Lupi A, Buffon A, Finocchiaro ML, Conti E, Maseri A, Crea F. Mechanisms of adenosine-induced epicardial coronary artery dilatation. Eur Heart J. 1997;18(4):614–7.
8. Feigl EO. Coronary physiology. Physiol Rev. 1983;63:1–205.
9. Rushmer RF, Thal N. The mechanics of ventricular contraction; a cinefluorographic study. Circulation. 1951;4:219–28.
10. Bell JR, Fox AC. Pathogenesis of subendocardial ischemia. Am J Med Sci. 1974;268:3–13.
11. Kobayashi Y, Fearon WF. Invasive coronary microcirculation assessment. Circ J. 2014;78(5):1021–8.
12. Chan SY, Brunken RC, Czernin J, Porenta G, Kuhle W, Krivokapich J, Phelps ME, Schelbert HR. Comparison of maximal myocardial blood flow during adenosine infusion with that of intravenous dipyridamole in normal men. J Am Coll Cardiol. 1992;20:979–85.
13. Prior JO, Schindler TH, Facta AD, Hernandez-Pampaloni M, Campisi R, Dahlbom M, Schelbert HR. Determinants of myocardial blood flow response to cold pressor testing and pharmacologic vasodilation in healthy humans. Eur J Nucl Med Mol Imaging. 2007;34:20–7.

14. Krivokapich J, Huang SC, Schelbert HR. Assessment of the effects of dobutamine on myocardial blood flow and oxidative metabolism in normal human subjects using nitrogen-13 ammonia and carbon-11 acetate. Am J Cardiol. 1993;71:1351–6.

15. Bigler MR, Ashraf A, Seiler C, Praz F, Ueki Y, Windecker S, Kadner A, Räber L, Gräni C. Hemodynamic relevance of anomalous coronary arteries originating from the opposite sinus of Valsalva-in search of the evidence. Front Cardiovasc Med. 2021;7:591326.

16. Angelini P, Flamm SD. Newer concepts for imaging anomalous aortic origin of the coronary arteries in adults. Catheter Cardiovasc Interv. 2007;69:942–54.

17. Grani C, Chappex N, Fracasso T, Vital C, Kellerhals C, Schmied C, Saguner AM, Trachsel LD, Eser P, Michaud K, Wilhelm M. Sports related sudden cardiac death in Switzerland classified by static and dynamic components of exercise. Eur J Prev Cardiol. 2016;23:1228–36.

18. Driesen BW, Warmerdam EG, Sieswerda GT, Schoof PH, Meijboom FJ, Haas F, Stella PR, Kraaijeveld AO, Evens FCM, Doevendans PAFM, Krings GJ, van Dijk APJ, Voskuil M. Anomalous coronary artery originating from the opposite sinus of Valsalva (ACAOS), fractional flow reserve–and intravascular ultrasound-guided management in adult patients. Catheter Cardiovasc Interv. 2018;92:68–75.

19. Cheitlin MD, MacGregor J. Congenital anomalies of coronary arteries: role in the pathogenesis of sudden cardiac death. Herz. 2009;34:268–79.

20. Lee SE, Yu CW, Park K, Park KW, Suh JW, Cho YS, Youn TJ, Chae IH, Choi DJ, Jang HJ, Park JS, Na SH, Kim HS, Kim KB, Koo BK. Physiological and clinical relevance of anomalous right coronary artery originating from left sinus of Valsalva in adults. Heart. 2016;102(2):114–9.

Myocardial Bridge(s)

4

Alberto Barioli, Flavia Belloni,
and Giuseppe Tarantini

Introduction

A myocardial bridge (MB) is defined as an anatomical variant in which a segment of a coronary artery (referred to as a tunneled artery) deepens into the myocardium for a variable distance, before returning to the epicardial surface. The presence of a band of myocardial fibers (i.e. the "myocardial bridge") overlying the coronary artery may result in compression of the artery during the systolic phase of the cardiac cycle. This anatomic variant, despite being traditionally considered a benign condition, has been associated with various clinical presentations, such as silent ischemia, exertional angina, acute coronary syndromes, Takotsubo cardiomyopathy, and sudden cardiac death [1–5].

Supplementary Information The online version contains supplementary material available at https://doi.org/10.1007/978-3-031-36966-7_4.

A. Barioli
Cardiology Unit, Cardio-Neuro-Vascular Department, Ca' Foncello Hospital, Treviso, Italy
e-mail: alberto.barioli@aulss2.veneto.it

F. Belloni
Division of Cardiology, Santo Spirito Hospital, Rome, Italy
e-mail: flavia.belloni@aslroma1.it

G. Tarantini (✉)
Department of Cardiac, Thoracic, Vascular Science and Public Health, University of Padua, Padua, Italy

The prevalence of this congenital coronary anomaly is highly variable, and depends largely on the techniques used to detect its presence and on patient's condition. In necropsy series, the reported rate of MB varies between 5 and 86% [1, 6], with a mean frequency of 25%. Recently, a meta-analysis of 15 autopsy studies reported an average prevalence of 42% [7]. These numbers are consistent with those observed in studies involving coronary-computed tomography (CCT) [8, 9]. Conversely, these rates are considerably higher than those found in angiographic studies, where the reported prevalence of MBs varies from 0.5% to 12% in basal conditions to 40% if provocative tests or intracoronary injection of nitroglycerin are used [10]. The observed rates of MBs increase to 23% when intravascular ultrasound (IVUS) is performed [11]. Prevalence of MBs has been reported to be higher in patients with hypertrophic cardiomyopathy and in cardiac transplant recipients [1, 12, 13].

The differences between the rates observed at necropsy or CCT and those detected at coronary angiography may lie in the different sensitivity of the investigative methods. As a matter of fact, if autopsy and CCT permit the direct visualization of the anatomy and course of the bridged segment, coronary angiography allows only the visualization of the "milking effect" (i.e. the dynamic narrowing of the coronary artery during systole). Intuitively, small intramyocardial courses with no hemodynamic significance can-

G. Butera, A. Frigiola (eds.), *Congenital Anomalies of Coronary Arteries*,
https://doi.org/10.1007/978-3-031-36966-7_4

not be detected with the latter method. In turn, the hemodynamic significance of MBs depends upon several factors, including the length of the bridged segment, the thickness of the myocardium overlying the tunneled artery, the nature and characteristics of the tissue surrounding the vessel, the orientation between myocardial fibers and the coronary artery, the presence of a coronary stenosis proximal to the MB, and observer experience [14].

Anatomy

The left anterior descending (LAD) artery is the most common coronary artery affected by MBs, although bridging can be found less frequently in the other major epicardial coronary arteries. Eventually, diagonal and marginal branches may be involved in 18% and 40% of cases, respectively [1, 15].

LAD-MBs may significantly vary in depth (1–10 mm) and length of encasement (10–30 mm) [16]. These characteristics, along with the degree of systolic diameter reduction and secondary branches involvement, are key elements for the evaluation of the hemodynamic significance of MBs. Ferreira et al. proposed a classification of LAD-MBs into two subtypes, according to the depth of embedment of the coronary artery: a more common superficial bridge (75% of cases), in which the myocardial fibers cross the artery transversely towards the apex of the heart at an acute angle or perpendicularly; and a deep variant (25% of cases), in which the LAD deviates towards the right ventricle and deepens into the interventricular septum, where it is crossed transversely, obliquely or helically by a muscle bundle arising from the apex of the right ventricle [17]. While the superficial variant rarely results in systolic compression of the artery, the deep variant is supposed to cause myocardial ischemia due to the distortion and twisting of the bridged segment induced by the overlying muscle bundle, resulting in impaired coronary blood flow.

Pathophysiology

The physiology of MBs is substantially different both from that of fixed defects and from the dynamic phenomenon of coronary vasospasm. Therefore, in the last decades, numerous studies have been carried out to understand the mechanism by which the presence of a MB can cause myocardial ischemia.

It is known that myocardial perfusion occurs mainly during the diastolic phase of the cardiac cycle. How the presence of a MB should impair diastolic coronary blood flow, since extravascular compression of the tunneled artery occurs during systole? It has been shown that the systolic narrowing of the bridged segment can extend into the early diastolic phase, resulting in the so-called "spillover" phenomenon [18]. In general, the more severe the systolic compression, the more likely the luminal area will be compromised in the early and even mid-diastole, where a persistent reduction of 34–51% in the bridged segment has been observed [19]. This phenomenon is further exacerbated by an increased heart rate, which causes a reduction of the diastolic perfusion time and an increase in epicardial coronary vasoconstriction and contraction of the MB [20, 21]. The resulting reduction in diastolic coronary blood flow may cause subendocardial ischemia downstream of severe arterial bridge compression, as the shortened diastolic perfusion time may exacerbate the normal time delay in early diastolic subendocardial hyperemia compared to the subepicardial layers. More often, MBs can trigger septal ischemia by the "branch steal" mechanism, whereby increased flow velocity in the compressed artery results in depressurization of septal branches within the MB [22].

MBs are thought to be protective against the formation of atherosclerotic plaques within the bridged segment. As a matter of fact, it has been postulated that the characteristics of the intima of the tunneled segment, which contains a predominance of the contractile subtype of smooth muscle cells, the separation of the bridged segment from epicardial perivascular adipose tissue and the absence of foam cells may play a role in this anti-atherosclerotic effect [23–25]. On the other hand, MBs are associated with up to 90% increased atherogenesis at the vessel segment proximal to the bridge [26]. This could be explained by the fact that systolic compression of the tunneled artery results in retrograde flow in the segment proximal to MB entrance, causing disturbance in systolic wall shear stress that has been linked to coronary plaques formation at this site [27, 28]. In addition, the altered hemodynamic pattern at the level of the MB has also been associated with other potential complications, including plaque vulnerability/thrombosis [27], increase in vasospasticity [29], and intimal injury possibly leading to dissection [30].

Clinical Presentation

Most MBs are clinically silent and usually represent an incidental finding on angiography, CCT, or autopsy. Patients with MB may present with stable symptomatic or silent myocardial ischemia, as well as with acute coronary syndromes. Other reported clinical presentations are coronary spasm, myocardial stunning, transient ventricular dysfunction, stress cardiomyopathy, syncope, exercise-induced dysrhythmias like supraventricular tachycardia, atrioventricular conduction block, and life-threatening ventricular arrhythmias possibly leading to sudden death [1–5, 10, 31, 32]. Previously silent MBs may become symptomatic over time. Pathophysiological factors that may reveal or exacerbate symptoms are age, heart rate, left ventricular hypertrophy, and coronary atherosclerosis [33].

Diagnosis

Morphological Assessment

CCT is a prime important, non-invasive tool in the diagnosis of MBs, being reported superior to coronary angiography in terms of detection rates [1]. CCT provides three-dimensional images with high spatial and contrast resolution, allowing identification of morphological features of MBs, including the length and the degree of encasement of the bridged artery, as well as the length and thickness of the MB over the tunneled segment [34, 35] (Fig. 4.1). The technique also allows the classification of the vessel intramyocardial course in superficial or deep. Recently, the use of new post-processing algorithms for the derivation of functional information from the anatomic assessment provided by CCT, such as transluminal attenuation gradient and CCT-based fractional flow reserve (FFR), has brought encouraging, albeit initial, results [36–39].

With coronary angiography, the MB appears as a systolic compression, or milking, of the tunneled artery, that reverses during diastole. A systolic narrowing is defined as a ≥50% systolic diameter stenosis not present or less evident during diastole, and can be enhanced by intracoronary administration of nitroglycerine [40, 41]. To note, the severity of systolic compression at angiography does not always correlate with the functional relevance of MBs [42]. In addition to coronary milking, a MB can be suspected when a characteristic "step-down" and "step-up" morphology, also known as the "U" sign, of the intramural course of the LAD is observed [40]. Several angiographic views, including the lateral projection, are usually obtained to better visualize and characterize the vessel course (Fig. 4.2) (Videos 4.1 and 4.2).

Given its ability to characterize the length, thickness, and location of the MB, IVUS assessment can be an adjunctive valuable tool to increase the detection rate of this coronary anomaly. Imaging with IVUS may display the reduced vessel area within the MB segment, the loss of the circular morphology of the artery under the compression of the bridge, as well as the characteristic, hypoechogenic "half-moon" sign over the bridged segment [43] (Fig. 4.3) (Video 4.3). Although the etiology of this last phenomenon is still a matter of debate, it appears to be highly specific as it can only be found in the bridged segment and not in adjacent reference segments or other coronary arteries [26]. Lastly, IVUS examination can provide useful

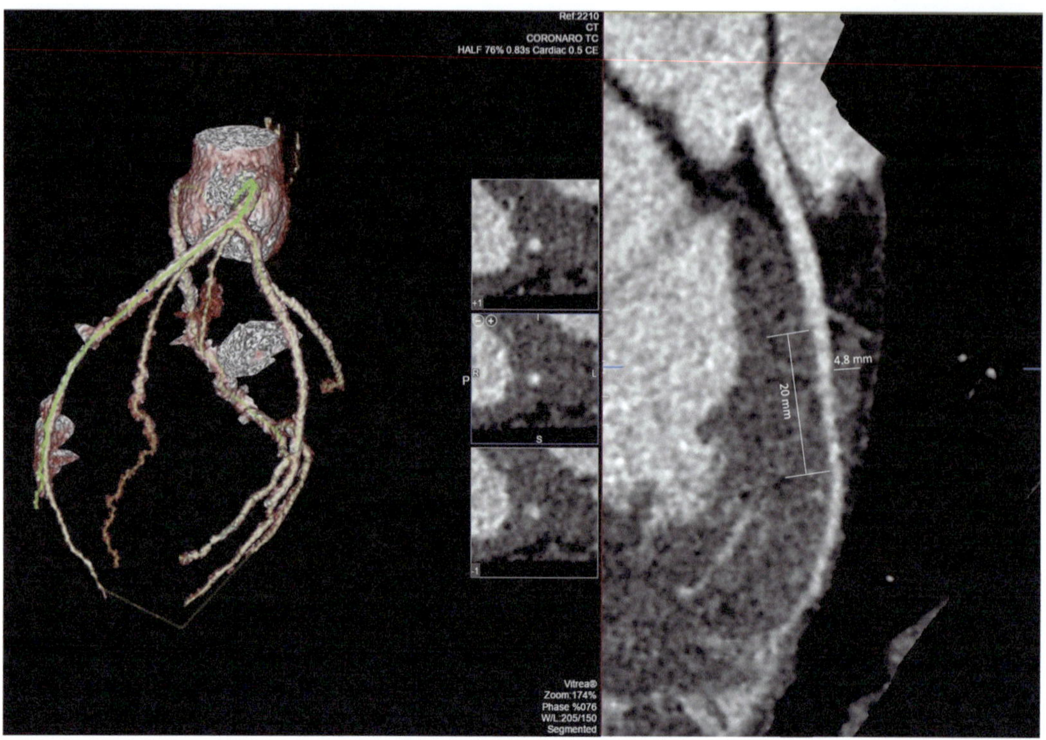

Fig. 4.1 Volume rendering 3D image showing myocardial bridging of the LAD. The intramyocardial course involves the middle third of the vessel and shows overlying myocardial tissue. Therefore, the MB can be addressed as deep. *LAD* left anterior descending artery. *MB* myocardial bridge

information on the presence, severity, and distribution of subangiographic atherosclerosis [43], in order to guide treatment (e.g. appropriate stent selection and placement). Other intravascular imaging techniques, such as optical coherence tomography (OCT), may theoretically improve the characterization of the vessel wall within the bridged segment, but existing evidence is still scarce [44, 45].

Functional Assessment

An appropriate diagnostic workup of MBs should include the hemodynamic assessment of the bridged coronary artery. As previously mentioned, physiology of MBs is rather different to that of fixed lesions. Because the dynamic stenoses in the context of MBs are dependent on extravascular compression and intramyocardial tension, their functional assessment should not be limited to resting conditions and thus should include chronotropic and inotropic stimulation. Also, during systole, the vascular compression causes distal pressure overshooting due to milking of blood against a highly restrictive circulation. This translates into higher intracoronary over aortic pressures distal to the MB, or, in other words, in negative pressure systolic gradients across the MB [46] (Fig. 4.4). Distal pressure overshooting and systolic pressure gradient inversion may lead to an underestimation of the functional impact of the MB when assessed with conventional FFR, this being an average of systolic and diastolic gradients. In view of these considerations, the use of diastolic-FFR during dobutamine challenge or after intracoronary adenosine administration has been shown to be a better alternative approach to test MB functional significance [42]. However, the acquisition of diastolic rather than mean FFR is complex and more vulnerable to measurement errors, and

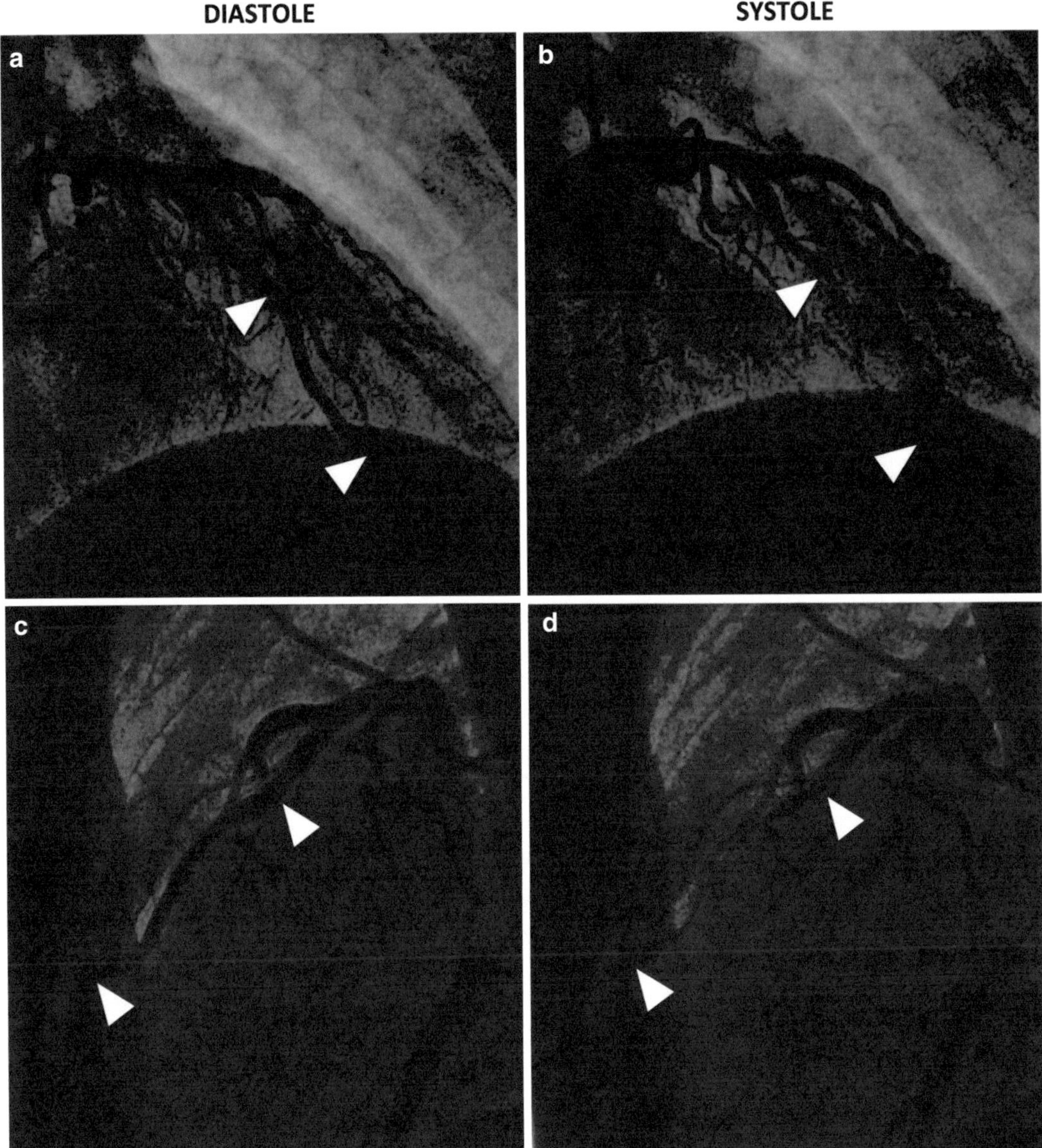

Fig. 4.2 Angiographic appearance of a LAD-MB in a patient with hypertrophic cardiomyopathy, both in diastole (**a** and **c**) and systole (**b** and **d**). The lateral projection enhances the step-down (top arrow) and step-up (bottom arrow) of the bridged LAD (**c** and **d**). *LAD* left anterior descending artery. *MB* myocardial bridge

therefore is not routinely performed in most cardiac laboratories [47].

More recently, the introduction of a lesion-specific, non-hyperemic diastolic index, the instantaneous wave-free ratio (iFR®, Volcano corporation, San Diego, Ca, USA), has shed new light on functional assessment of MBs. This index measures the translesional pressure gradient in a specific phase of the cardiac diastole (the wave-free period), in which coronary flow is maximal and microcirculatory resistances are low and stable. As such, it might not be hampered by systolic pressure overshooting and negative systolic pressure gradient caused by extravascular compression of the tunneled artery. Moreover, iFR allows anatomic mapping

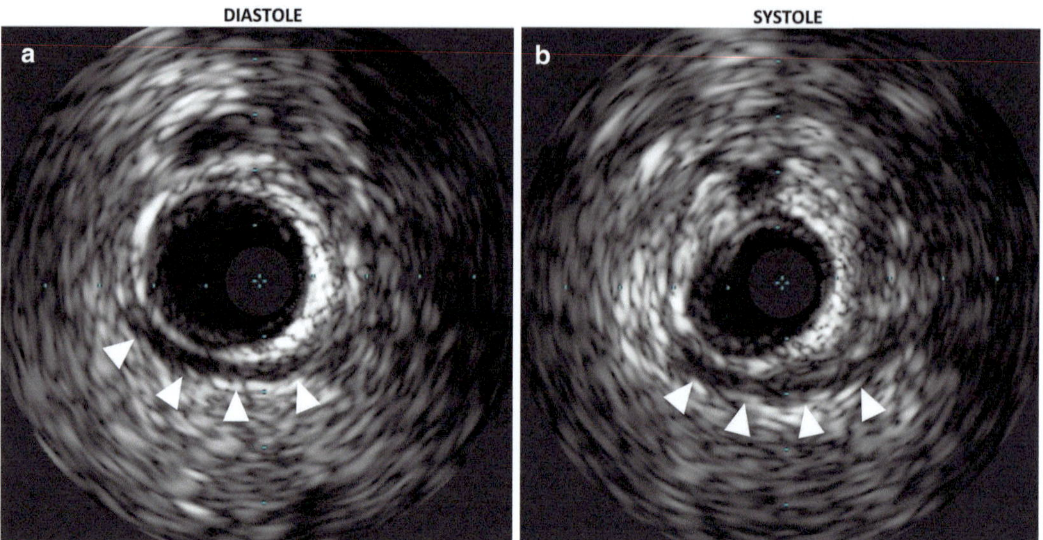

Fig. 4.3 IVUS imaging of a LAD-MB during diastole (**a**) and systole (**b**). An hypoechogenic "half-moon" image surrounding the bridge is present during the entire cardiac cycle (arrows). IVUS: intravascular ultrasound. LAD: left anterior descending artery. MB: myocardial bridge

Fig. 4.4 Intracoronary pressure tracings at baseline and during inotropic challenge in MB. Pressure overshooting during dobutamine challenge occurs because of systolic milking of blood distal to the MB, causing higher intracoronary (Pd – blue tracing) over aortic (Pa – red tracing) pressures. *MB* myocardial bridge

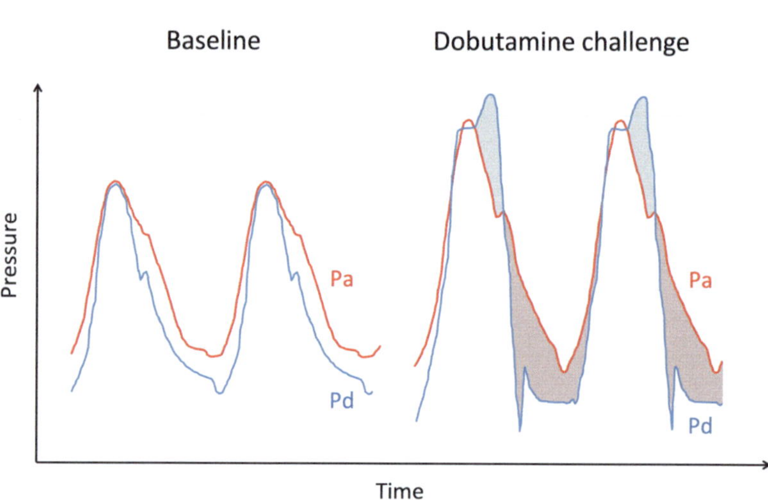

of the vessel by guidewire pullback (iFR Scout), providing information on the ischemic contribution of the MB [48]. iFR has been shown to have greater correlation to patients' symptoms or presence of myocardial ischemia than FFR. In a series of 20 patients with angina, no significant coronary artery disease (CAD), silent ischemia confirmed by non-invasive stress test, and angiographic or CCT evidence of MB, iFR at rest was abnormal in 65% of cases (with a clear step-up across the MB at iFR pullback), whereas FFR at rest was negative in all patients. In addition, after inotropic stimulus by intravenous dobutamine infusion, iFR dropped in all cases, while conventional FFR did not significantly change. The discrepancy between FFR and iFR correlated with the reduction or negativization of the systolic pressure gradient both at rest and after dobutamine challenge, further supporting the hypothesis that systolic pressure gradient inversion observed in significant MBs can invariably affect FFR measurements [49]. A typical clinical example of LAD-MB functional evaluation is shown in Fig. 4.5.

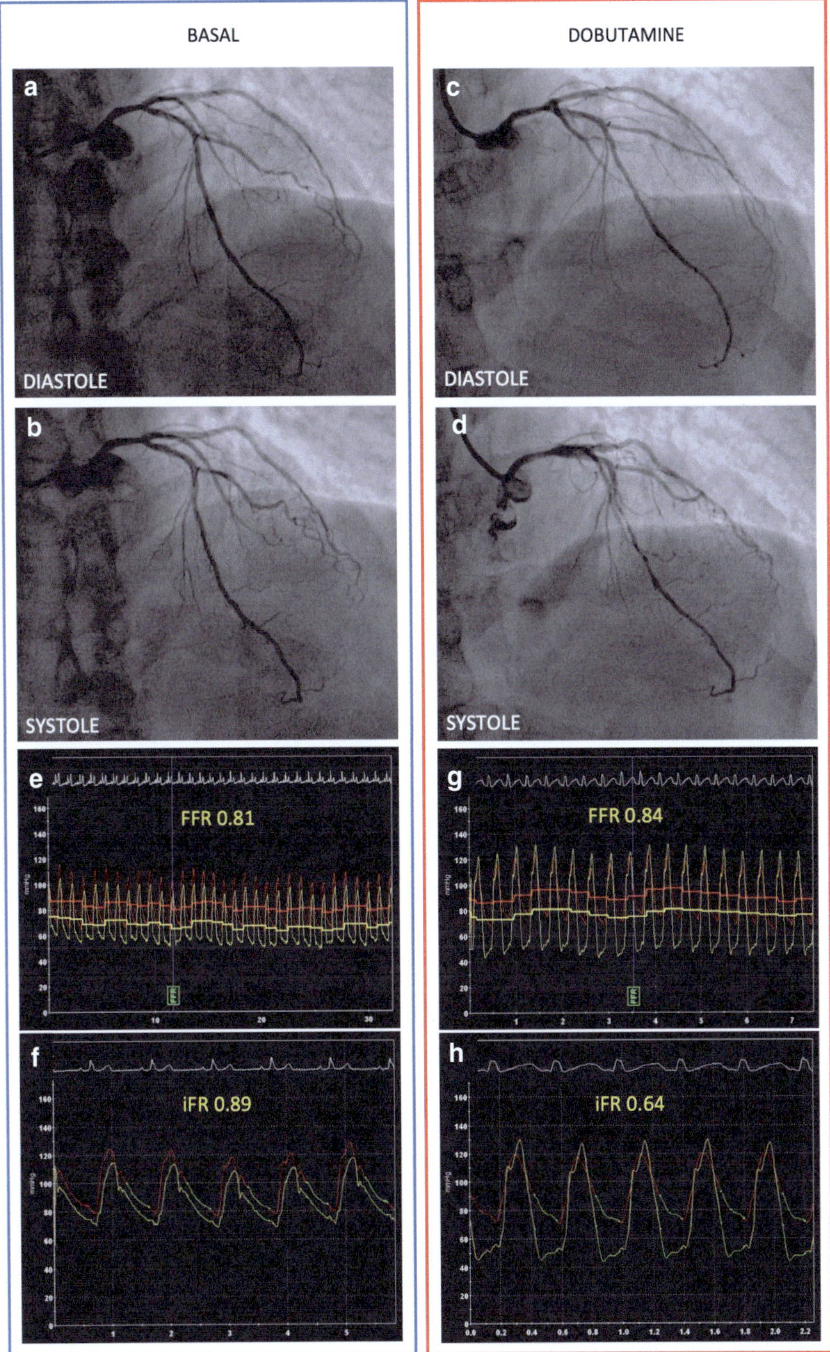

Fig. 4.5 Morphological and functional assessment of a patient with LAD-MB. (**a** and **b**) Diastolic and systolic angiographic appearance of the MB at resting conditions and (**c** and **d**) after dobutamine administration (20 μ/kg/min). Hemodynamic assessment shows near-cutoff values for both FFR (e) and iFR (f) in basal conditions. FFR values increase during dobutamine infusion (**g**). Conversely, iFR measurements become more positive after dobutamine challenge (**h**). Red and yellow tracings indicate proximal (Pa) and distal (Pd) pressures, respectively. *LAD* left anterior descending artery, *MB* myocardial bridge, *FFR* fractional flow reserve, *iFR* instantaneous wave-free ratio

The use of Doppler-tipped guidewires to assess intracoronary flow velocity and coronary flow reserve is by far a less diffuse tool to evaluate MB functional significance. The analysis of flow velocity in vessels with MB revealed a systolic flow reversal proximal to the bridged segment and a characteristic "spike and dome" pattern or "fingertip phenomenon", due to abrupt early diastolic flow acceleration, rapid mid-diastolic flow deceleration and mid to late diastolic plateau [26, 50]. An impaired coronary flow reserve has been observed when measured distal to the MB [19].

Among functional non-invasive imaging tests, stress echocardiography, stress cardiac magnetic resonance, single-photon emission-computed tomography and positron emission tomography are the most widely used [51]. As already mentioned, transluminal attenuation gradient and CCT-derived FFR are emerging as new post-processing techniques to derive functional information from CCT [36–39].

Treatment

Medical Therapy

The treatment of MBs should be reserved only for patients with symptoms and/or objective signs of ischemia, and should focus on relieving potential triggers and hemodynamic disturbances that aggravate the MB, such as hypertension/hypertrophy, increased heart rate, reduced diastolic coronary filling period, and inappropriate compression of the artery. Although evidence is limited, symptomatic patients seem to respond well to pharmacological treatment with beta-blockers or non-dihydropyridine calcium-channel blockers (CCB), which are therefore considered as first-line therapy [52–54]. By reducing heart rate and myocardial contractility, beta-blockers have been shown to restore base-line pressure tracings in patients with significant overshooting induced by inotropic challenge, providing evidence of treatment efficacy [42, 49, 52]. Given the similar hemodynamic effect of beta-blockers and the additional benefit in reduc-

ing concomitant vasospasm, CCB can be used as an alternative to beta-blockers when they are not tolerated or contraindicated [54]. Pure vasodilators, such as nitrates, are contraindicated in patients with functional significant MBs, as they may exacerbate symptoms by augmentation of the systolic narrowing and increase in vessel wall compliance [41]. Ivabradine, which acts by slowing the heart rate and thereby prolonging the diastolic period, may be considered as a second-line therapy for patients who cannot tolerate beta-blockers or CCB, or in combination with lower doses of these drugs [10]. Patients with concomitant atherosclerotic disease may benefit from aggressive risk factor modification and treatment with antiplatelet and statin therapy.

Percutaneous Coronary Intervention

No randomized studies between optimal medical treatment and medical therapy plus percutaneous coronary intervention (PCI) in patients with MB have been reported so far. Nevertheless, percutaneous stent implantation may be considered in selected patients refractory to maximal medical therapy. Although some initial experiences had shown an improvement in hemodynamic abnormalities and symptoms [50, 55], further studies have raised concerns by reporting higher rates of target lesion revascularization after PCI of the bridged segments [56]. In addition, stent implantation in MBs has been associated with higher rates of complications, including coronary perforation [57], stent fracture [58, 59], in-stent restenosis [56], and stent thrombosis [60]. An elegant study using IVUS reported increased rates of late events after stenting of the LAD when the stent extended unintentionally into the MB, compared to patients who underwent stent implantation only in the epicardial obstructive lesion [61]. Given these unfavorable outcomes, revascularization using drug-eluting stents should be considered only for severely symptomatic patients who are refractory to optimal medical therapy and who are not amenable for surgery. Bioresorbable scaffolds, when implanted in MBs, have recently been shown to be superior to everolimus-eluting stents in terms of angiographic late loss and tissue proliferation, suggesting a potential benefit of vascular restoration in this setting [62].

Surgery

Surgical options for MBs include supra-arterial myotomy (i.e. surgical unroofing of the bridged LAD) and coronary artery bypass grafting (CABG). Isolated supra-arterial myotomy can be performed in the absence of severe atherosclerotic disease, and involves dissection of the myocardial fibers overlying the bridged segment with complete exposure of the coronary artery [63–65]. This procedure is not without risk, and may result in wall perforation, ventricular aneurism formation, and post-operative bleeding [64]. In this regard, intraoperative high-frequency epicardial echocardiography may help to identify the course of the vessel thereby reducing the risk of complications [66]. CABG has been shown to be superior to myotomy in cases of extensive (>25 mm) or deep (>5 mm) MBs, and might be a better option for patients with significant atherosclerotic disease proximal to the MB [67, 68]. However, graft failure rates have been reported to be high due to potential competitive flow [69].

Surgical treatment should be considered for patients with persistent symptoms despite optimal medical therapy and with proven inducible ischemia, especially for those who have experienced myocardial infarction, life-threatening arrhythmias, and resuscitated cardiac arrest. A recent meta-analysis of 18 studies comparing different therapeutic strategies for patients with MB showed that, among invasively treated patients, surgery was superior to percutaneous treatment in terms of symptoms relief and major cardiovascular events related to target vessel revascularization [70].

References

1. Möhlenkamp S, Hort W, Ge J, Erbel R. Update on myocardial bridging. Circulation. 2002;106:2616–22.
2. Migliore F, Maffei E, Perazzolo Marra M, Bilato C, Napodano M, Corbetti F, Zorzi A, Andres AL, Sarais C, Cacciavillani L, Favaretto E, Martini C, Seitun S, Cademartiri F, Corrado D, Iliceto S, Tarantini G. LAD coronary artery myocardial bridging and apical ballooning syndrome. JACC Cardiovasc Imaging. 6:32–41.
3. Migliore F, Zorzi A, Marra MP, Basso C, Corbetti F, De Lazzari M, Tarantini G, Buja P, Lacognata C, Thiene G, Corrado D, Iliceto S. Myocardial edema underlies dynamic T-wave inversion (Wellens' ECG pattern) in patients with reversible left ventricular dysfunction. Heart Rhythm. 2011;8:1629–34.
4. Feld H, Guadanino V, Hollander G, Greengart A, Lichstein E, Shani J. Exercise-induced ventricular tachycardia in association with a myocardial bridge. Chest. 1991;99:1295–6.
5. Desseigne P, Tabib A, Loire R. Pont myocardique Sur l'interventriculaire antérieure et mort subite. A propos de 19 cas autopsiés [myocardial bridging on the left anterior descending coronary artery and sudden death. Apropos of 19 cases with autopsy]. Arch Mal Coeur Vaiss. 1991;84:511–6.
6. Rossi L, Dander B, Nidasio GP, Arbustini E, Paris B, Vassanelli C, Buonanno C, Poppi A. Myocardial bridges and ischemic heart disease. Eur Heart J. 1980;1:239–45.
7. Hostiuc S, Negoi I, Rusu MC, Hostiuc M. Myocardial bridging: a meta-analysis of prevalence. J Forensic Sci. 2018;63:1176–85.
8. La Grutta L, Runza G, Lo Re G, Galia M, Alaimo V, Grassedonio E, Bartolotta TV, Malagò R, Tedeschi C, Cademartiri F, De Maria M, Cardinale AE, Lagalla R, Midiri M. Prevalence of myocardial bridging and correlation with coronary atherosclerosis studied with 64-slice CT coronary angiography. Radiol Med. 2009;114:1024–36.
9. Hwang JH, Ko SM, Roh HG, Song MG, Shin JK, Chee HK, Kim JS. Myocardial bridging of the left anterior descending coronary artery: depiction rate and morphologic features by dual-source CT coronary angiography. Korean J Radiol. 2010;11:514–21.
10. Tarantini G, Migliore F, Cademartiri F, Fraccaro C, Iliceto S. Left anterior descending artery myocardial bridging: a clinical approach. J Am Coll Cardiol. 2016;68:2887–99.
11. Tsujita K, Maehara A, Mintz GS, Doi H, Kubo T, Castellanos C, Liu J, Yang J, Oviedo C, Franklin-Bond T, Dasgupta N, Biro S, Dani L, Dangas GD, Mehran R, Kirtane AJ, Lansky AJ, Kreps EM, Collins MB, Stone GW, Moses JW, Leon MB. Comparison of angiographic and intravascular ultrasonic detection of myocardial bridging of the left anterior descending coronary artery. Am J Cardiol. 2008;102:1608–13.
12. Sorajja P, Ommen SR, Nishimura RA, Gersh BJ, Tajik AJ, Holmes DR. Myocardial bridging in adult patients with hypertrophic cardiomyopathy. J Am Coll Cardiol. 2003;42:889–94.
13. Wymore P, Yedlicka JW, Garcia-Medina V, Olivari MT, Hunter DW, Castañeda-Zúñiga WR, Amplatz K. The incidence of myocardial bridges in heart transplants. Cardiovasc Intervent Radiol. 1989;12:202–6.

14. Alegria JR, Herrmann J, Holmes DR Jr, Lerman A, Rihal CS. Myocardial bridging. Eur Heart J. 2005;26:1159–68.

15. Polacek P, Kralove H. Relation of myocardial bridges and loops on the coronary arteries to coronary occlusions. Am Heart J. 1961;61:44–52.

16. Angelini P, Trivellato M, Donis J, Leachman RD. Myocardial bridges: a review. Prog Cardiovasc Dis. 1983;26:75–88.

17. Ferreira AG Jr, Trotter SE, König B Jr, Décourt LV, Fox K, Olsen EG. Myocardial bridges: morphological and functional aspects. Br Heart J. 1991;66:364–7.

18. Sivananthan M. Coronary anatomy. In: Vasan RS, Sawyer DB, editors. Encyclopedia of Cardiovascular Research and Medicine. Amsterdam: Elsevier; 2018.

19. Schwarz ER, Klues HG, vom Dahl J, Klein I, Krebs W, Hanrath P. Functional characteristics of myocardial bridging. A combined angiographic and intracoronary Doppler flow study. Eur Heart J. 1997;18:434–42.

20. Bourassa MG, Butnaru A, Lespérance J, Tardif JC. Symptomatic myocardial bridges: overview of ischemic mechanisms and current diagnostic and treatment strategies. J Am Coll Cardiol. 2003;41:351–9.

21. Gould KL, Johnson NP. Imaging coronary blood flow in AS: let the data talk, again. J Am Coll Cardiol. 2016;67:1423–6.

22. Lin S, Tremmel JA, Yamada R, Rogers IS, Yong CM, Turcott R, McConnell MV, Dash R, Schnittger I. A novel stress echocardiography pattern for myocardial bridge with invasive structural and hemodynamic correlation. J Am Heart Assoc. 2013;2:e000097.

23. Risse M, Weiler G. Die koronare Muskelbrücke und ihre Beziehungen zu lokaler Koronarsklerose, regionaler Myokardischämie und Koronarspasmus. Eine morphometrische Studie [coronary muscle bridge and its relations to local coronary sclerosis, regional myocardial ischemia and coronary spasm. A morphometric study]. Z Kardiol. 1985;74:700–5.

24. Verhagen SN, Rutten A, Meijs MF, Isgum I, Cramer MJ, van der Graaf Y, Visseren FL. Relationship between myocardial bridges and reduced coronary atherosclerosis in patients with angina pectoris. Int J Cardiol. 2013;167:883–8.

25. Ishii T, Asuwa N, Masuda S, Ishikawa Y. The effects of a myocardial bridge on coronary atherosclerosis and ischaemia. J Pathol. 1998;185:4–9.

26. Ge J, Jeremias A, Rupp A, Abels M, Baumgart D, Liu F, Haude M, Görge G, von Birgelen C, Sack S, Erbel R. New signs characteristic of myocardial bridging demonstrated by intracoronary ultrasound and Doppler. Eur Heart J. 1999;20:1707–16.

27. Ishikawa Y, Akasaka Y, Suzuki K, Fujiwara M, Ogawa T, Yamazaki K, Niino H, Tanaka M, Ogata K, Morinaga S, Ebihara Y, Kawahara Y, Sugiura H, Takimoto T, Komatsu A, Shinagawa T, Taki K, Satoh H, Yamada K, Yanagida-Iida M, Shimokawa R, Shimada K, Nishimura C, Ito K, Ishii T. Anatomic properties of myocardial bridge predisposing to myocardial infarction. Circulation. 2009;120:376–83.

28. Uusitalo V, Saraste A, Pietilä M, Kajander S, Bax JJ, Knuuti J. The functional effects of intramural course of coronary arteries and its relation to coronary atherosclerosis. JACC Cardiovasc Imaging. 2015;8:697–704.

29. Kim JW, Park CG, Suh SY, Choi CU, Kim EJ, Rha SW, Seo HS, Oh DJ. Comparison of frequency of coronary spasm in Korean patients with versus without myocardial bridging. Am J Cardiol. 2007;100:1083–6.

30. Wu S, Liu W, Zhou Y. Spontaneous coronary artery dissection in the presence of myocardial bridge causing myocardial infarction: an insight into mechanism. Int J Cardiol. 2016;206:77–8.

31. den Dulk K, Brugada P, Braat S, Heddle B, Wellens HJ. Myocardial bridging as a cause of paroxysmal atrioventricular block. J Am Coll Cardiol. 1983;1:965–9.

32. Ural E, Bildirici U, Celikyurt U, Kilic T, Sahin T, Acar E, Kahraman G, Ural D. Long-term prognosis of non-interventionally followed patients with isolated myocardial bridge and severe systolic compression of the left anterior descending coronary artery. Clin Cardiol. 2009;32:454–7.

33. Corban MT, Hung OY, Eshtehardi P, Rasoul-Arzrumly E, McDaniel M, Mekonnen G, Timmins LH, Lutz J, Guyton RA, Samady H. Myocardial bridging: contemporary understanding of pathophysiology with implications for diagnostic and therapeutic strategies. J Am Coll Cardiol. 2014;63:2346–55.

34. Konen E, Goitein O, Sternik L, Eshet Y, Shemesh J, Di Segni E. The prevalence and anatomical patterns of intramuscular coronary arteries: a coronary computed tomography angiographic study. J Am Coll Cardiol. 2007;49:587–93.

35. Forsdahl SH, Rogers IS, Schnittger I, Tanaka S, Kimura T, Pargaonkar VS, Chan FP, Fleischmann D, Tremmel JA, Becker HC. Myocardial bridges on coronary computed tomography angiography-correlation with intravascular ultrasound and fractional flow reserve. Circ J. 2017;81:1894–900.

36. Stuijfzand WJ, Danad I, Raijmakers PG, Marcu CB, Heymans MW, van Kuijk CC, van Rossum AC, Nieman K, Min JK, Leipsic J, van Royen N, Knaapen P. Additional value of transluminal attenuation gradient in CT angiography to predict hemodynamic significance of coronary artery stenosis. JACC Cardiovasc Imaging. 2014;7:374–86.

37. Yoon YE, Choi JH, Kim JH, Park KW, Doh JH, Kim YJ, Koo BK, Min JK, Erglis A, Gwon HC, Choe YH, Choi DJ, Kim HS, Oh BH, Park YB. Noninvasive diagnosis of ischemia-causing coronary stenosis using CT angiography: diagnostic value of transluminal attenuation gradient and fractional flow reserve computed from coronary CT angiography compared to invasively measured fractional flow reserve. JACC Cardiovasc Imaging. 2012;5:1088–96.

38. Zhou F, Wang YN, Schoepf UJ, Tesche C, Tang CX, Zhou CS, Xu L, Hou Y, Zheng MW, Yan J, Lu MJ, Lu GM, Zhang DM, Zhang B, Zhang JY, Zhang LJ. Diagnostic performance of machine learning

based CT-FFR in detecting ischemia in myocardial bridging and concomitant proximal atherosclerotic disease. Can J Cardiol. 2019;35:1523–33.

39. Koo HJ, Yang DH, Kim YH, Kang JW, Kang SJ, Kweon J, Kim HJ, Lim TH. CT-based myocardial ischemia evaluation: quantitative angiography, transluminal attenuation gradient, myocardial perfusion, and CT-derived fractional flow reserve. Int J Cardiovasc Imaging. 2016;32(Suppl 1):1–19.

40. Juilliére Y, Berder V, Suty-Selton C, Buffet P, Danchin N, Cherrier F. Isolated myocardial bridges with angiographic milking of the left anterior descending coronary artery: a long-term follow-up study. Am Heart J. 1995;129:663–5.

41. Hongo Y, Tada H, Ito K, Yasumura Y, Miyatake K, Yamagishi M. Augmentation of vessel squeezing at coronary-myocardial bridge by nitroglycerin: study by quantitative coronary angiography and intravascular ultrasound. Am Heart J. 1999;138:345–50.

42. Escaned J, Cortés J, Flores A, Goicolea J, Alfonso F, Hernández R, Fernández-Ortiz A, Sabaté M, Bañuelos C, Macaya C. Importance of diastolic fractional flow reserve and dobutamine challenge in physiologic assessment of myocardial bridging. J Am Coll Cardiol. 2003;42:226–33.

43. Ge J, Erbel R, Rupprecht HJ, Koch L, Kearney P, Görge G, Haude M, Meyer J. Comparison of intravascular ultrasound and angiography in the assessment of myocardial bridging. Circulation. 1994;89:1725–32.

44. Cao HM, Jiang JF, Deng B, Xu JH, Xu WJ. Evaluation of myocardial bridges with optical coherence tomography. J Int Med Res. 2010;38:681–5.

45. Bose D, Philipp S. Images in clinical medicine. High-resolution imaging of myocardial bridging. N Engl J Med. 2008;358:392.

46. Hakeem A, Cilingiroglu M, Leesar MA. Hemodynamic and intravascular ultrasound assessment of myocardial bridging: fractional flow reserve paradox with dobutamine versus adenosine. Catheter Cardiovasc Interv. 2010;75:229–36.

47. Abe M, Tomiyama H, Yoshida H, Doba N. Diastolic fractional flow reserve to assess the functional severity of moderate coronary artery stenoses: comparison with fractional flow reserve and coronary flow velocity reserve. Circulation. 2000;102:2365–70.

48. Sen S, Asrress KN, Nijjer S, Petraco R, Malik IS, Foale RA, Mikhail GW, Foin N, Broyd C, Hadjiloizou N, Sethi A, Al-Bustami M, Hackett D, Khan MA, Khawaja MZ, Baker CS, Bellamy M, Parker KH, Hughes AD, Francis DP, Mayet J, Di Mario C, Escaned J, Redwood S, Davies JE. Diagnostic classification of the instantaneous wave-free ratio is equivalent to fractional flow reserve and is not improved with adenosine administration. Results of CLARIFY (Classification Accuracy of Pressure-Only Ratios Against Indices Using Flow Study). J Am Coll Cardiol. 2013;61:1409–20.

49. Tarantini G, Barioli A, Nai Fovino L, Fraccaro C, Masiero G, Iliceto S, Napodano M. Unmasking myocardial bridge-related ischemia by intracoronary functional evaluation. Circ Cardiovasc Interv. 2018;11:e006247.

50. Klues HG, Schwarz ER, vom Dahl J, Reffelmann T, Reul H, Potthast K, Schmitz C, Minartz J, Krebs W, Hanrath P. Disturbed intracoronary hemodynamics in myocardial bridging: early normalization by intracoronary stent placement. Circulation. 1997;96:2905–13.

51. Danad I, Szymonifka J, Twisk JWR, Norgaard BL, Zarins CK, Knaapen P, Min JK. Diagnostic performance of cardiac imaging methods to diagnose ischaemia-causing coronary artery disease when directly compared with fractional flow reserve as a reference standard: a meta-analysis. Eur Heart J. 2017;38:991–8.

52. Schwarz ER, Klues HG, vom Dahl J, Klein I, Krebs W, Hanrath P. Functional, angiographic and intracoronary Doppler flow characteristics in symptomatic patients with myocardial bridging: effect of short-term intravenous beta-blocker medication. J Am Coll Cardiol. 1996;27:1637–45.

53. Nair CK, Dang B, Heintz MH, Sketch MH. Myocardial bridges: effect of propranolol on systolic compression. Can J Cardiol. 1986;2:218–21.

54. Alessandri N, Dei Giudici A, De Angelis S, Urciuoli F, Garante MC, Di Matteo A. Efficacy of calcium channel blockers in the treatment of the myocardial bridging: a pilot study. Eur Rev Med Pharmacol Sci. 2012;16:829–34.

55. Prendergast BD, Kerr F, Starkey IR. Normalisation of abnormal coronary fractional flow reserve associated with myocardial bridging using an intracoronary stent. Heart. 2000;83:705–7.

56. Haager PK, Schwarz ER, vom Dahl J, Klues HG, Reffelmann T, Hanrath P. Long term angiographic and clinical follow up in patients with stent implantation for symptomatic myocardial bridging. Heart. 2000;84:403–8.

57. Ernst A, Bulum J, Šeparović Hanževački J, Lovrić Benčić M, Strozzi M. Five-year angiographic and clinical follow-up of patients with drug-eluting stent implantation for symptomatic myocardial bridging in absence of coronary atherosclerotic disease. J Invasive Cardiol. 2013;25:586–92.

58. Tandar A, Whisenant BK, Michaels AD. Stent fracture following stenting of a myocardial bridge: report of two cases. Catheter Cardiovasc Interv. 2008;71:191–6.

59. Srinivasan M, Prasad A. Metal fatigue in myocardial bridges: stent fracture limits the efficacy of drug-eluting stents. J Invasive Cardiol. 2011;23:E150–2.

60. Agirbasli M, Hillegass WB Jr, Chapman GD, Brott BC. Stent procedure complicated by thrombus formation distal to the lesion within a muscle bridge. Catheter Cardiovasc Diagn. 1998;43:73–6.

61. Tsujita K, Maehara A, Mintz GS, Doi H, Kubo T, Castellanos C, Liu J, Yang J, Oviedo C, Franklin-Bond T, Sugirtharaj DD, Dangas GD, Lansky AJ, Stone GW, Moses JW, Leon MB, Mehran R. Impact of myocardial bridge on clinical outcome after coronary stent placement. Am J Cardiol. 2009;103:1344–8.

62. Kameda R, Okada K, Kitahara H, Hollak MB, Yock PG, Popma J, Kusano H, Cheong WF, Sudhir K, Honda Y, Kimura T. TCT-311. Long-term vascular response to bioresorbable scaffolds versus metallic stents in coronary lesions with myocardial bridging: a potential benefit of vascular restoration under dynamic compression force. J Am Coll Cardiol. 2018;72(13_Supplement):B128.

63. Katznelson Y, Petchenko P, Knobel B, Cohen AJ, Kishon Y, Schachner A. Myocardial bridging: surgical technique and operative results. Mil Med. 1996;161:248–50.

64. Iversen S, Hake U, Mayer E, Erbel R, Diefenbach C, Oelert H. Surgical treatment of myocardial bridging causing coronary artery obstruction. Scand J Thorac Cardiovasc Surg. 1992;26:107–11.

65. Ochsner JL, Mills NL. Surgical management of diseased intracavitary coronary arteries. Ann Thorac Surg. 1984;38:356–62.

66. Hiratzka LF, McPherson DD, Brandt B 3rd, Lamberth WC Jr, Marcus ML, Kerber RE. Intraoperative high-frequency epicardial echocardiography in coronary revascularization: locating deeply embedded coronary arteries. Ann Thorac Surg. 1986;42(6 Suppl):S9–11.

67. Attaran S, Moscarelli M, Athanasiou T, Anderson J. Is coronary artery bypass grafting an acceptable alternative to myotomy for the treatment of myocardial bridging? Interact Cardiovasc Thorac Surg. 2013;16:347–9.

68. Murtaza G, Mukherjee D, Gharacholou SM, Nanjundappa A, Lavie CJ, Khan AA, Shanmugasundaram M, Paul TK. An updated review on myocardial bridging. Cardiovasc Revasc Med. 2020;21:1169–79.

69. Boyd JH, Pargaonkar VS, Scoville DH, Rogers IS, Kimura T, Tanaka S, Yamada R, Fischbein MP, Tremmel JA, Mitchell RS, Schnittger I. Surgical Unroofing of hemodynamically significant left anterior descending myocardial bridges. Ann Thorac Surg. 2017;103:1443–50.

70. Cerrato E, Barbero U, D'Ascenzo F, Taha S, Biondi-Zoccai G, Omedè P, Bianco M, Echavarria-Pinto M, Escaned J, Gaita F, Varbella F. What is the optimal treatment for symptomatic patients with isolated coronary myocardial bridge? A systematic review and pooled analysis. J Cardiovasc Med (Hagerstown). 2017;18:758–70.

Isolated Coronary Artery Fistulas

5

M. Rebonato, G. Butera, S. Qureshi,
and M. Carminati

Introduction

Coronary artery fistulas (CAF) are rare anomalies of the cardiovascular system first described by Krause in 1865. A CAF is defined as an abnormal connection that bypasses the myocardial capillary bed between a normally originating coronary artery and another cardiovascular structure, which can be a cardiac chamber, the coronary sinus, vena cava, or a pulmonary artery or even a bronchial artery or vein. They are the most common of hemodynamically significant coronary lesions and comprise nearly half of all coronary artery anomalies [1].

Haller and Little [2] described the diagnostic triad for CAFs: an abnormal location for a to-and-fro murmur thought to be due to a patent ductus arteriosus; a left to right shunt at the atrial or ventricular level; and a large, tortuous coronary artery at coronary angiography. Bjork and Crafoord reported the first successfully corrected CAFs in 1947 [3], and the first successful transcatheter closure of a CAF was reported in 1983 [4].

The site and size of the fistulous communication may determine in large part the clinical and hemodynamic consequences. Their clinical importance, usually in adult life, is due to an increased risk of complications including heart failure, myocardial ischemia, infective endocarditis, arrhythmias, and rupture. Fortunately, clinically important coronary arteriovenous fistulas are uncommon in childhood.

The natural history of CAF is not associated with a normal life expectancy, due to the eventual development of either congestive heart failure, myocardial ischemia, subacute bacterial endocarditis, aneurysm formation with rupture or embolization, or the development of pulmonary hypertension.

Epidemiology

The exact incidence of CAFs is unknown because the undiagnosed rate still remains high, but may represent about 0.2–0.4% of all cardiac malformations and 14% of all coronary anomalies.

Frequently isolated (80%), several studies report the presence of CAF in 0.3% of patients

M. Rebonato · G. Butera (✉)
Department of Cardiac Surgery, Cardiology, Heart
and Lung Transplantation, Bambino Gesù Children's
Hospital, Rome, Italy
e-mail: Micol.rebonato@opbg.net;
Gianfranco.butera@opbg.net

S. Qureshi
Paediatric and Adult Cardiology, Evelina London
Children's Hospital, London, UK
e-mail: Shakeel.qureshi@gstt.nhs.uk

M. Carminati
Children and Adults Congenita Heart disease,
Policlinico San Donato, Milan, Italy
e-mail: Mario.carminati@grupposandonato.it

© Springer Nature Switzerland AG 2023
G. Butera, A. Frigiola (eds.), *Congenital Anomalies of Coronary Arteries*,
https://doi.org/10.1007/978-3-031-36966-7_5

presenting with congenital heart disease, in 0.06% of children undergoing echocardiography, and in 0.13–0.22% of adults undergoing coronary angiography.

Multiple fistulas are present in 10.7–16% of all CAFs with single fistula being far more common, occurring in up to 90% of the cases.

The embryologic origin of these fistulous communications is likely due to persistence of sinusoids in the coronary system and abnormalities in coronary capillary differentiation. Normally, the intramyocardial sinusoids become narrowed and persist only as thebesian vessels in the adult. If obliteration of the intramyocardial trabecular sinusoids fails, a fistulous communication persists between the coronary arteries and a cardiac chamber [5].

Although in the past, CAF was usually congenital, over the years the development and dissemination of interventional and surgical techniques have resulted in a change of its etiology, with a higher prevalence of the acquired forms, [6] which may include those secondary to infective endocarditis, aortic dissection, previous surgery, endomyocardial biopsy, coronary angioplasty and bypass surgery, valve replacement, cardiac transplantation, trauma, permanent pacemaker placement, closed-chest ablation of accessory pathways, neoplasms, and iatrogenic management of Kawasaki disease.

Anatomy

The majority of coronary fistulas arise from the right coronary arteries or the left anterior descending; the circumflex coronary artery is rarely involved. Several case series report that the right coronary artery, or its branches, is the site of the fistula in about 55% of cases; the left coronary artery in about 35%; and both coronary arteries in 5% [7].

However, this was contradicted by a review of 12 case series including 227 patients, which revealed half of the CAFs to involve the left coronary artery, 38% involving the right coronary artery, and the remaining 12% involving both left and right coronary arteries [8].

Over 90% of the CAFs drain into the venous circulation. Low-pressure structures are the most common sites of drainage of the fistulas. These include right-sided chambers, pulmonary artery, superior vena cava, and coronary sinus [9]. Fistulous communication to the left-sided chambers is less frequent. Fistulous drainage occurs into the right ventricle in 41%, right atrium in 26%, pulmonary artery in 17%, left ventricle in 3%, and superior vena cava in 1%. Coronary artery dilatation is usual, and the degree of dilatation does not always depend on the shunt size. When the fistulous communication arises in the distal part of a coronary artery, the arterial diameter may remain small.

The more proximal the feeding artery originates from the main coronary artery, the more dilated it tends to be (Fig. 5.1). If the fistula drains to the right atrium with a proximally arising feeding artery, it tends to be considerably dilated but less tortuous. If there is a more distal origin of the feeding artery, and in particular when the fistulas originate from the left coronary artery and drain to the left ventricle, they may be very tortuous, presenting a challenge for catheter closure. However, in the less frequently encountered right coronary artery to coronary sinus drainage, the fistula vessel may be large and very tortuous. It is

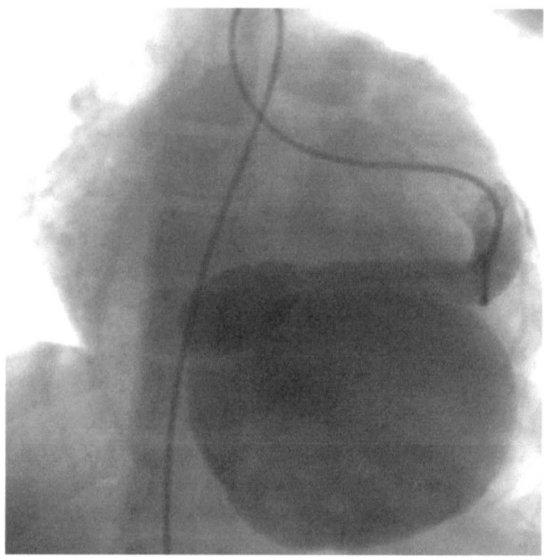

Fig. 5.1 Example of a huge fistula originating from left anterior descending coronary artery

important to note that there may be multiple feeding arteries to a single coronary arterial fistula drainage point or there may be multiple drainage sites [10].

Pathophysiology

The pathophysiology of a CAF depends on the resistance of the fistulous connection and on the site of fistulous termination, the hemodynamic consequences depend on the size of the fistula, the pressure gradient along the fistula, and the volume of the shunt flow.

When the fistula drains to the right side of the heart, the volume load is increased to the right heart as well as to the pulmonary vascular bed, the left atrium, and the left ventricle and may present with a continuous flow for the whole duration of the cardiac cycle, because the pressure is lower than the one encountered in myocardial arterioles and capillaries.

A left-to-right shunt exists in over 90% of the cases [11]. In these conditions, especially in CAF with a large caliber, it could allow the well-known phenomenon of the coronary steal, in which blood with a diastolic run-off is directed away from the normal coronary circulation and myocardial microcirculation.

Coronary "steal phenomenon" is believed to be the primary pathophysiological problem seen in CAF without outflow obstruction. The mechanism is related to the run-off from the high-pressure coronary vasculature to a low-resistance receiving cavity due to a diastolic pressure gradient. Eventually, there is a high risk of ischemia in the myocardium beyond the site of the origin of the fistula, which is most frequently evident in association with increased myocardial oxygen demand during exercise or activity [12].

When the fistula drains into the left atrium or the left ventricle, there is volume overloading of these chambers but no increase in the pulmonary blood flow, that, over time, could lead to dilatation of the heart chambers. The clinical consequences of this volume overload may be heart failure, atrial and ventricular tachyarrhythmias.

Clinical Presentation

Most CAFs are small, and patients are asymptomatic because myocardial blood flow is not compromised. Symptoms tend to occur more in the older age groups (aged >20 years).

The diagnosis of a CAF is often suspected on auscultation when a continuous murmur is noted. Newborns can present with signs and symptoms of congestive heart failure immediately after birth due to the volume load on the left heart. Most pediatric patients, however, are asymptomatic at the time of diagnosis. Whilst only 10–20% of pediatric patients will be symptomatic, adults are more likely to report symptoms.

Small CAFs in children tend to grow with age. If untreated, fistulas cause clinical symptoms in 19% of patients aged younger than 20 years and in 63% of older patients [1].

Complications of CAFs include excessive load on the cardiac chambers which give rise to increased left ventricular end-diastolic pressure, left ventricular hypertrophy, and in older patients, congestive cardiac failure [13].

With increased flow, the coronary artery branches proximal to the shunt site become significantly enlarged. Symptoms and sequelae of coronary complications include chronic myocardial ischemia and angina, cardiomyopathy, and myocardial infarction. Coronary steal, producing myocardial ischemia due to diversion of blood, is commonly expected [14].

Thrombosis within the fistula is rare but may cause acute myocardial infarction, and atrial and ventricular arrhythmias. Persistent high flow in coronary arteries can give rise to massive dilatation and aneurysm formation. Premature coronary atherosclerosis is also reported.

Valvar regurgitation, secondary to papillary muscle dysfunction, has been described in children and adults with CAF. Hemopericardium can result from the rupture of an associated aneurysm [15].

The exact percentage of spontaneous closure of the CAFs remains unknown but relatively rare in consideration of the uncertain natural history. Review of the literature shows that fistulae draining into the right ventricle have some chances to close spontaneously [16]. Gewillig and colleagues reported six cases of full spontaneous closure of congenital CAFs monitored by color Doppler echocardiography. Their series is the first to describe patients whose follow-up by color Doppler echocardiography permitted monitoring of spontaneous CAF closure by non-invasive techniques [17].

Diagnosis

Prenatal diagnosis of isolated CAF is rare but can be made in fetal life by cross-sectional and color Doppler echocardiography. It is possible to detect CAFs prenatally, which may indicate fistulas with large left-to-right shunts, and thus may predispose the patients to the early onset of congestive cardiac failure and the need for early intervention [18].

The divert of blood from the aorta through the shunts into the right ventricular cavity during diastole possibly leads to a "steal" effect with partial ischemia of the myocardium that is insufficiently supplied by its coronary artery; occasionally, fetal hydrops may develop [19].

Most cases of CAF are asymptomatic and diagnosed incidentally during a routine clinical examination. During a physical examination, an atypical systolic, diastolic, or continuous murmur can be heard occasionally. Some patients with large shunts may present with signs of congestive cardiac failure and angina, usually at the two extremes of life.

The electrocardiogram and chest X-ray are unhelpful usually, although the electrocardiogram may show the effects of left ventricular volume overload and occasionally ischemic changes. When the electrocardiogram is normal and if the patient is old enough to exercise on the treadmill with electrocardiographic monitoring, ischemic ST segment changes may become apparent. Generally, the chest X-ray is normal, but occasionally moderate cardiomegaly may be present when there is a large left-to-right shunt.

Two-dimensional and color Doppler echocardiography is helpful in visualizing volume overload of the chambers, decreased regional or global dysfunction as a consequence of myocardial ischemia, and in some cases, dilatation of the affected coronary artery and coronary artery aneurysms. Echocardiography may show the site of drainage, but it is difficult to visualize detailed anatomy of the fistula. Three-dimensional echocardiography may be more superior in this aspect.

On color Doppler flow imaging, large flow may be seen at the origin or even along the length of the vessel and indeed flow into the right heart chambers may also be visualized.

Catheter angiography is invasive in nature. Although it delineates the origin and proximal course of CAFs well, demonstration of distal drainage may be suboptimal. This is attributed to the contrast dilution that occurs at the distal drainage sites, usually low-pressure chambers of the heart. Previously, cardiac catheterization was usually performed pre-operatively to confirm the anatomy and in planning the surgical treatment. However, with advances in non-invasive imaging modalities, nowadays it is only used as an adjunct to endovascular management in these lesions [20].

Magnetic resonance (MR) imaging has also been used in the preoperative evaluation of CAFs. Newer MRI sequences allow improvement in image quality along with better anatomical demarcation. Cine MR sequences demonstrate the flow dynamics, especially the turbulence observed at the fistulous communication site, whilst the black-blood sequences permit excellent visualization of the vessel lumen and its wall [21]. MRI has evolved into an imaging substitute to assess anatomic, flow-related, and functional aspects of the lesion with no ionizing radiation burden [22]. Its greatest limitation, however, is the determination of distal coronary course. Therefore, this technique is not so helpful in evaluating CAFs, collateral vessels, and coronary origin outside the normal sinuses.

Coronary CTA is a relatively new imaging modality that has been used for non-invasive coronary artery imaging. With the introduction of multi-detector computed tomography (MDCT), many problems with image quality have been overcome. ECG-gated dual tube 128-slice MDCT is capable of producing high-quality images with the ECG-gated image reconstruction algorithms allowing phase-correlated image data sets [23]. In this manner, Coronary CTA clearly delineates the cardiac chambers, the coronary arteries, and coronary veins. It has been used as the technique of choice in demonstrating anomalous coronary artery anatomy and similarly is ideally suited to imaging patients with suspected CAFs. Multiplanar reconstruction with 3D volume-rendered imaging yields excellent anatomic information, including the origin, course, and drainage site of CAFs—even in cases of complex anomalies—and thus has the potential to serve as a basic guide for treatment planning [24].

Management of Coronary Artery Fistula

The best management of a patient with a CAF should provide the greatest probability of event-free survival over a lifetime.

According to the American College of Cardiology/American Heart Association (ACC/AHA) guidelines, "percutaneous or surgical closure is a Class I recommendation" for large fistulas regardless of symptoms and for small- to moderate-sized fistulas with evidence of myocardial ischemia, arrhythmia, ventricular dysfunction, left ventricular enlargement, or endarteritis [25]. Indication for closure also includes a pulmonary to systemic blood flow ratio >1.5–1.7 or right ventricular volume overload, signs of ischemia, or volume overload in the right ventricle on echocardiography, progression of pulmonary hypertension, or congestive heart failure.

Small, asymptomatic fistulas, which are clinically silent, may best be observed over time since the risks of complications or symptoms appear to be low and spontaneous closure is a possibility.

With regard to children, especially those older than 5 years, elective closure of any clinically apparent fistula should be performed, even if the patient remains asymptomatic. Late stenosis, secondary to intimal hyperplasia, represents a very important complication that has been reported in children, which could increase the risk of myocardial infarction later in life.

While the traditional approach to coronary fistulas in the past was surgical closure, coronary fistulas are now best closed in the cardiac catheterization laboratory.

The choice of the technique for CAF closure depends on its morphology, its course, tortuosity, and the presence of an aneurysmal dilatation of the vessel that supplies and the vessel which is being considered for occlusion. The results of all techniques for CAF closure are comparable with a total mortality of <1% and low rates of complications.

Surgical Treatment

The surgical obliteration of the fistula by epicardial and endocardial ligations is the cornerstone of surgical treatment, first described by Bjorck in 1947.

Surgical treatment has been reported with excellent short- and long-term results, even in childhood, despite complications including myocardial infarction and valve insufficiency, especially of the tricuspid valve, occurring in up to 11% of patients [26].

Surgical treatment is generally reserved for single, large, symptomatic fistulas that are present with angina, cardiac decompensation, or complications characterized by high-fistula flow, multiple communications, very tortuous pathways, multiple terminations, significant aneurysmal formation, or need for simultaneous distal bypass [27].

Some authors have reported successful surgical occlusion of CAF on beating heart off-pump [28].

Ligation of the CAF may be performed outside the heart without cardiopulmonary bypass when there is a simple and easily accessible CAF. Surgical ligation at the fistula drainage site should be the preferable way of treatment, avoiding the occurrence of myocardial ischemia.

Depending on the anatomical morphology of the fistula and the consequent involvement of the chambers, the most appropriate technique has to be chosen.

An interesting series of cases, spanning over 37 years of medical practice, comes from the Texas Heart Institute. Following that experience, several techniques may be considered: internal closure of the fistula, proximal and distal ligation or the latest alone, tangential arterial suture, ligation and bypass (simple or with Dacron graft required), or closure within an aneurysm [29].

From recent reports, the overall operative mortality for surgical treatment is about 2%.

Mortality related to surgical closure of isolated CAF should be rare (<1%).

Said et al. from the Mayo Clinic observed perioperative Myocardial Infarction (MI) in three of their patients (6.5%), and late MI was documented in two other patients. The common factors noted were the presence of a large and significant fistulous communication and dilated or aneurysmal CA. The infarction occurred in the distribution of the involved CA. Residual fistulas were detected in three patients (6%), with no reintervention needed [30].

Data from Wang et al. showed that TCC had a higher rate of residual shunt compared to the surgical group. At follow-up, they demonstrated that 10 (6.9%) patients in TCC group had a residual shunt versus 2 (3.6%) patients in surgical closure (SC) group, suggesting that SC had a better long-term efficacy, as was better long-term safety.

Another series by Schumacher and colleagues shows similar results with a very low morbidity and mortality rate (0–4%) when fistulas are operated on in infancy and childhood [31].

Transcatheter Closure

Transcatheter CAF closure has emerged as a feasible alternative to surgical closure with associated shorter hospitalization and recovery, and reported efficacy and safety in several small single-center series [7–10].

However, due to the rarity of CAF, the reported experience remains relatively limited. As a result, anatomic and procedural factors that may lead to unsuccessful closure, complications, or recanalization of CAF are unclear.

Due to its low rate of major complications, transcatheter closure has been promoted as treatment of choice, even in neonates and infants [32].

Small single-center studies have suggested that transcatheter CAF closure is associated with a high rate of procedural success (82–93%) and relatively low morbidity in select patients [33].

Similar rates of procedural success and complications were observed in a multicenter series [34]. Different transcatheter closing techniques (TCC) and different devices can be used safely with good long-term results, even in small infants. The choices of TCC and device selection vary, and are primarily determined by the heterogeneous anatomic characteristics of the fistulas. The aim of catheter closure is to occlude the fistula feeding artery as distally and as close to its termination point as possible, so as to avoid any possibility of occluding branches to the normal myocardium.

The techniques for transcatheter closure of CAFs include various types of occlusion devices such as Amplatzer duct occluder and Amplatzer vascular plug (St Jude/AGA Medical, Golden Valley); detachable coils (PFM Medical, Germany; Cook Gianturco patent ductus arteriosus coil, Cook Cardiology, Bloomington,); free coil (Cook coil, Cook Cardiology, Bloomington); and detachable balloon (Goldbal, Balt, France).

There are three major access approaches for percutaneous closure. One is the venous approach, one is arteriovenous loop, and the other is the arterial approach. Arterial approach is suitable for smaller fistulas that can be closed with coils (Fig. 5.2). When the fistula is large requiring a device or a plug, the venous approach is preferable (Fig. 5.3). Also, when the fistula is tortuous and long and can be approached easily through the venous side, the venous approach is preferable. Creating an AV loop allows a most distal positioning of the implantation sheath from the venous site without compromising coronary arterial blood flow during the procedure.

The choice of equipment and technique depends on the morphology of the fistulas. The factors include their tortuosity, the presence of high flow in the fistula, aneurysmal dilation of the

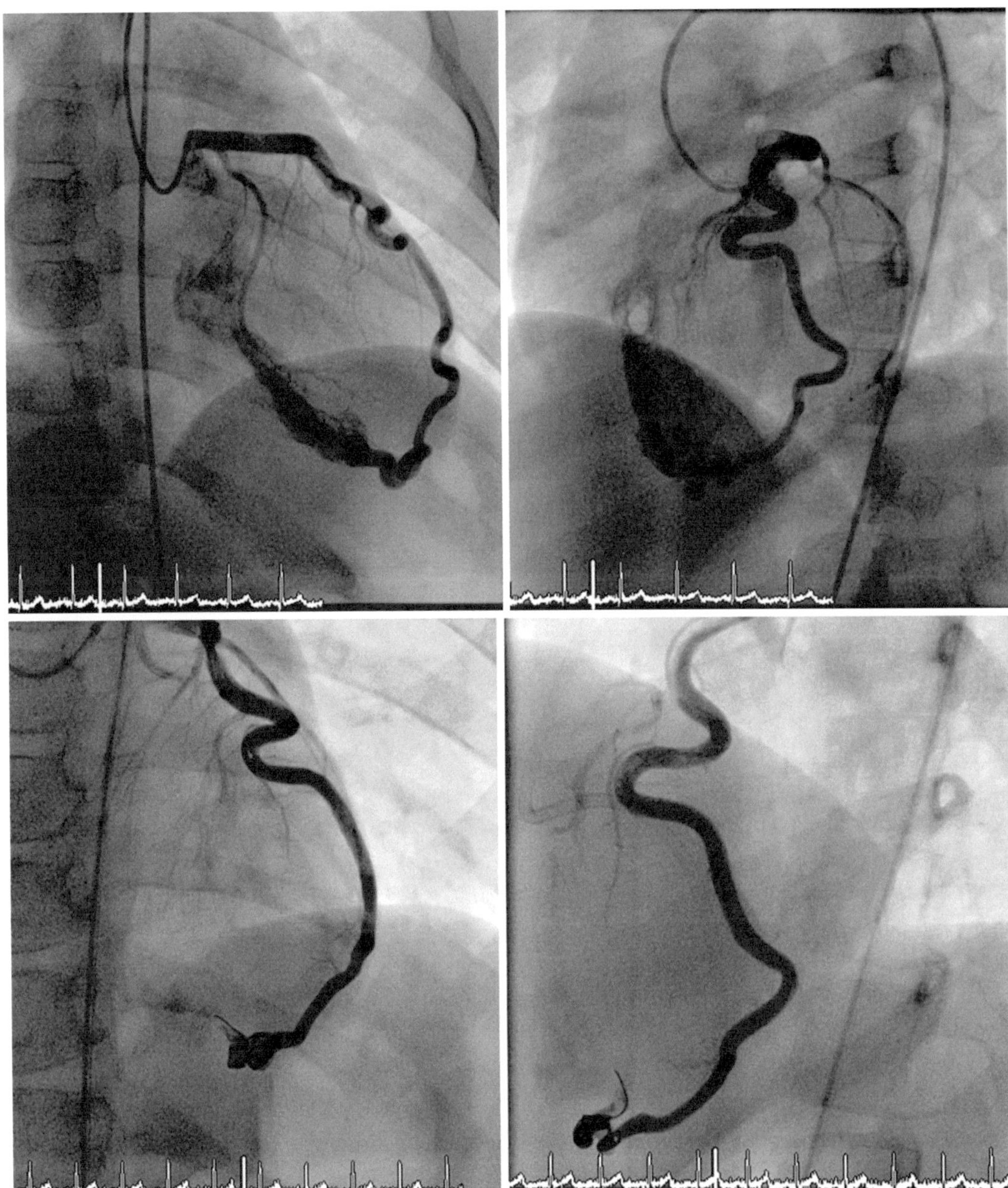

Fig. 5.2 Left coronary angiogram reveals dilated and tortuous left anterior descending coronary artery with distal fistulous communication with the right ventricle. Insertion of microcatheter and anterograde fistula closure with Concerto coils

feeding vessel, and the point of intended occlusion. Other important determinants include the age and size of the patient, the catheter size that can be used in the patient, the size of the vessel to be occluded, and the tortuosity of the catheter course to reach the intended point of occlusion.

Mavroudis et al. outlined the requirements for satisfactory embolization of a CAF as follows: the ability to cannulate safely the branch coronary artery that supplies the fistula, the absence of large and significant myocardial branches that can be inadvertently embolized or occluded, the

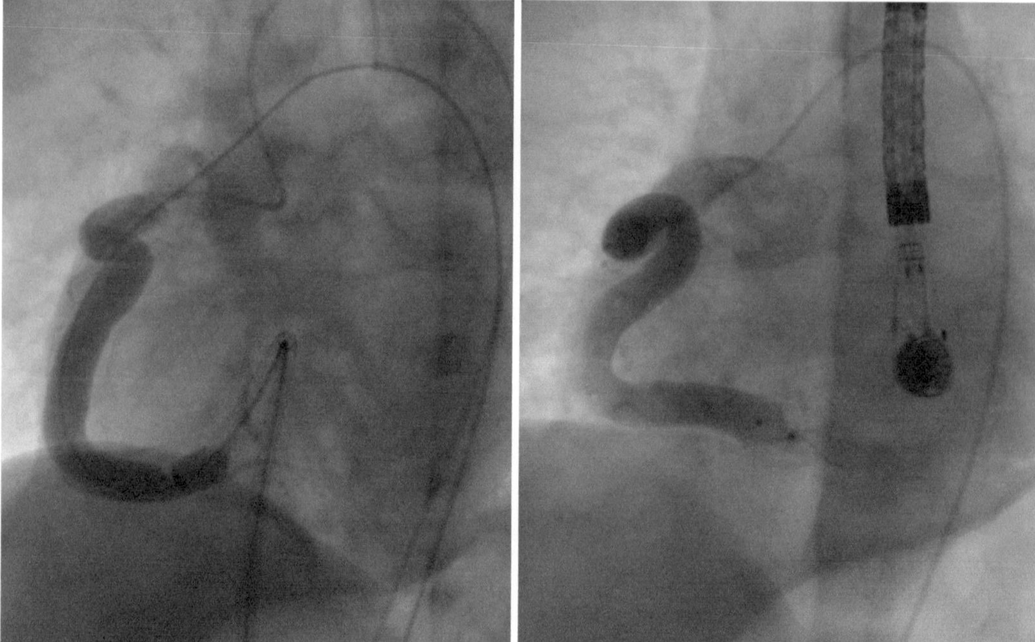

Fig. 5.3 Right coronary fistula closed with plug

presence of single, narrow restrictive drainage site into the cardiac chamber or vessel, and the absence of multiple fistulous communications [35].

Ischemic complications represent the main risk during TCC of CAFs; coronary thrombosis, and early or late STEMI have been reported in some studies [36].

Other important procedural risks include ventricular arrhythmias, coronary spasm, coronary perforation or fistula dissection, and device embolization.

Due to the potential long-term risk of recanalization with residual flow and potential thrombotic complications, close follow-up with periodic noninvasive imaging or angiography should be routinely performed after CAF closure as repeat procedure may be occasionally needed.

In a retrospective series of 76 patients with mean follow-up of 12.2 years, Valente et al. also identified anastomosis in the coronary sinus as a risk factor for long-term morbidity after closure [37]. This is because these fistulas tend to be very large, tortuous, and prone to challenging procedures and complications.

Antithrombotic treatment is usually recommended to prevent thrombus extension from the CAF to the nearby coronary artery branches, although it is not clear whether antiplatelet or anticoagulant therapy should be used. Latson has advised long-term oral anticoagulation and then anatomical reassessment in case of large CAF and antiplatelet therapy (aspirin) for the patients without residual coronary dilatation [38].

Prognosis

The prognosis of CAFs depends on the severity of the shunt and complications that sometimes occur, such as heart failure, pulmonary hypertension, and bacterial endocarditis.

The transcatheter and surgical approaches have similar early effectiveness, morbidity, and mortality.

Sequelae after closure of the fistula include persistent coronary dilatation, residual leak, thrombosis with or without myocardial infarction, and coronary artery stenosis with perfusion defects [39]. Patients who undergo a closure procedure may have a recurrence rate of up to 20–30%. Intermediate and longer-term follow-up of these thin-walled, ectatic coronary arteries after either surgical or transcatheter repair appears mandated.

References

1. Mavroudis C, Backer CL, Rocchini AP, Muster AJ, Gevitz M. Coronary artery fistulas in infants and children: a surgical review and discussion of coil embolization. Ann Thorac Surg. 1997;63:1235–42.
2. Haller JA, Little JA. Diagnosis and surgical correction of congenital coronary artery–coronary sinus fistula. Circulation. 1963;27:939.
3. Bjork G, Crafoord C. Arteriovenous aneurysm on the pulmonary artery simulating patent ductus arteriosus botalli. Thorax. 1947;2:65.
4. Reidy JF, Sowton E, Ross DN. Transcatheter occlusion of coronary to bronchial anastomosis by detachable balloon combined with coronary angioplasty at same procedure. Br Heart J. 1983;49:284–7.
5. Rittenhouse EA, Doty DB, Ehrenhaft JL. Congenital coronary artery—cardiac chamber fistula: review of operative management. Ann Thorac Surg. 1975;20:468–85.
6. Said SA, El Gamal LI, Van der Werf T. Coronary arteriovenous fistulas: collective review and management of six new case: changing etiology, presentation, and treatment strategy. Clin Cardiol. 1997;20:748–52.
7. McNamara JJ, Gross RE. Congenital coronary artery fistula. Surgery. 1969;65:59–69.
8. Ceresnak S, Gray RG, Altmann K, Chen JM, Glickstein JS, Hellenbrand WE. Coronary artery fistulas: a review of the literature and presentation of two cases of coronary fistulas with drainage into the left atrium. Congenit Heart Dis. 2007;2(3):208–13.
9. Levin DC, Fellows KE, Abrams HL. Hemodynamically significant primary anomalies of the coronary arteries. Circulation. 1978;58:25–34.
10. Qureshi SA. Coronary arterial fistulas. Orphanet J Rare Dis. 2006;1:51.
11. Gowda RM, Vasavada BC, Khan IA. Coronary artery fistulas: clinical and therapeutic considerations. Int J Cardiol. 2006;107:7–10.
12. Dimitrakakis G, Von Oppell U, Luckraz H, Groves P. Surgical repair of triple coronary-pulmonary artery fistulae with associated atrial septal defect and aortic valve regurgitation. Interact Cardiovasc Thorac Surg. 2008;7(5):933–4. https://doi.org/10.1510/icvts.2008.181388. Epub 2008 Jun 10.
13. Liberthson RR, Sagar K, Berkoben JP, Weintraub RM, Levine FH. Congenital coronary arteriovenous fistula. Report of 13 patients, review of the literature and delineation of management. Circulation. 1979;59:849–54.
14. Kugelmass AD, Manning WJ, Piana RN, Weintraub RM, Baim DS, Grossman W. Coronary arteriovenous fistula presenting as congestive heart failure. Catheter Cardiovasc Diagn. 1992;26:19–25.
15. Bauer HH, Allmendinger PD, Flaherty J, Owlia D, Rossi MA, Chen C. Congenital coronary arteriovenous fistula: spontaneous rupture and cardiac tamponade. Ann Thorac Surg. 1996;62:1521–3.
16. Santoro G, Formigari R, Di Carlo D, Ballerini L. Spontaneous closure of coronary fistulas: a possible prognostic role of the site of drainage. G Ital Cardiol. 1994;24(10):1223–6.
17. Schleich J, Rey C, Gewillig M, et al. Spontaneous closure of congenital coronary artery fistulas. Heart. 2001;85:6e.
18. Sharland GK, Konta L, Qureshi SA. Prenatal diagnosis of isolated coronary artery fistulas: progression and outcome in five cases. Cardiol Young. 2016;26(5):915–20.
19. Oztunc F, Gokalp S, Yuksel MA, Imamoglu M, Madazli R. Prenatal diagnosis of left coronary artery to right ventricle fistula. J Clin Ultrasound. 2015;43(2):129–31.
20. Schmitt R, Froehner S, Brunn J, Wagner M, Brunner H, Cherevatyy O, Gietzen F, Christopoulos G, Kerber S, Fellner F. Congenital anomalies of the coronary arteries: imaging with contrast-enhanced, multidetector computed tomography. Eur Radiol. 2005;15(6):1110–21.
21. Parga JR, Ikari NM, Bustamante LN, Rochitte CE, de Avila LF, Oliveira SA. Case report: MRI evaluation of congenital coronary artery fistulae. Br J Radiol. 2004;77(918):508–11.
22. Duerinckx AJ, Shaaban A, Lewis A, Perloff J, Laks H. 3D MR imaging of coronary arteriovenous fistulas. Eur Radiol. 2000;10:1459–63. https://doi.org/10.1007/s003309900273.
23. Schroeder S, Achenbach S, Bengel F, Burgstahler C, Cademartiri F, De Feyter P, George R, Kaufmann P, Kopp AF, Knutti J, Ropers D, Schuijf J, Tops LF, Bax JJ. Cardiac computed tomography: indications, applications, limitations and training requirements. Eur Heart J. 2008;29:531–56.
24. Dodd JD, Ferencik M, Liberthson RR, et al. Evaluation of efficacy of 64-slice multidetector computed tomography in patients with congenital coronary fistulas. J Comput Assist Tomogr. 2008;32(2):265–70.
25. Warnes CA, Williams RG, Bashore TM, et al. ACC/AHA 2008 guidelines for the Management of Adults with congenital heart disease: executive summary: a report of the American College of Cardiology/American Heart Association task force on practice guidelines writing committee to develop guidelines for the management of adults with congenital heart disease. Circulation. 2008;118(23):2395–451.
26. Mangukia CV. Coronary artery fistula. Ann Thorac Surg. 2012;93:2084–92.
27. Said SA, Nijhuis RL, Akker JW, Takechi M, Slart RH, Bos JS, et al. Unilateral and multilateral congenital coronary-pulmonary fistulas in adults: clinical pre-

sentation, diagnostic modalities, and management with a brief review of the literature. Clin Cardiol. 2014;37:536–45.

28. Hoendermis ES, Waterbolk TW, Willems TP, Zijlstra F. Large common left and right coronary artery to coronary sinus fistula. Interact Cardiovasc Thorac Surg. 2006;5(6):788–9.

29. Reul R, Cooley D, Hallman G, Reul G. Surgical treatment of coronary artery anomalies: report of a 371/2-year experience at the Texas heart institute. Tex Heart Inst J. 2002;29:299–307.

30. Said SM, Burkhart HM, Schaff HV, Connolly HM, Phillips SD, Suri RM, Eidem B, Rihal CS, Dearani JA. Late outcome of repair of congenital coronary artery fistulas–a word of caution. J Thorac Cardiovasc Surg. 2013;145(2):455–60.

31. Schumacher G, Roithmaier A, Lorenz HP, et al. Congenital coronary artery fistula in infancy and childhood: diagnostic and therapeutic aspects. Thorac Cardiovasc Surg. 1997;45:287–94.

32. Ilkay E, Celebi OO, Kacmaz F, Ozeke O. Percutaneous closure of coronary artery fistula: long-term follow-up results. Postepy Kardiol Interwencyjnej. 2015;11:318–22.

33. Armsby LR, Keane JF, Sherwood MC, Forbess JM, Perry SB, Lock JE. Management of coronary artery fistulae. Patient selection and results of transcatheter closure. J Am Coll Cardiol. 2002;39:1026–32.

34. Mottin B, Baruteau A, Boudjemline Y, et al. Transcatheter closure of coronary artery fistulas in infants and children: a French multicenter study. Catheter Cardiovasc Interv. 2016;87:411–8.

35. Mavroudis C, Backer CL, Rocchini AP, et al. Coronary artery fistulas in infants and children: a surgical review and discussion of coil embolization. Ann Thorac Surg. 1997;63:1235–42.

36. Kharouf R, Cao QL, Hijazi ZM. Transcatheter closure of coronary artery fistula complicated by myocardial infarction. J Invasive Cardiol. 2007;19:E146–9.

37. Valente AM, Lock JE, Gauvreau K, Rodriguez-Huertas E, Joyce C, et al. Predictors of long-term adverse outcomes in patients with congenital coronary artery fistulae. Circ Cardiovasc Interv. 2010;3:134–9.

38. Latson LA. Coronary artery fistulas: how to manage them. Catheter Cardiovasc Interv. 2007;70:110–6.

39. Gowda ST, Forbes TJ, Singh H, Kovach JA, Prieto L, Latson LA, et al. Remodeling and thrombosis following closure of coronary artery fistula with review of management: large distal coronary artery fistula – to close or not to close? Catheter Cardiovasc Interv. 2013;82:132–42.

Coronary Artery Abnormalities Associated to Congenital or Non-congenital Heart Disease

Roberto Formigari and Micol Rebonato

Coronary Artery Abnormalities Associated to Congenital Heart Disease

The anatomic variations of the coronary artery system are a well-known feature of many congenital cardiac malformations, and their precise recognition is mandatory to provide optimal care and to avoid potentially ominous consequences. The embryology of the coronary system is discussed elsewhere and will not be the focus of this chapter.

Knowledge of all the issues bound to the relationship of the great arteries, the number of coronary ostia and their locations within the sinuses, the proximal courses of vessels, branching patterns, and regions of supply is very important for the congenital cardiologist and cardiac surgeon, allowing the precise planning and conduction of surgical and interventional procedures, and avoiding unnecessary diagnostic workouts. Because of the variability of the coronary system and the geometry of the aortic and pulmonary roots in congenital heart defects, the ordinary concepts of "right" and "left" coronary branches may be misleading. Thus, for decades, the nomenclature of the coronary anatomy has been a matter of discussion and controversies between surgeons and imaging cardiologists [1]. Several coding systems have been proposed (Yacoub, Leiden, and others) which can be adopted for the morphological description of the coronaries; nevertheless, shorthand descriptive terminology is still commonly accepted in many institutions.

Pulmonary Atresia with Intact Ventricular Septum

Coronary anatomy in pulmonary atresia with intact ventricular septum (PA-IVS) has a profound influence on surgical management and outcomes. PA-IVS features a wide spectrum of underdevelopment of the tricuspid valve (TV) and the right ventricle (RV). A proportion of patients with PA and IVS may have unique coronary artery abnormalities, ranging from clinically unimportant myocardial sinusoids to the presence of an RV-dependent coronary circulation [2, 3]. Right ventricle-to-coronary artery connections (RVCAC) are thick-walled structures with myointimal hyperplasia, thought to be a consequence of repeated injury to the intima from the high-pressure, turbulent, RV systolic flow [4]. The frequency of RV coronary artery fistulas has

Supplementary Information The online version contains supplementary material available at https://doi.org/10.1007/978-3-031-36966-7_6.

R. Formigari (✉) · M. Rebonato
Interventional Cardiology, Bambino Gesù Pediatric Hospital, Rome, Italy
e-mail: micol.rebonato@opbg.net

© Springer Nature Switzerland AG 2023
G. Butera, A. Frigiola (eds.), *Congenital Anomalies of Coronary Arteries*,
https://doi.org/10.1007/978-3-031-36966-7_6

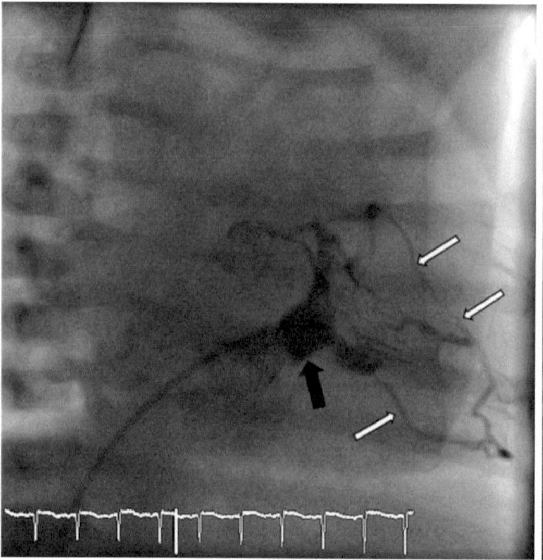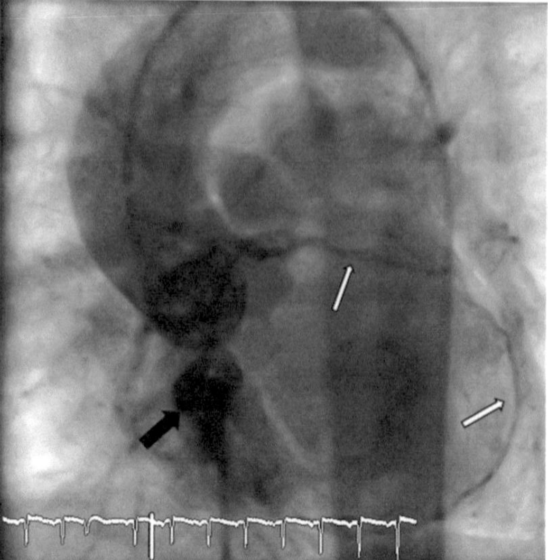

Fig. 6.1 Right-ventricular angiogram without (left panel) and with simultaneous injection in the aorta (right panel). Sinusoids (white arrows) are connecting a hypoplastic RV (black arrow) with the aorta

been reported to be 45% [2, 5, 6] and there is an inverse correlation between the diameter of the TV annulus, and therefore also to the RV size, and the probability of RVCAC [6], ranging from 98% for a TV annulus Z-value of −5 to 5% at a Z-value of 0.

A subset of these patients may demonstrate RV-dependent coronary circulation secondary to aortocoronary discontinuity with stenosis and/or interruption, or major coronary-cameral fistulae with the myocardium being supplied by the low O_2-saturated, predominantly systolic flow from the hypertensive RV. Thus, not only there is a clear substrate for myocardial ischemia, but the potential of a two-ventricle repair is doomed to failure because the RV cannot be decompressed and there is no way to provide antegrade pulmonary flow.

Therefore, complete recognition of coronary artery anatomy is of the utmost priority in the early management of these infants, as this directly impacts the decision to proceed with a single ventricle palliation pathway as opposed to biventricular repair (Fig. 6.1) [7].

Usually, the presence of RVCAC may be suspected by color-Doppler echocardiography (online video), which may provide some initial clues concerning the potential dependency of the coronary supply from the hypertensive RV [8].

However, in cases with a potentially recruitable RV and suspected major coronary anomalies, cardiac catheterization is mandatory and is still the gold standard [9], with the potential to perform interventional procedures of pulmonary perforation and/or ductal stenting. Computed tomography (CT) may be considered as a possible adjunctive tool [10].

Tetralogy of Fallot

Coronary artery abnormalities are common in tetralogy of Fallot (ToF), with a reported incidence between 4% and 6% [11, 12]. The spectrum varies from a prominent conal branch (7%) to a left anterior descending artery (LAD) originating from the right coronary artery (RCA) (3%), to the so-called "double left anterior descending artery" (2%), where a normal LAD from the left common trunk is paralleled by a supplemental LAD from the RCA. These vessels may run across the right-ventricular outflow tract (RVOT), preventing the complete resection of the subpulmonary infundibulum without jeopardizing the coronary perfusion. Indeed, the great majority of ToF patients have some component of their supply to the LAD territory coming from the RCA by a vessel crossing the RV-free wall at a variable distance below the pulmonary annulus, which may even be concealed in the muscle or the epicardial fat. This may be explained by the clockwise rotation of the aortic root, as viewed from the apex, which is a classic hallmark of conotruncal anomalies. This, and so more in case of a side-by-side arrangement of the great arteries in patients with double outlet right ventricle and/or mitro-aortic discontinuity, brings the right anterior-facing sinus into a leftward and more anterior position, much closer to the LAD. In patients with a LAD crossing the RVOT, anatomic repair is sometimes delayed, eventually with the creation of a more stable pulmonary blood supply by means of palliative surgical or interventional procedures. If relief of the annular/infundibular obstruction is deemed impossible without the risk of transection of a coronary artery, a prosthetic conduit is usually the only solution for definitive repair. Therefore, timely recognition of coronary vessels crossing the RVOT is extremely important to avoid a nasty surprise in the operating theatre with the potential need for an unplanned bailout surgical strategy, a potentially hazardous situation in neonates or young toddlers. For decades, coronary imaging of ToF has been the realm of cardiac catheterization and angiography (Fig. 6.2) but echocardiography [13] and CT [14] have progressively taken over, offering a safe, reliable, and non-invasive tool of imaging.

With the increasing popularity of percutaneous pulmonary valve replacement (PPVR), the importance of coronary artery anatomy has gained even more relevance for the interventional cardiologist, who needs to be familiar with the surgical techniques of RVOT repair and the spatial relationship with the coronary course. These patients typically undergo magnetic resonance imaging to evaluate right-ventricular volume and function with simultaneous evaluation of the coronary anatomy, as compression by an ill-placed stent or valve within the RVOT can be a fatal complication [15] (Fig. 6.3).

In patients with pulmonary atresia with ventricular septal defect (PA-VSD), the coronary system may provide collateral arteries to the pul-

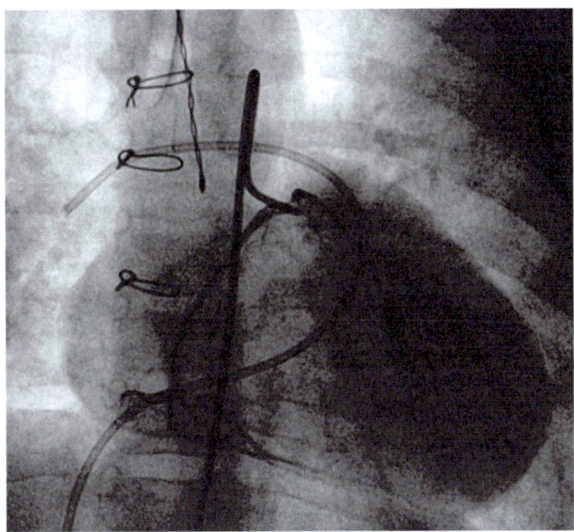

Fig. 6.2 Right coronary anteroposterior selective angiogram of a patient with ToF. Origin of the LAD (black arrow) from the RCA. The LAD crosses the RVOT, marked by a diagnostic catheter (white arrow)

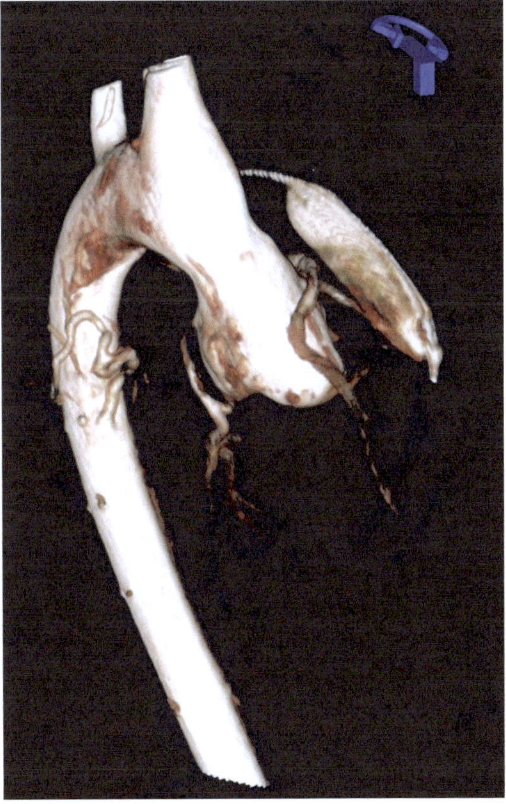

Fig. 6.3 3D rotational angiography of a patient with ToF and RV to pulmonary artery conduit. A balloon has been inflated into the conduit while contrast has been simultaneously injected into the ascending aorta. The RCA runs between the aorta and the balloon

monary circulation which needs to be embolized before any type of surgical pulmonary augmentation or unifocalization procedure.

Transposition of the Great Arteries

Transposition of the great arteries (TGA) can be considered as the prototype of congenital heart defects where treatment has been conditioned by the native anatomy of the coronary system. Indeed, the coronary arteries were regarded a little more than an anatomic curiosity in patients undergoing a Senning/Mustard operation until the first successful arterial switch procedure by Jatene in 1975. The feasibility of anatomic repair of TGA compelled pediatric cardiologists to refine their diagnostic skills in order to make surgeons confident enough to carry out a successful coronary translocation, still a risky affair until the mid-1990s, when complex coronary patterns were considered a major contraindication for anatomic repair. Even if no longer such a crucial issue in the current era, nevertheless, the timely recognition of major coronary anomalies still plays a significant role in the preoperative assessment of neonates with TGA and may impact surgical outcome [16]. Because of the high variability of aortopulmonary spatial relation-

ships, the concept of "facing sinus" is commonly used in clinical and surgical practice [1]. In this description, the observer places themselves in the nonadjacent aortic sinus looking toward the pulmonary valve. The anterior sinus on the left hand is labeled "1" and the posterior sinus on the right hand is labeled "2" (Fig. 6.4).

Coronary branching can be described as normal, looping, or intramural. In the "normal" pattern, which accounts for 60–70% of cases, sinus 1 gives rise to the anterior descending and circumflex arteries. Sinus 2 gives rise to the right coronary artery. The "looping" pattern results when one or more of the three major coronary arteries run in front of or behind the major arterial trunks. The classification of the different patterns of coronary anatomy has been extensively studied [17] and echocardiography is still the mainstay of the preoperative assessment (Fig. 6.5) [18].

Branching patterns giving rise to double loops are not uncommon and occasionally there is no true circumflex coronary artery, but separate branches arise from the left coronary to supply the corresponding portion of the left ventricle. A single coronary orifice is another possible occurrence (Fig. 6.6).

Finally, a coronary artery may cross through the media of the aortic wall behind the valve

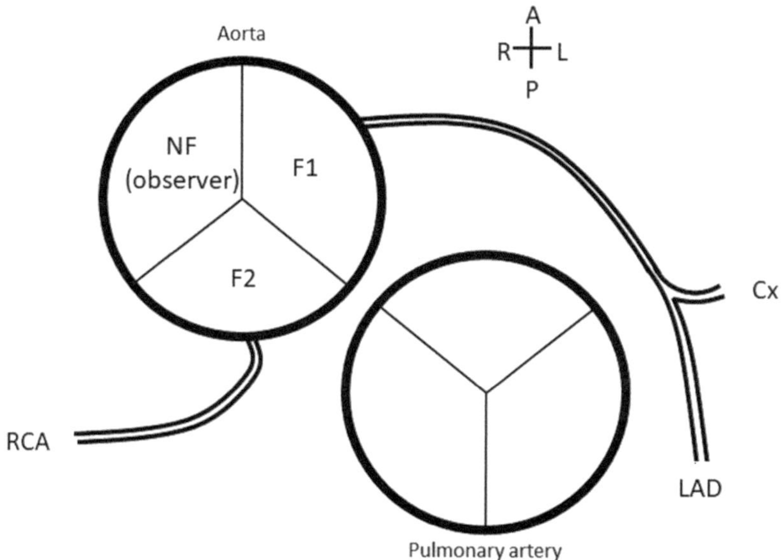

Fig. 6.4 Drawing of the concept of "facing sinuses" in TGA as seen by echocardiography. *F* facing, *NF* non facing

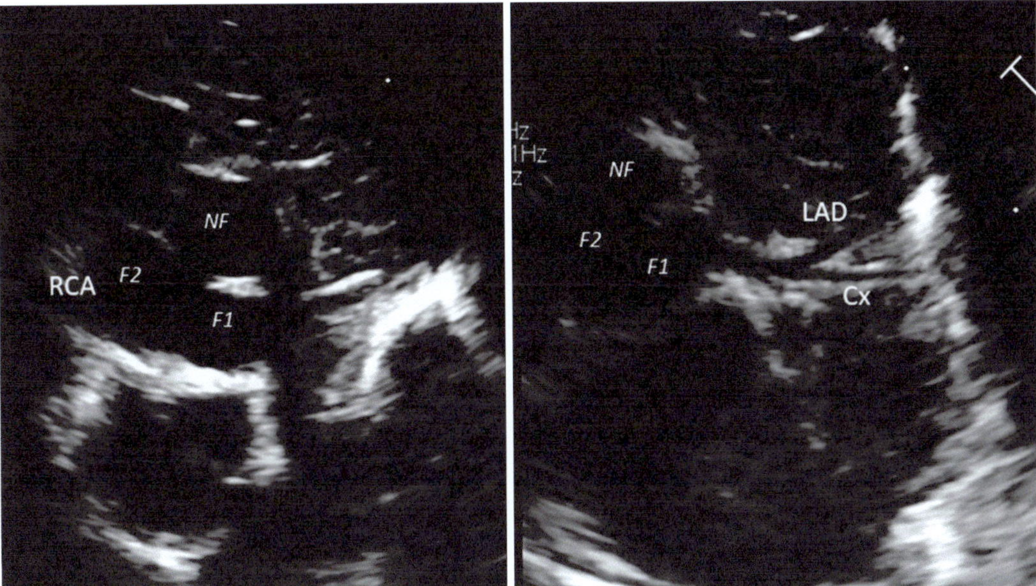

Fig. 6.5 Coronary artery origin as seen by echocardiography in a TGA with an anterior aorta. Note the rotation of the facing sinuses

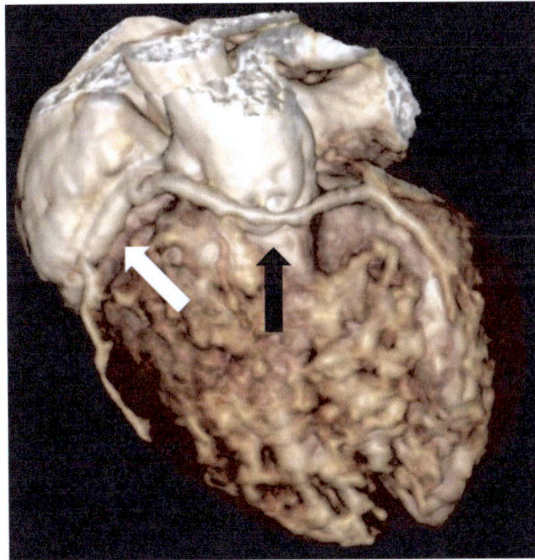

Fig. 6.6 CT scan of a patient with TGA and single right coronary orifice, giving rise to the LAD (black arrow), RCA (white arrow), and circumflex arteries

Other Types of Congenital Heart Defects Associated with Abnormal Coronary Artery Anatomy

In patients with congenitally corrected transposition of the great arteries (ccTGA) the morphology of the coronary system is said to "follow" that of the ventricle. Thus, when there is a leftward-anterior aorta, the coronary connecting to the right anterior-facing sinus has the distribution of a morphologically left coronary artery, while the coronary connecting to the left posterior-facing sinus runs in the left atrioventricular groove and supplies the RV and posterior interventricular septum [20]. In patients with ccTGA who are candidates for double switch procedures, the coronary anatomy should be thoroughly investigated by coronary angiography or CT scan. Moreover, the sinus node artery may arise from the circumflex artery, crossing the medial side of the morphologic right atrial wall, thus jeopardizing atriotomy or baffling for the atrial switch procedure. Patients with common arterial trunk exhibit a high incidence of slit-like coronary orifices, often with higher take-off from

commissure, arising from the other adjacent aortic sinus, with a so-called "intramural" course which can be suspected by echocardiography [19] and still poses a challenge for surgical repair.

the aortic wall. Hypoplastic left heart syndrome with mitral stenosis and aortic atresia may show the presence of left ventricle-coronary connections whose impact on prognosis has yet to be understood. Anomalous coronary origin from the pulmonary artery has been reported in patients with aortopulmonary window [21].

Inflammatory Diseases of the Coronary System

Coronary artery vasculitis (CAV) is an emerging field of diseases featured by the propensity of younger population groups and with multiple complications including the development of coronary artery aneurysms, coronary stenotic lesions, and thrombosis, all of which may result in acute coronary syndromes. More recently, the COVID-19 pandemic witnessed the outbreak of several cases of children with a multi-inflammatory disease with coronary and myocardial involvement [22]. Other types of CAV diseases are Kawasaki disease (KD) and Takayasu arteritis (TA). KD is a predominant vasculitis of childhood that primarily affects the coronary arteries (~25% of patients) and is the most common cause of coronary artery aneurysms which may be complicated by endoluminal thrombosis or late stenosis (Fig. 6.7) [23]. Prompt recognition of coronary aneurysm in the acute phase by echocardiography is mandatory as intravenous administration of gamma globulin has been proved as highly effective in preventing the formation of coronary aneurysms. In TA the most common lesions are stenosis or occlusion of the coronary ostia, diffuse or focal coronary arteritis, and aneurysms. These findings are detected in up to 60% of patients on coronary angiography (<20% symptomatic cases) [24].

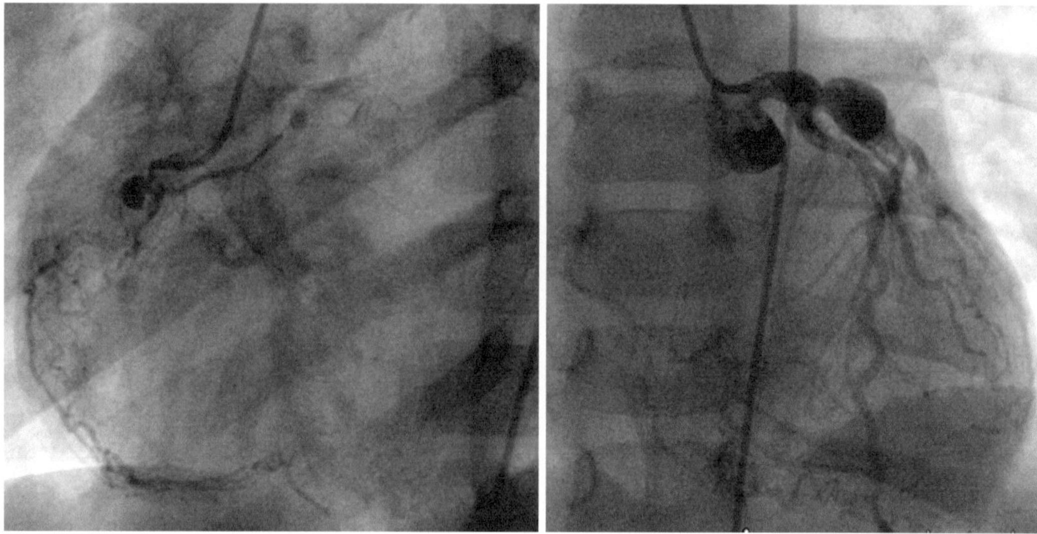

Fig. 6.7 Coronary angiography in a child after KD. Aneurysm and complete occlusion of the RCA (left panel). Giant aneurysm of the Cx artery (right panel)

References

1. Gittenberger-de Groot AC, Koenraadt WMC, Bartelings MM, Bökenkamp R, DeRuiter MC, Hazekamp MG, Bogers AJJC, Quaegebeur JM, Schalij MJ, Vliegen HW, Poelmann RE, Jongbloed MRM. Coding of coronary arterial origin and branching in congenital heart disease: the modified Leiden convention. J Thorac Cardiovasc Surg. 2018;156(6):2260–9. https://doi.org/10.1016/j.jtcvs.2018.08.009. Epub 2018 Aug 18. PMID: 30243713.
2. Daubeney PE, Delany DJ, Anderson RH, Sandor GG, Slavik Z, Keeton BR, Webber SA. United Kingdom and Ireland collaborative study of pulmonary atresia with intact ventricular septum. Pulmonary atresia with intact ventricular septum: range of morphology in a population-based study. J Am Coll Cardiol. 2002;39(10):1670–9. https://doi.org/10.1016/s0735-1097(02)01832-6. PMID: 12020496.
3. Freedom RM, Anderson RH, Perrin D. The significance of ventriculo-coronary arterial connections in the setting of pulmonary atresia with an intact ventricular septum. Cardiol Young. 2005;15(5):447–68. https://doi.org/10.1017/S1047951105001319. PMID: 16164782.
4. Gittenberger-de Groot AC, Tennstedt C, Chaoui R, et al. Ventriculo coronary arterial communications (VCAC) and myocardial sinusoids in hearts with pulmonary atresia with intact ventricular septum: two different diseases. Prog Pediatr Cardiol. 2001;13:157–64.
5. Calder AL, Peebles CR, Occleshaw CJ. The prevalence of coronary arterial abnormalities in pulmonary atresia with intact ventricular septum and their influence on surgical results. Cardiol Young. 2007;17:387–96.
6. Giglia TM, Jenkins KJ, Matitiau A, Mandell VS, Sanders SP, Mayer JE Jr, Lock JE. Influence of right heart size on outcome in pulmonary atresia with intact ventricular septum. Circulation. 1993;88(5 Pt 1):2248–56. https://doi.org/10.1161/01.cir.88.5.2248. PMID: 8222119.
7. Hanley FL, Sade RM, Blackstone EH, Kirklin JW, Freedom RM, Nanda NC. Outcomes in neonatal pulmonary atresia with intact ventricular septum. A multiinstitutional study. J Thorac Cardiovasc Surg. 1993;105(406–423):24–7.
8. Peterson RE, Freire G, Marino CJ, Jureidini SB. Transthoracic echocardiographic assessment of coronary flow in the diagnosis of right ventricular-dependent coronary circulation in pulmonary atresia with intact ventricular septum. Pediatr Cardiol. 2018;39(5):967–75. https://doi.org/10.1007/s00246-018-1846-3.
9. Qureshi SA. Catheterization in neonates with pulmonary atresia with intact ventricular septum. Catheter Cardiovasc Interv. 2006;67(6):924–31. https://doi.org/10.1002/ccd.20690. PMID: 16649237.
10. Séguela PE, Houyel L, Loget P, Piot JD, Paul JF. Critical stenosis of a right ventricle to coronary artery fistula seen at dual-source CT in a newborn with pulmonary atresia and intact ventricular septum. Pediatr Radiol. 2011;41:1069–72.
11. Fellows KE, Freed MD, Keane JF, Praagh R, Bernhard WF, Castaneda AC. Results of routine preoperative coronary angiography in tetralogy of Fallot. Circulation. 1975;51:561–6.
12. Koppel CJ, Jongbloed MRM, Kiès P, Hazekamp MG, Mertens BJA, Schalij MJ, Vliegen HW. Coronary anomalies in tetralogy of Fallot—a meta-analysis. Int J Cardiol. 2020;306:78–85. https://doi.org/10.1016/j.ijcard.2020.02.037.
13. Need LR, Powell AJ, del Nido P, Geva T. Coronary echocardiography in tetralogy of fallot: diagnostic accuracy, resource utilization and surgical implications over 13 years. J Am Coll Cardiol. 2000;36(4):1371–7.
14. Vastel-Amzallag C, Le Bret E, Paul JF, Lambert V, Rohnean A, El Fassy E, Sigal-Cinqualbre A. Diagnostic accuracy of dual-source multislice computed tomographic analysis for the preoperative detection of coronary artery anomalies in 100 patients with tetralogy of Fallot. J Thorac Cardiovasc Surg. 2011;142(1):120–6. https://doi.org/10.1016/j.jtcvs.2010.11.016. Epub 2011 Feb 3. PMID: 21292283.
15. Fraisse A, Assaidi A, Mauri L, Malekzadeh-Milani S, Thambo JB, Bonnet D, Iserin L, Mancini J, Boudjemline Y. Coronary artery compression during intention to treat right ventricle outflow with percutaneous pulmonary valve implantation: incidence, diagnosis, and outcome. Catheter Cardiovasc Interv. 2014;83(7):E260–8. https://doi.org/10.1002/ccd.25471. Epub 2014 Mar 19. PMID: 24619978.
16. Moll M, Michalak KW, Sobczak-Budlewska K, Moll JA, Kopala M, Szymczyk K, Dryżek P, Moll JJ. Coronary artery anomalies in patients with transposition of the great arteries and their impact on postoperative outcomes. Ann Thorac Surg. 2017;104(5):1620–8. https://doi.org/10.1016/j.athoracsur.2017.03.078. Epub 2017 Jun 23. PMID: 28648541.
17. Yacoub MH, Radley-Smith R. Anatomy of the coronary arteries in transposition of the great arteries and methods for their transfer in anatomical correction. Thorax. 1978;33(4):418–24. https://doi.org/10.1136/thx.33.4.418.
18. Pasquini L, Sanders SP, Parness IA, Colan SD. Diagnosis of coronary artery anatomy by two-dimensional echocardiography in patients with transposition of the great arteries. Circulation. 1987;75(3):557–64. https://doi.org/10.1161/01.cir.75.3.557. PMID: 3815768.
19. Pasquini L, Parness IA, Colan SD, Wernovsky G, Mayer JE, Sanders SP. Diagnosis of intramural coronary artery in transposition of the great arteries using two-dimensional echocardiography. Circulation. 1993;88(3):1136–41. https://doi.org/10.1161/01.cir.88.3.1136. PMID: 8353875.

20. McKay R, Anderson RH, Smith A. The coronary arteries in hearts with discordant atrioventricular connections. J Thorac Cardiovasc Surg. 1996;111:988–97.
21. Alhadlaq A, Dhillon S, Hancock-Friesen CL, Hussain A. A hidden culprit for ventricular dysfunction in aortopulmonary window repair: anomalous origin of left coronary artery. Case report and review of literature. J Thorac Cardiovasc Surg. 2016;152(6):e123–6. https://doi.org/10.1016/j.jtcvs.2016.07.055. Epub 2016 Aug 5. PMID: 27576371.
22. Verdoni L, Mazza A, Gervasoni A, Martelli L, Ruggeri M, Ciuffreda M, Bonanomi E, D'Antiga L. An outbreak of severe Kawasaki-like disease at the Italian epicentre of the SARS-CoV-2 epidemic: an observational cohort study. Lancet. 2020;395(10239):1771–8. https://doi.org/10.1016/S0140-6736(20)31103-X. Epub 2020 May 13. PMID: 32410760; PMCID: PMC7220177.
23. McCrindle BW, Rowley AH, Newburger JW, Burns JC, Bolger AF, Gewitz M, Baker AL, Jackson MA, Takahashi M, Shah PB, Kobayashi T, Wu MH, Saji TT, Pahl E, American Heart Association Rheumatic Fever, Endocarditis, and Kawasaki Disease Committee of the Council on Cardiovascular Disease in the Young; Council on Cardiovascular and Stroke Nursing; Council on Cardiovascular Surgery and Anesthesia; and Council on Epidemiology and Prevention. Diagnosis, Treatment, and Long-Term Management of Kawasaki Disease: a Scientific Statement for Health Professionals From the American Heart Association. Circulation. 2017;135(17):e927–99. https://doi.org/10.1161/CIR.0000000000000484. Epub 2017 Mar 29.
24. Matsubara O, Kuwata T, Nemoto T, Kasuga T, Numano F. Coronary artery lesions in Takayasu arteritis: pathological considerations. Heart Vessels Suppl. 1992;7:26–31. https://doi.org/10.1007/BF01744540. PMID: 1360966

Anomalous Origin of the Coronary Arteries from the Pulmonary Artery: ALCAPA and ARCAPA

Alessandro Giamberti, Massimo Chessa,
Martina Evangelista, and Federica Caldaroni

Introduction

The first descriptions of anomalous coronary arteries (CA) from the pulmonary artery (PA) were performed by Krause in 1865 and by Brooks in 1885. They reported the presence of accessory arteries originating from the anterior side of the PA and joining a network of thoraco-mediastinal thoracic vessels, including CAs branches normally originating from the aorta. The first adult report of anomalous left CA (LCA) from PA (ALCAPA) came in 1908 from Maude Abbott's contribution to Osler's Modern Medicine. Thereby, she reported the case of an asymptomatic 60-year-old woman with a dilated and aneurysmal right coronary artery (RCA) giving off branches that anastomosed with venous-like vessels running in the normal territory of the LCA, but originating from the posterior sinus of the PA. Such autoptic finding became known as Bland-White-Garland syndrome in 1933, with the landmark publication of a 3-month-old infant with autopsy confirmed ALCAPA [1].

A. Giamberti (✉) · M. Evangelista · F. Caldaroni
Department of Pediatric and Adult Cardiac Surgery,
IRCCS- Policlinico San Donato, Milan, Italy
e-mail: alessandro.giamberti@grupposandonato.it;
martina.evangelista@grupposandonato.it;
federica.caldaroni@grupposandonato.it

M. Chessa
ACHD Unit, IRCCS- Policlinico San Donato and
Vita Salute San Raffaele University, Milan, Italy

Epidemiology

Anomalous origin of right coronary artery (ARCAPA) anatomy was found in 0.002% of patients undergoing coronary angiography, but, given the inherent bias related to the cohort of patients undergoing the procedure and the possible asymptomatic course of some patients with ARCAPA, the true incidence is unknown [2]. A slight predominance of male has been reported for ARCAPA [3], as compared to a greater than 2:1 predominance of females for ALCAPA [4]. The estimated incidence of ALCAPA is 1/300000 live births, representing 0.24–0.46% of congenital cardiac disease [2, 5, 6]. If untreated, approximately 90% of infants die within the first year of life. Since it predominantly presents in the first year of life, diagnosis in adult age is extremely rare, and the majority of information comes from case reports or from pediatric case series. Over the past two decades, the number of reported patients with ALCAPA over 50 years old has increased. This might correlate with advances in echocardiography and wide diffusion of cardiac computed tomography (CT) and magnetic resonance imaging (MRI). Early autopsy studies reported that SCD among untreated adult ALCAPA patients occurs at 35 years old on average, thereby requiring surgical treatment in all diagnosed adults [7, 8]. Nevertheless, with the increased diagnostic rate of adult ALCAPA cases,

© Springer Nature Switzerland AG 2023
G. Butera, A. Frigiola (eds.), *Congenital Anomalies of Coronary Arteries*,
https://doi.org/10.1007/978-3-031-36966-7_7

the true association between ALCAPA and SCD may be lower than estimated, especially among older patients.

Anatomy

The anomalous connection of a CA from the PA is included in the major anomalies of the coronary arteries (APOC-Anomalous Pulmonary Origin of the Coronaries, in the accepted classification of the STS database and Nomenclature project Fig. 7.1) [9].

The morphological spectrum accounts for Four different variants: (1) ALCAPA, (2) ARCAPA, (3) anomalous origin of both CAs from the PA, and (4) anomalous origin of the circumflex artery from the PA. Among these variants, ALCAPA and ARCAPA are the most frequent and clinically relevant, since only a few cases of anomalous origin of both CAs or an "accessory" artery from the PA have been described [3, 9, 10] and the anatomical variants are depicted as follows.

1. Anomalous origin of the left main CA from the pulmonary artery (ALCAPA)
    1.1. From right-handed sinus (sinus 1)
    1.2. From non-facing pulmonary sinus
    1.3. From left-handed sinus (sinus 2)
    1.4. From commissure between sinus 1 and non-facing sinus
    1.5. From commissure between sinus 2 and non-facing sinus
    1.6. From commissure between sinus 1 and sinus 2
    1.7. High takeoff from left or right pulmonary arteries
2. Anomalous origin of the right coronary artery (ARCAPA)
3. Anomalous origin of the circumflex coronary artery from the PA (ACxPA)
4. Anomalous right and left coronaries from the PA (both)

The ALCAPA is the most frequent form; however, the anatomy can be variable, influencing the technique of surgical correction [11, 12]. Most frequently, the anomalous CA arises from the left or posterior sinus of Valsalva of the PA, rarely from the right sinus, and usually gives branches (LAD and Cx) 5–6 mm after its origin. Collateral circula-

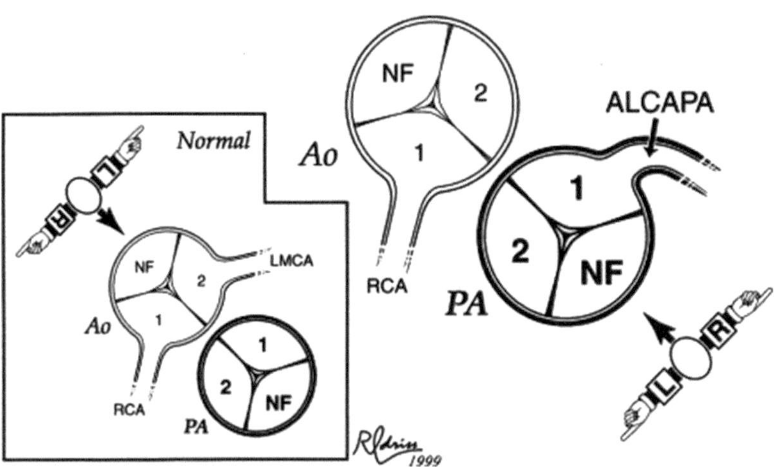

Fig. 7.1 Diagrammatic representation of aortic and pulmonary artery origins of the left main coronary artery in normal and anomalous conditions. Cephalic views depict a person in the non-facing sinus with the right hand always signifying sinus 1 and the left hand always signifying sinus 2. [The sinuses of the pulmonary valve are designated right hand (sinus number 1), and left hand (sinus number 2), as viewed from the non-facing sinus of the pulmonary trunk toward the aorta. Sinus 1 of the aorta faces sinus 2 of the pulmonary trunk and vice versa; both non-facing sinuses are at the two extremities]. Reproduced with permission from Dodge/Khatami et al.

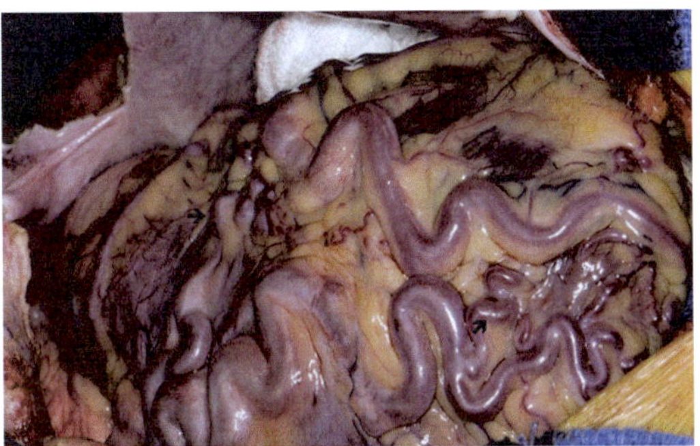

Fig. 7.2 Intraoperative image showing multiple large collaterals (arrows) arising from the right coronary artery from anomalous origin of left coronary artery from pulmonary artery. Reproduced with permission from Rajbanshi et al. [13]

tion, more represented in adults, gives origin to a network of collateral vessels of technical importance during surgery [3, 13] (Fig. 7.2). The left ventricle is usually dilated, with impaired function and myocardial fibrosis, in response to a maladaptive remodeling secondary to chronic ischemic insult [3, 6, 12]. The result is often secondary mitral regurgitation with the underlying mechanism being annular dilation, chordal tethering, and papillary muscle fibrosis and dysfunction [14].

Clinical Presentation/Diagnosis

In fetal and early neonatal life, the origin of one CA from the PA is well tolerated because pulmonary artery pressure (PAP) equals systemic pressure, leading to adequate anterograde flow in both the anomalous and the normal CA. After birth, when PAP decreases, flow in the anomalous CA decreases and eventually reverses, therefore leading to myocardial ischemia (MI) and infarction. The long-term consequence of reverse flow is volume overload caused by left-to-right shunt; the left-to-right shunt is also known as the steal phenomenon. The development of collateral circulation between the RCA and LCA during the critical period, when PAP gradually decreases, determines the extent of MI. Patients without collateral vessels have the infant type of the disease, and

those with well-established collateral vessels have the adult type (Fig. 7.3). These two disease types have different manifestations and outcomes. In the infant type, symptoms onset usually occurs about 8 weeks after birth: with the establishment of reversal of flow in the anomalous CA, the limited blood supply to the myocardium due to the absence of coronary collateral development leads to congestive heart failure (HF) and mitral insufficiency secondary to MI [6]. Infants present with failure to thrive, profuse sweating, dyspnea, pallor, and atypical chest pain while eating or crying. Without surgical repair, death ensues in up to 90% of patients within weeks or months of life [4, 15]. In the adult type, chronic LV sub-endocardial ischemia ensues despite the development of significant collateral circulation from the normal to the anomalous CA. As a result, patients may develop malignant ventricular arrhythmia (VA). Symptoms upon ALCAPA presentation are angina, dyspnea, palpitations, or fatigue in 66% of patients; 17% present with VAs, syncope, or SCD and only a minority remain asymptomatic until adulthood (14%) [4, 15–17]. Out of patients with life-threatening presentations, more than a half (62%) have no antecedent symptoms.

ARCAPA is frequently diagnosed incidentally, and patients may be completely asymptomatic (38% of patients), or may present with angina (22%), dyspnea (17%), HF (10%), or SCD (2,7%) [3]. Both CAs arising from the PA is an extremely rare condition. In such cases, symptoms manifest within a few days after birth, and death follows within 2 weeks; this condition is compatible with life only if associated with pulmonary hypertension [6].

Associated congenital abnormalities may be present. In patients with ALCAPA, the most common abnormalities are extracardiac collateral circulation, including bronchial artery collaterals. The most common abnormality in patients with ARCAPA is aorto-pulmonary window (10.8%) followed by ventricular septal defect (6.3%) and atrial septal defect (4.9%) [3, 4].

Abnormalities on physical examination are frequent findings, and the most common is a sys-

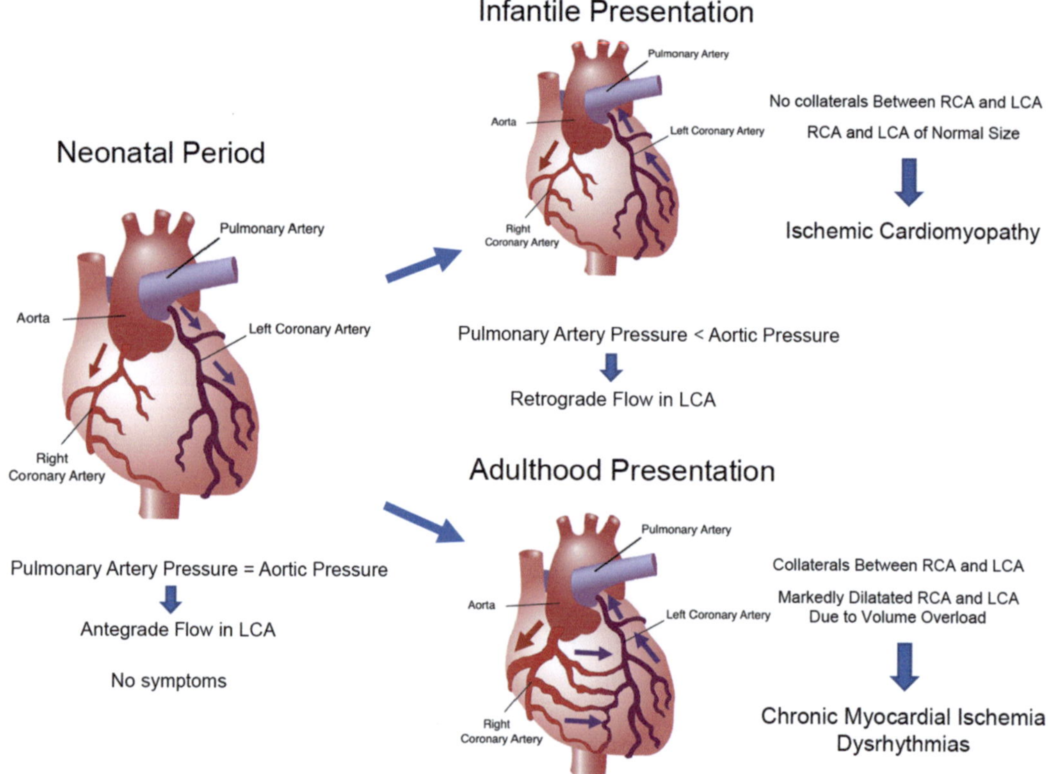

Fig. 7.3 Pathophysiology of APOC. In the neonatal period, the anomaly does not cause any perfusion abnormality, nor any clinical signs. Progressively the pulmonary artery pressure decreases leading to changes in the coronary artery perfusion, therefore to the Infantile or the Adulthood presentation

tolic or continuous or "to-and-fro" murmur, predominantly localized to the left sternal border or apical region (87% of patients). The electrocardiography (ECG) frequently reveals infarct patterns with Q-waves (50%), otherwise it may present LV hypertrophy (28%) or left axis deviation (15%), and it is normal in only a minority of cases (4%) [4]. Noninvasive diagnosis of coronary abnormalities has always been challenging [18, 19]. Echocardiographic markers of ALCAPA have been identified, highlighting differences between infant and adulthood presentation. The most common markers in infants include mildly dilated RCA, prominent fibrotic changes of papillary muscles, secondary fibroelastosis of endocardium, severely dilated LV, abnormal myocardial contractility especially of the anterior and lateral walls, and severe LV systolic dysfunction. In adulthood presentation, the most frequent markers are severely dilated RCA and prominent septal flow from collateralization, without LV dilatation or dysfunction [19]. In 46% of the exams, echocardiography findings are diagnostic or suggestive of ALCAPA; 44% of echocardiography exams are abnormal but do not indicate ALCAPA (predominantly mitral regurgitation and segmental ventricular dysfunction). Echocardiography may be normal in 10% of patients. Stress tests may be useful to identify ischemia. Stress ECG and stress imaging studies have been reported to detect ischemia respectively in 85% and 87% of the cases.

The development of cardiac CT and MRI has improved noninvasive evaluation of the coronary anatomy [15, 20, 21]. CT and MRI findings of ALCAPA in adults include direct visualization of the origin of the LCA from the posterior aspect of the PA, dilated and tortuous RCA, and visualization of dilated inter-coronary collateral arteries along the external surface of the heart or within the interventricular septum. Both modalities may be used to assess LV systolic function. MRI has the additional advantage of demonstrating and assessing flow from the LCA into the PA, and to determine myocardial viability with delayed gadolinium enhancement.

Surgical Indications

Anomalous LCA from the PA (ALCAPA), if left unrepaired has a mortality rate up to 90% [22]. Surgery, however, has good early and long-term results [23–25], proving to be effective and resolutive, restoring a two-coronary system [10, 26]. Diagnosis itself is a surgical indication, so that the currently and generally accepted standards include urgent surgical repair soon after diagnosis, with establishment of a dual-CA system, regardless of age or degree of inter-coronary collateralization [10, 15, 24, 27]. In fact, in neonates or infants who have little or no coronary collateral development, the surgical treatment is lifesaving and the best results are achieved with the availability of postoperative mechanical assist devices [23, 28]. Adults, on the other hand, in whom a developed network of collateral circulation is generally already established, even if asymptomatic, continue to have a significant left-to-right shunt and poor coronary reserve (steal phenomenon), and will therefore be predisposed to ischemia, arrhythmia, and sudden death [4, 13, 15, 17].

ARCAPA and other variants (single LAD or Cx arising from the PA) are considerably rarer and less malignant than ALCAPA and are often underdiagnosed because of the absence of clinical manifestations. However, operation is likewise indicated upon the diagnosis for all these variants [13, 29].

Surgical Technique

Several surgical procedures have been described, including simple ligation, various forms of bypass grafting, subclavian artery graft, intrapulmonary baffle, and, the most frequently used, direct coronary reimplantation to the aorta [4, 12–15, 20, 24, 26, 28, 30–33].

Usually, the discriminant for the choice of the technique is the position of the anomalous CA, when it is on the right side of the PA or arises from the posterior wall (i.e. from a pulmonary sinus facing the aortic wall, direct anastomosis with mobilization of the left coronary is recognized as the simplest and best choice) [12, 24, 32]. In case of origin from the left side of the PA, a baffle type of technique can be considered (Takeuchi-type repair) [24, 32, 33] (Fig. 7.4).

In adult patients, in case of technical issues or presence of associated CAD, CA bypass grafting techniques, with ligation of the origin of anomalous CA, deem feasible [4, 13].

Cardiopulmonary bypass is routinely established with high aortic and bi-caval or single right atrial venous cannulation. Myocardial protection, of utmost importance, is performed with antegrade root cardioplegia, taking care of manually occluding the anomalous origin of CA or the main or the branches of pulmonary arteries, to prevent cardioplegia steal into the pulmonary bed [10, 13, 24, 26, 32].

 A. Giamberti et al.

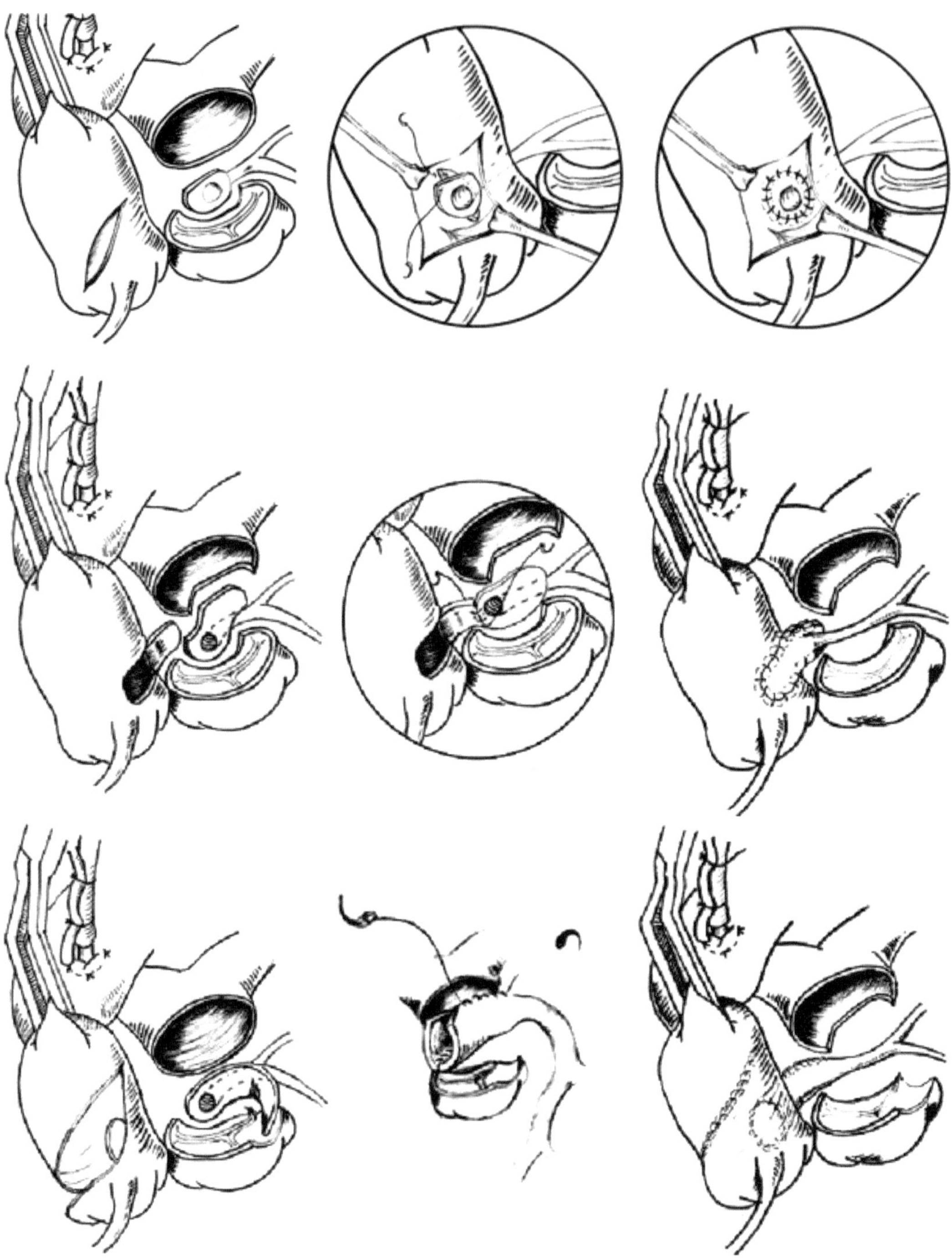

Fig. 7.4 Surgical technique, reproduced with permission from Alsoufi et al. Ann Thorac Surg. 2008 [12]

Postoperatively, a left atrial pressure monitoring is advisable and the use of mechanical assist devices ranges from 25% to 36% [23, 24, 26, 28, 30].

Complications

The reported early mortality rate after ACAPA correction varies from 0% to 16% [10, 26, 34]. Presumably, after hospital discharge, there is a sharp decrease in the hazard, but a low risk remains constant, mostly conditioned by the amount of residual ischemic left ventricle. In fact, the onset of malignant VAs, induced by the presence of areas of ischemic myocardium, represents the substrate for sudden death. In most patients, however, the left ventricular function recovers to almost normal after several months [7, 8, 10, 12].

Management of mitral regurgitation is controversial. In most cases, insufficiency is deemed to be reversible, and therefore should not be addressed at the time of surgery [12, 14, 23, 35]. In addition, some studies demonstrate that, in ALCAPA, even preoperatively severe MR fully regresses after reperfusion alone, while MV replacement or repair during ALCAPA correction could potentially be harmful by prolonging the ischemic time and by acutely increasing the afterload in an already-damaged ventricle. Therefore, the primary goal of the initial surgery should be to establish antegrade coronary perfusion [23, 35]. However, significant mitral regurgitation persists in at least one-third of patients, despite good recovery of LV function [23, 24, 28, 30]. This usually reflects the presence of irreversible papillary muscle infarction and scarring [23]. In that case, with a completely different underlying mechanism of mitral regurgitation, reoperation is required to address the valve insufficiency and reduce its impact on ventricular dysfunction [14, 16, 30, 31, 36].

Even though surgical results are satisfactory, there is potential for postoperative complications such as ischemia due to anastomosis or conduit restenosis or aortic valve or pulmonary valve injury [12, 13, 30]. Some cases of RVOT obstruction have also been reported after Takeuchi repair [10, 30, 33, 37].

Follow-up

Although early diagnosis and prompt surgical intervention lead to excellent results, the possibility of postoperative complications necessitates long-term follow-up imaging [14, 24, 30, 32]. Cardiac CT and MRI offer prognostic information, allow for risk stratification, and should be used for long-term follow-up. MRI also allows functional assessment of the heart and evaluation of MI and viability [4, 15]. Currently, there are no clear indications for the follow-up evaluation of these patients. According to the authors of the chapter, a reasonable approach is to schedule the first clinical evaluation 1 month after the discharge and in the same context, to perform an ECG and an echocardiography. The clinical evaluation has to be focused on signs and symptoms of HF and of MI; the ECG has to highlight new ischemic modifications and the echocardiography has to asses myocardial function as well as the improvement or the worsening of MR. Whenever feasible, we suggest scheduling a coronary CT scan 6 months after the operation, mainly to evaluate the anastomosis between the CA and the aorta or the anastomosis of the baffle, in case a Takeuchi-type repair has been performed. If the coronary CT scan shows any abnormalities or a doubtful result in patients who refer to typical or atypical symptoms of MI, a coronary angiogram should be performed.

An exercises stress test should be scheduled as soon as feasible, according to the growing-up rate of the patient.

In case signs or symptoms of MI appear at the follow-up, we suggest performing a functional test, above all stress-MRI, to asses inducible MI, myocardial viability, and myocardial fibrosis.

References

1. Bland EF, White PD, Garland J. Congenital anomalies of the coronary arteries: report of an unusual case associated with cardiac hypertrophy. Am Heart J. 1933;8(6):787–801. https://doi.org/10.1016/s0002-8703(33)90140-4.
2. Yamanaka O, Hobbs RE. Coronary artery anomalies in 126,595 patients undergoing coronary arteriography. Catheter Cardio Diagn. 1990;21(1):28–40. https://doi.org/10.1002/ccd.1810210110.
3. Guenther TM, Sherazee EA, Wisneski AD, Gustafson JD, Wozniak CJ, Raff GW. Anomalous origin of the right coronary artery from the pulmonary artery: a systematic review. Ann Thorac Surg. 2020;110(3):1063–71. https://doi.org/10.1016/j.athoracsur.2020.01.082.
4. Yau JM, Singh R, Halpern EJ, Fischman D. Anomalous origin of the left coronary artery from the pulmonary artery in adults: a comprehensive review of 151 adult cases and a new diagnosis in a 53-year-old woman. Clin Cardiol. 2011;34(4):204–10. https://doi.org/10.1002/clc.20848.
5. Frescura C, Basso C, Thiene G, et al. Anomalous origin of coronary arteries and risk of sudden death: a study based on an autopsy population of congenital heart disease. Hum Pathol. 1998;29(7):689–95. https://doi.org/10.1016/s0046-8177(98)90277-5.
6. Hauser M. Congenital anomalies of the coronary arteries. Heart. 2005;91(9):1240. https://doi.org/10.1136/hrt.2004.057299.
7. Moodie DS, Fyfe D, Gill CC, et al. Anomalous origin of the left coronary artery from the pulmonary artery (Bland-White-Garland syndrome) in adult patients: long-term follow-up after surgery. Am Heart J. 1983;106(2):381–8. https://doi.org/10.1016/0002-8703(83)90207-7.
8. Lampe CFJ, Verheugt APM. Anomalous left coronary artery. Adult type. Am Heart J. 1960;59(5):769–76. https://doi.org/10.1016/0002-8703(60)90518-4.
9. Dodge-Khatami A, Mavroudis C, Backer CL. Congenital heart surgery nomenclature and database project: anomalies of the coronary arteries. Ann Thorac Surg. 2000;69(3):270–97. https://doi.org/10.1016/s0003-4975(99)01248-5.
10. Dodge-Khatami A, Mavroudis C, Backer CL. Anomalous origin of the left coronary artery from the pulmonary artery: collective review of surgical therapy. Ann Thorac Surg. 2002;74(3):946–55. https://doi.org/10.1016/s0003-4975(02)03633-0.
11. Smith A, Arnold R, Anderson RH, et al. Anomalous origin of the left coronary artery from the pulmonary trunk anatomic findings in relation to pathophysiology and surgical repair. J Thorac Cardiovasc Surg. 1989;98(1):16–24. https://doi.org/10.1016/s0022-5223(19)34455-1.
12. Alsoufi B, Sallehuddin A, Bulbul Z, et al. Surgical strategy to establish a dual-coronary system for the Management of Anomalous Left Coronary Artery Origin from the pulmonary artery. Ann Thorac Surg. 2008;86(1):170–6. https://doi.org/10.1016/j.athoracsur.2008.03.032.
13. Rajbanshi BG, Burkhart HM, Schaff HV, Daly RC, Phillips SD, Dearani JA. Surgical strategies for anomalous origin of coronary artery from pulmonary artery in adults. J Thorac Cardiovasc Surg. 2014;148(1):220–4. https://doi.org/10.1016/j.jtcvs.2013.08.026.
14. Kudumula V, Mehta C, Stumper O, et al. Twenty-year outcome of anomalous origin of left coronary artery from pulmonary artery: Management of Mitral Regurgitation. Ann Thorac Surg. 2014;97(3):938–44. https://doi.org/10.1016/j.athoracsur.2013.11.042.
15. Peña E, Nguyen ET, Merchant N, Dennie G. ALCAPA syndrome: not just a pediatric Disease1. Radiographics. 2009;29(2):553–65. https://doi.org/10.1148/rg.292085059.
16. Boutsikou M, Shore D, Li W, et al. Anomalous left coronary artery from the pulmonary artery (ALCAPA) diagnosed in adulthood: varied clinical presentation, therapeutic approach and outcome. Int J Cardiol. 2018;261:49–53. https://doi.org/10.1016/j.ijcard.2018.02.082.
17. Cannata' A, Pareek N, Cannata S, et al. Out-of-hospital cardiac arrest caused by ALCAPA syndrome in adulthood. Eur Heart J. 2020;42(11):1118. https://doi.org/10.1093/eurheartj/ehaa827.
18. Frommelt MA, Miller E, Williamson J, Bergstrom S. Detection of septal coronary collaterals by color flow Doppler mapping is a marker for anomalous origin of a coronary artery from the pulmonary artery. J Am Soc Echocardiogr. 2002;15(3):259–63. https://doi.org/10.1067/mje.2002.115658.
19. Yang Y, Nanda NC, Wang X, et al. Echocardiographic diagnosis of anomalous origin of the left coronary artery from the pulmonary artery. Echocardiogr. 2007;24(4):405–11. https://doi.org/10.1111/j.1540-8175.2006.00406.x.
20. Kothari J, Lakhia K, Solanki P, Parmar D, Boraniya H, Patel S. Anomalous origin of the left coronary artery from the pulmonary artery in adulthood: challenges and outcomes. Korean J Thorac Cardiovasc Surg. 2016;49(5):383–6. https://doi.org/10.5090/kjtcs.2016.49.5.383.
21. Horisaki T, Yamashita T, Yokoyama H, Urasawa K, Kitabatake A. Three-dimensional reconstruction of computed tomographic images of anomalous origin of the left main coronary artery from the pulmonary trunk in an adult. Am J Cardiol. 2003;92(7):898–9. https://doi.org/10.1016/s0002-9149(03)00913-5.
22. Wesselhoeft H, Fawcett JS, Johnson AL. Anomalous origin of the left coronary artery from the pulmonary

trunk. Circulation. 1968;38(2):403–25. https://doi.org/10.1161/01.cir.38.2.403.

23. Cochrane AD, Coleman DM, Davis AM, Brizard CP, Rory WP, Karl TR. Excellent long-term functional outcome after an operation for anomalous left coronary artery from the pulmonary artery. J Thorac Cardiovasc Surg. 1999;117(2):332–42. https://doi.org/10.1016/s0022-5223(99)70431-9.

24. Naimo PS, Fricke TA, d'Udekem Y, et al. Surgical intervention for anomalous origin of left coronary artery from the pulmonary artery in children: a long-term follow-up. Ann Thorac Surg. 2016;101(5):1842–8. https://doi.org/10.1016/j.athoracsur.2015.11.020.

25. Azakie A, Russell JL, McCrindle BW, et al. Anatomic repair of anomalous left coronary artery from the pulmonary artery by aortic reimplantation: early survival, patterns of ventricular recovery and late outcome. Ann Thorac Surg. 2003;75(5):1535–41. https://doi.org/10.1016/s0003-4975(02)04822-1.

26. Backer CL, Hillman N, Dodge-Khatami A, Mavroudis C. Anomalous origin of the left coronary artery from the pulmonary artery: successful surgical strategy without assist devices. Seminars Thorac Cardiovasc Surg Pediatric Cardiac Surg Annu. 2000;3(1):165–72. https://doi.org/10.1053/tc.2000.6516.

27. Baumgartner H, Backer JD, Babu-Narayan SV, et al. ESC guidelines for the management of adult congenital heart diseaseThe task force for the management of adult congenital heart disease of the European Society of Cardiology (ESC). Eur heart J. 2020;42(6):ehaa554. https://doi.org/10.1093/eurheartj/ehaa554.

28. del Nido PJ, Duncan BW, Mayer JE, Wessel DL, LaPierre RA, Jonas RA. Left ventricular assist device improves survival in children with left ventricular dysfunction after repair of anomalous origin of the left coronary artery from the pulmonary artery. Ann Thorac Surg. 1999;67(1):169–72. https://doi.org/10.1016/s0003-4975(98)01309-5.

29. Radke PW, Messmer BJ, Haager PK, Klues HG. Anomalous origin of the right coronary artery: preoperative and postoperative hemodynamics. Ann Thorac Surg. 1998;66(4):1444–9. https://doi.org/10.1016/s0003-4975(98)00716-4.

30. Schwartz ML, Jonas RA, Colan SD. Anomalous origin of left coronary artery from pulmonary artery: recovery of left ventricular function after dual coronary repair. J Am Coll Cardiol. 1997;30(2):547–53. https://doi.org/10.1016/s0735-1097(97)00175-7.

31. Lange R, Cleuziou J, Krane M, et al. Long-term outcome after anomalous left coronary artery from the pulmonary artery repair: a 40-year single-Centre experience. Eur J Cardio-thorac. 2017;53(4):732–9. https://doi.org/10.1093/ejcts/ezx407.

32. Cabrera AG, Chen DW, Pignatelli RH, et al. Outcomes of anomalous left coronary artery from pulmonary artery repair: beyond Normal function. Ann Thorac Surg. 2015;99(4):1342–7. https://doi.org/10.1016/j.athoracsur.2014.12.035.

33. Takeuchi S, Imamura H, Katsumoto K, et al. New surgical method for repair of anomalous left coronary artery from pulmonary artery. J Thorac Cardiovasc Surg. 1979;78(1):7–11. https://doi.org/10.1016/s0022-5223(19)38154-1.

34. Vouhé PR, Tamisier D, Sidi D, et al. Anomalous left coronary artery from the pulmonary artery: results of isolated aortic reimplantation. Ann Thorac Surg. 1992;54(4):621–7. https://doi.org/10.1016/0003-4975(92)91004-s.

35. Brown JW, Ruzmetov M, Parent JJ, Rodefeld MD, Turrentine MW. Does the degree of preoperative mitral regurgitation predict survival or the need for mitral valve repair or replacement in patients with anomalous origin of the left coronary artery from the pulmonary artery? J Thorac Cardiovasc Surg. 2008;136(3):743–8. https://doi.org/10.1016/j.jtcvs.2007.12.065.

36. Kwiatkowski DM, Mastropietro CW, Cashen K, et al. Characteristics and surgical outcomes of patients with late presentation of anomalous left coronary artery from the pulmonary artery: a multicenter study. Seminars Thorac Cardiovasc Surg. 2021;33(1):141–50. https://doi.org/10.1053/j.semtcvs.2020.08.014.

37. Regeer MV, Bondarenko O, Zeppenfeld K, Egorova AD. Anomalous left coronary artery from the pulmonary artery: a rare cause of an out-of-hospital cardiac arrest in an adult—a case report. European Hear J-Case Reports. 2020;4(3):1–5. https://doi.org/10.1093/ehjcr/ytaa061.

Coronary Artery Anomalies: An Updated Discussion on Nomenclature, Pathophysiology, and Screening

Paolo Angelini and Carlo Uribe

Introduction

In this chapter, we provide updates on several critical issues that experts on coronary artery anomalies (CAAs) are currently discussing: (a) A rational nomenclature scheme for CAAs is urgently needed and is potentially available. (b) A core parameter of CAA pathophysiology was recently established, such that the severity of coronary stenosis can now be confidently and consistently established as the single essential factor for evaluating clinical manifestations and risk in CAAs. (c) Prospective screening to detect CAAs in athletes and military recruits is achievable and may substantially lower sudden cardiac death (SCD) rates in these populations.

CAA Nomenclature

Nomenclature is particularly relevant in view of the persistent hodge-podge of terms and acronyms that too frequently confuses clinical service providers. In this regard, for the past 20 years, our group has supported a specific and descriptive staged nomenclature scheme for CAAs (in an initialism style) that brings new clarity to the subject. In particular:

1. The initialism begins with the letter indicating the coronary artery involved, either right (R-) or left (L-).
2. The presence of ectopic origin of the coronary artery, ie, anomalous origin from the right sinus of Valsalva (ACAOS-), follows.
3. The initialism ends with the path the ectopic artery takes to cross to the destination territory, which may be intramural (IM, the only prognostically serious course), prepulmonic (PP), intraseptal (IS), retroaortic (RA), or retrocardiac (RC). See Figs. 8.1 and 8.2. The CAA type and its implicit risk are defined more by this path than by ectopy.

ACAOS-IM is characterized by: (1) a tangential origin (usually, but not always, ectopic from the opposite sinus: see also the cases of high-origin and the proper site of origin with IM course [1]); (2) frequently a slit-like orifice; and (3) a constant proximal course within the aortic wall, where the vessel becomes compressed at varying degrees during the cardiac cycle, in different individuals and at different times in their lives. On the contrary, L-ACAOS-IS always implies a straight-down initial epicardial course (a partial interarterial course that is always extramural) directed towards the supraventricular crista of the right ventricle, and then the

P. Angelini (✉) · C. Uribe
Department of Cardiology, Texas Heart Institute, Houston, TX, USA
e-mail: pangelini@texasheart.org;
curibe@texasheart.org

© Springer Nature Switzerland AG 2023
G. Butera, A. Frigiola (eds.), *Congenital Anomalies of Coronary Arteries*,
https://doi.org/10.1007/978-3-031-36966-7_8

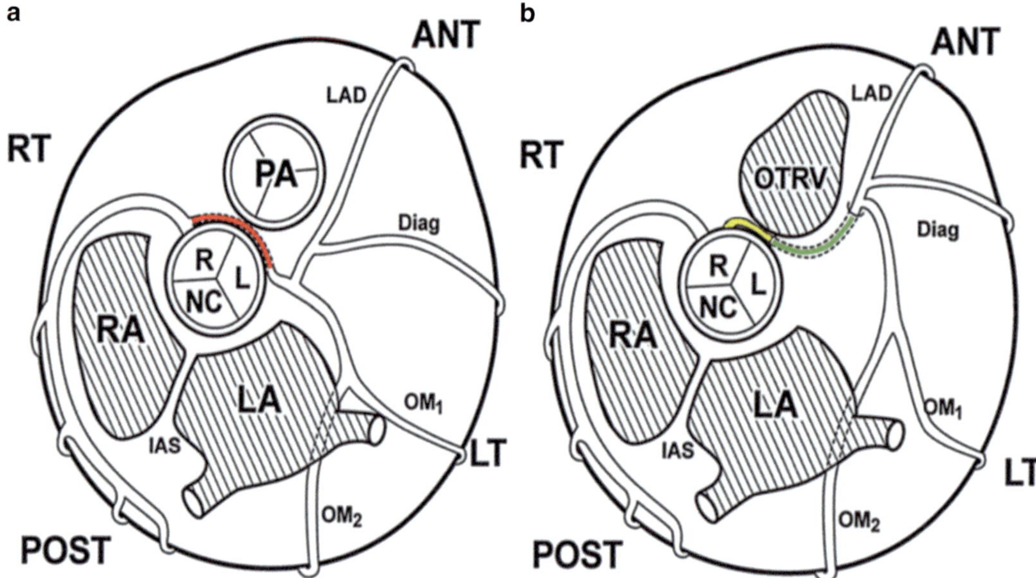

Fig. 8.1 Schematic illustrations of L-ACAOS-IM and L-ACAOS-IS on a coronal plane. (**a**) An intramural course features a proximal left main coronary artery trunk "attached" (intramural) to the aortic wall (segment in red), whereas (**b**) in an intraseptal course, the proximal segment of the left main coronary artery is initially extramural/off the aortic root (in yellow) and then intramyocardial at the supraventricular crista and intraventricular septum (in green). *ANT* anterior side, *DIAG* diagonal branch of the LAD, *IAS* interatrial septum, *L* left sinus of Valsalva, *L-ACAOS-IM* left coronary artery with anomalous origin from the right sinus of Valsalva and intramural course, *L-ACAOS-IS* left coronary artery with anomalous origin from the right sinus of Valsalva and intraseptal course, *LA* left atrium, *LAD* left anterior descending coronary artery, *LT* left side, *NC* noncoronary sinus, *OM* obtuse marginal coronary artery, *OTRV* right ventricular outflow tract, *PA* pulmonary artery, *POST* posterior side, *R* right sinus of Valsalva, *RA* right atrium, *RT* right side

interventricular septum, before emerging epicardially at the anterior interventricular sulcus and joining the epicardial left anterior descending and circumflex coronary arteries. This anomaly is mostly benign (see Figs. 8.1 and 8.2). An early origin of the first septal branch off the left main coronary artery is a distinctive pathognomonic sign in angiography. The other anomalous courses are essentially benign and extramural.

These concise initialisms quickly and effectively convey essential initial clues as to the pathology involved. Conversely, alternative nomenclatures seem to be generally unhelpful in clarifying the nature of the CAA and its intrinsic prognostic risk. Initialisms like AAOCA (anomalous aortic origin of a coronary artery) or AOCA (anomalous origin of a coronary artery) are simplified versions of our common nomenclature scheme that may be more confusing than useful. Many current investigators prefer subdivisions into consistent clinical entities.

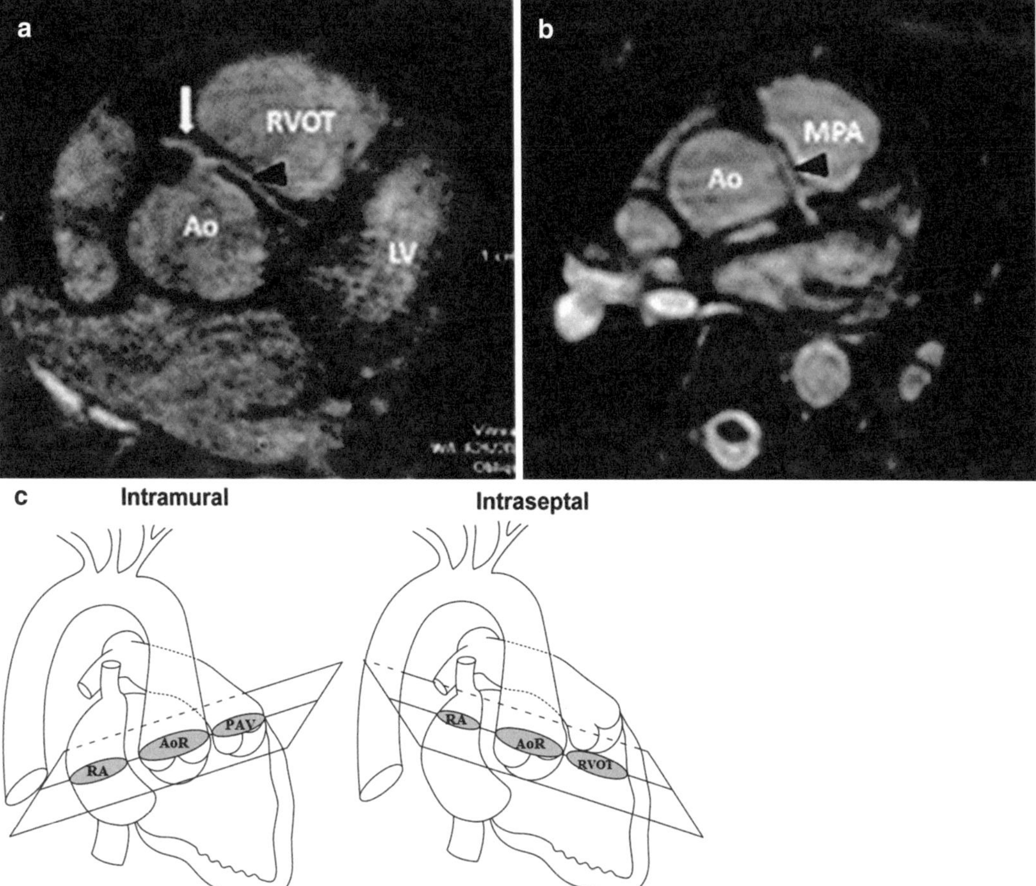

Fig. 8.2 Magnetic resonance imaging and preferred imaging planes for L-ACAOS-IS and L-ACAOS-IM. (**a**) In a case of L-ACAOS-IS, the long left main coronary artery trunk (black arrowhead) originates from a common niche with the right coronary artery (white arrow) and follows an oblique course (extramural, separated from the aortic wall) that eventually crosses the RVOT before entering the interventricular septum. (**b**) In L-ACAOS-IM, the long left main coronary artery trunk is shown to be adjacent to the aortic wall (black arrowhead) in this image taken at the sino-tubular junction, and its early bifurcation is seen. (**c**) Schematic drawings of the different preferred planes for computed tomography angiography of the L-ACAOS-IM course (left panel) and the L-ACAOS-IS course (right panel); the IM plane is at or about the level of the sino-tubular junction and the ostium of the ectopic artery (this plane also passes across the pulmonary valve), whereas the IS course is better seen in a plane that goes from the origin of the left coronary artery to the right ventricular outflow tract (infundibular). Mild variations are possible in individual cases, and the observer should follow the discipline of initially establishing the expected specific planes for each variant and then following the left main coronary artery above or below that plane (the specific plane is variable and usually not totally apparent in any single tomographic plane). *Ao* aorta, *AoR* aortic root, *L-ACAOS-IM* left coronary artery with anomalous origin from the right sinus of Valsalva and intramural course, *L-ACAOS-IS* left coronary artery with anomalous origin from the right sinus of Valsalva and intraseptal course, *LV* left ventricle, *MPA* main pulmonary artery, *PAV* pulmonary valve, *RA* right atrium, *RVOT* right ventricular outflow tract

CAA Screening

For several decades, cardiologists and medical organizations have debated and issued statements on the role of CAAs in precipitating SCD in athletes and military recruits and on the use of screening to prevent SCD in similar populations [2, 3]. Candidates for athletic or otherwise strenuous activity are uniquely amenable to routine, accurate preparticipation screening, given that syncopal emergencies and especially SCD are frequently the first symptoms of high-risk congenital conditions. Until such symptoms manifest, these candidates typically continue to train and compete, thereby progressively increasing their risk.

In order to be acceptable, preventive screening must be effective, affordable, and preferentially able to achieve definite primary diagnoses of potentially high-risk CAA(s) in 1 encounter. We have come to realize that prospective screening can indeed be done accurately, cost-effectively, and justifiably in large populations by using new, precise screening methods, such as cardiac magnetic resonance imaging (MRI) [4]. A key reason for MRI-based primary screening is that traditional screening programs (essentially based on history and physical examination plus occasional electrocardiography) generally perform too poorly to be justifiable as a primary program [4]. Indeed, history and physical alone are inadequate for identifying most high-risk cardiovascular conditions, and ACAOS-IM in particular. In contrast, MRI can be as accurate as an autopsy (and in fact has been termed *virtual autopsy*), requires only a 10–15 min acquisition time, is done without intravenous drugs or contrast agents, and does not induce significant complications.

A recent MRI-based screening study executed under the direction and supervision of the Texas Heart Institute in Houston may now enable the introduction of MRI as a novel basis for general primary screening of candidates for sports activities. In that study of 5169 adolescents (aged 11–18 years) examined by MRI, 1.5% were carriers of potentially high-risk cardiovascular conditions (cardiomyopathies, CAAs, or electrocardiographic abnormalities) [5]. We rec-

ognize that this initial study was preliminary, focusing only on the prevalence of high-risk cardiovascular conditions in sports candidates, and had no planned mortality endpoint [5, 6]. A historical study of US military recruits (6.3 million candidates) conducted by Eckart and colleagues [7] found that 33% of SCD events were caused by only one CAA type: L-ACAOS-IM. That population was screened by history and physical, and autopsy was performed on all.

Such new findings lay a strong foundation for restructuring screening programs for elite athletes and military recruits, who are under the supervision and responsibility of schools, sports organizations, or military administrations. Dedicated screening centers could eventually be organized within a comprehensive, integrated network of facilities with trained personnel who could in most cases complete a thorough screening without the need for extensive secondary expert evaluation, except for the rare cases in which a high-risk CAA is discovered at primary screening. In the unlikely event of a positive finding, the individual should be referred for specific expert evaluation (again, probably required in only 1.5% of total cases for the general population of sports candidates). The cost of a screening MRI in a dedicated high-volume center (organized to screen more than 20 cases/day) [4] was expected to be approximately US$200 [5]—the cost of a pair of basketball shoes.

Dedicated screening centers could facilitate the planning and execution of large-scale prospective and controlled studies on mortality risk in MRI-based screening aimed to acquire the evidence necessary to formulate and validate new protocols for effective screening to prevent SCD [6]. Such studies are vital for understanding the incidence of and mortality risk for each specific CAA and the circumstances that precipitate SCD.

Evaluating CAA Severity

If screening identifies potentially severe forms of L-ACAOS-IM, experts can be engaged electively to conduct secondary evaluations to determine the nature and severity of the anomaly. The information gained can be used to reliably advise candidates and to justify selective intervention or disqualification from sports activities.

Anatomical CAAs are numerous and dyshomogeneous (reported as present in 5.6% of patients undergoing cardiac catheterization [8]), but they are mostly clinically benign. Sports cardiologists are more likely to look for L-ACAOS-IM than for the generally benign myocardial bridges or other forms of ACAOS.

L-ACAOS-IM Pathophysiology

Given its inherent relation to intramural course, the term *L-ACAOS-IM* implies that a coronary artery has been irreversibly misplaced inside the aortic wall during its prenatal development. Under the radial force of the aortic wall, the coronary lumen cannot acquire a circular diameter, which is the most effective shape for a given circumference. After birth, an L-ACAOS-IM will always feature an ovaloid cross-section and will always be narrowed to some degree. The degree of luminal narrowing is at its least during the diastolic phase and at its worst in the systolic phase, even when the individual is at rest.

The simplest way to measure the severity of stenosis is by using the ratio of the widest and narrowest inner diameters in diastole: A ratio of more than 2:1 is indicative of potentially significant stenosis. The length of the stenotic segment is not usually a significant measure of severity, given that the critical site of maximal hemodynamic severity is usually short (less than 3 mm); it is the best site for measuring stenosis for interventional decisions.

Computerized axial tomography obtained at the aortopulmonary window (the Angelini-Cheong sign [9], see Fig. 8.3) can be useful for grossly quantifying the degree of stenosis. Intravascular ultrasound (IVUS) produces in-vivo video of great precision (30 images per second) and is therefore the most precise and useful method for measuring dynamic stenosis in L-ACAOS-IM in the selected patients. Transthoracic echocardiography produces less-precise measurements due to intrinsic limited

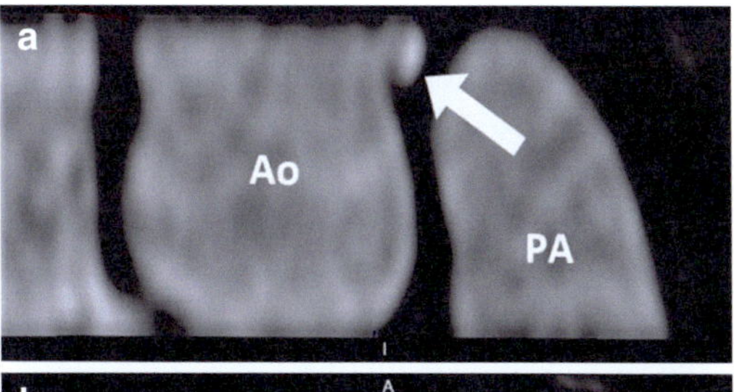

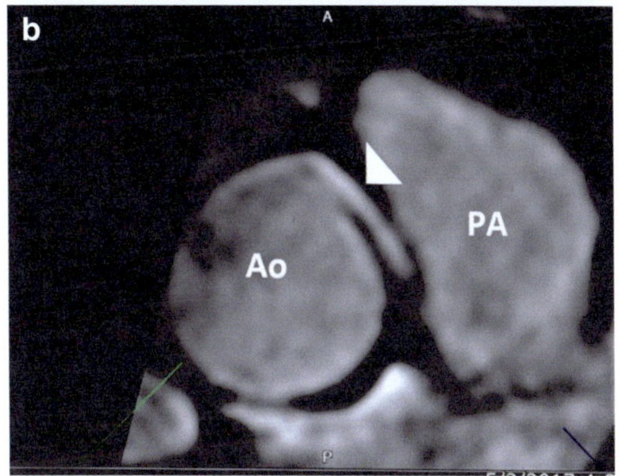

Fig. 8.3 Computed tomography angiograms from a young athlete with unrecognized L-ACAOS-IM who had syncope and chest pain during athletic activities. (**a**) A vertical cross-section at the level of the aortopulmonary window shows the passage of the ectopic left coronary artery above the sino-tubular junction (white arrow); this is highly suggestive of intramural lateral compression (the Angelini/Cheong sign). (**b**) A horizontal cross-section above the sino-tubular junction shows the proximal contiguous position of the left main coronary artery trunk (probable intramural course, white arrowhead). Intravascular ultrasound is the definitive method for quantifying severity in L-ACAOS-IM. *Ao* aorta, *L-ACAOS-IM* left coronary artery with anomalous origin from the right sinus of Valsalva and intramural course, *PA* pulmonary artery

precision, but especially because the position of a given planar sectioning is not known (ideally, it should be orthogonal to the luminal axis).

In practice, stenotic severity should be obtained during both end-systole and end-diastole [1, 10] and compared with distal reference values (the formula for stenotic area: distal cross-sectional area minus the proximal worse-stenosis cross-sectional area, divided by the distal cross-sectional area). The stenosis spectrum in diastole ranges from 20% to 80% in L-ACAOS-IM and 30–100% in R-ACAOS-IM, being about 10% worse in systole than in diastole. After observing more than 100 cases, including IVUS imaging correlated with symptomatology, we recently proposed that stenosis of more than 50% in L-ACAOS-IM or 60% in R-ACAOS-IM during diastole is suggestive of significant stenosis. Correlations between such data and clinical manifestations vary greatly (especially related to exercise habits); in borderline cases, the SAD test (bolus administration of 500 mL saline solution, plus infusion of atropine 0.5 mg and dobutamine up to 40 µg/kg/min) can be used to simulate actual exertion [10].

The elasticity of the aortic root varies from patient to patient and could be an important parameter to evaluate, especially to explain the progression of symptoms with aging. Systolic values are important to evaluate in athletes, especially because exercise (in the young, more than in the old) leads to significant relative increase in systolic time due to tachycardia (when the systolic time can increase from only 30% of total cardiac cycle time to 70%, as the heart rate reaches approximately 200 beats/min during maximal increase in oxygen demand). Aortic root size increases with aging and the onset of hypertension [1].

L-ACAOS-IS Pathophysiology

In cases of L-ACAOS-IS, the discussion is even more fundamental: (1) An IS (or infundibular) course does not feature stenosis, as can be shown by angiography or IVUS, if the diagnostic procedure is properly protected from guidewire-related spasm by administration of intracoronary nitroglycerin; (2) Advancing a relatively stiff, straight pressure-guidewire through the tortuous intramyocardial anatomy of the L-ACAOS-IS can frequently induce significant coronary spasm that is commonly visible on angiography and the corresponding pressure-wire recordings (Figs. 8.4 and 8.5). Tendency-to-spasm is clearly increased in cases of L-ACAOS-IS, while approximately 30% of these patients will have spontaneous angina that is responsive to nitroglycerin. Incidentally, clinical presentations of spontaneous spasms are relatively frequent in all ACAOS types [1]. We

have reviewed the few reported pilot cases of pressure-wire studies (mostly pediatric cases) [11, 12], and our impression is that the recently claimed "frequent" stenoses were not really present at baseline but were artifactual and would have resolved after nitroglycerin administration or wire removal [11, 13], as shown in Figs. 8.4 and 8.5.

We acknowledge that more experience with L-ACAOS-IS is needed, and prospective controlled studies will have to be performed before strong recommendations can be established. Cardiologists interested in coronary anomalies see L-ACAOS-IS fairly frequently in their adult patients, and they consider spontaneous spastic manifestations to be generally benign if treated with vasodilators [1].

Comments on Pathophysiological Differences Between L-ACAOS-IM and L-ACAOS-IS Studied by Pressure Wire

Recently, some authors have tentatively proposed that the severity of stenosis in L-ACAOS-IM and L-ACAOS-IS can be evaluated more simply by measuring intracoronary pressures (functional flow reserve [FFR] or instantaneous wave-free ratio [iFR]) [11, 12], but spastic complications can increase with this approach, especially in L-ACAOS-IS. Also, FFR (mean gradient through the full cardiac cycle) and iFR (gradient in diastole) have been initially validated only in patients who had atherosclerotic coronary artery disease and mild-to-moderate stenoses on angiography. The practical conclusion of such studies has been that an FFR <0.80 or an iFR <0.89 is associated with more frequent early clinical events in these patients [14–16]: Specifically, within a 1-year follow-up, the incidence of mortality, acute myocardial infarction, urgent percutaneous coronary intervention, and cardiac death globally increased in such patients with acquired coronary artery disease [14, 15]. A decreased maximal vasodilatory capacity is not equivalent to proof of resting ischemia, if not during maximal exertion.

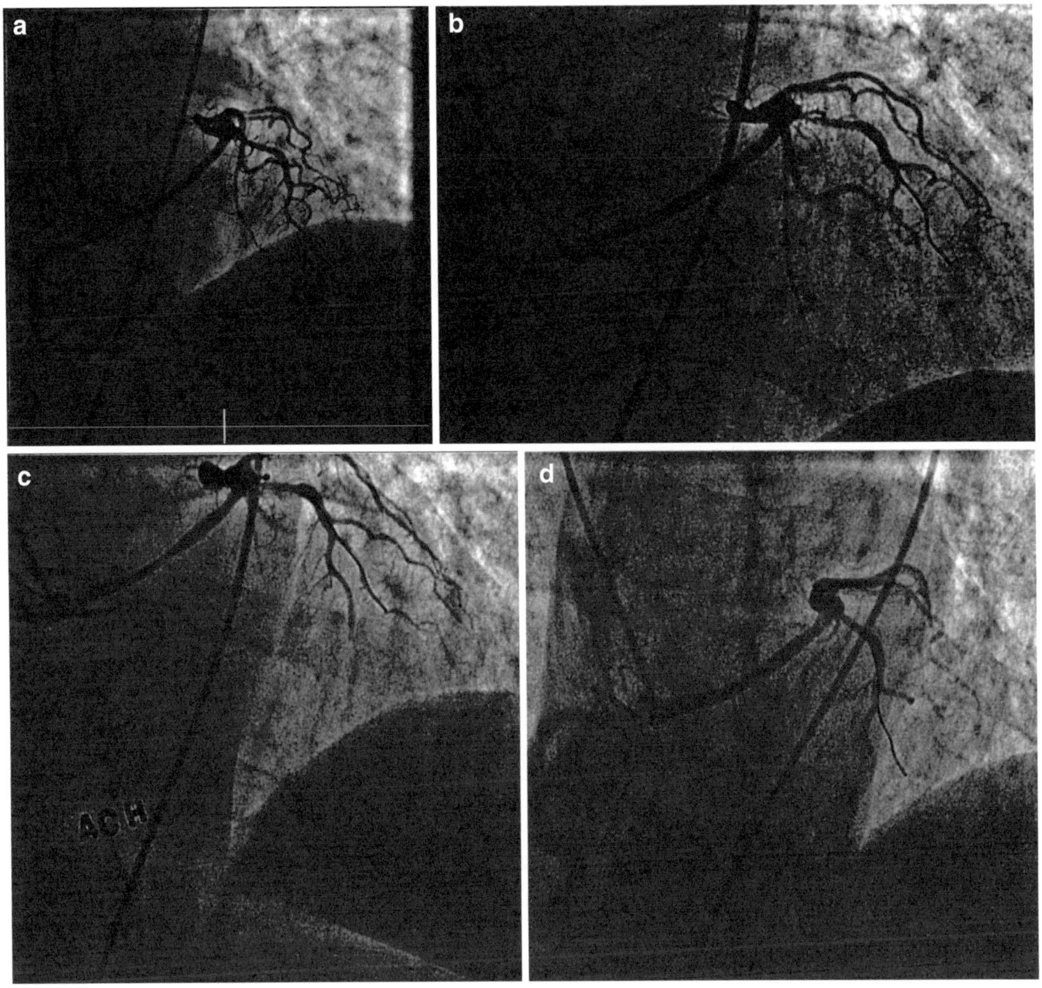

Fig. 8.4 Still images from coronary angiograms taken at four different times. (**a**) Baseline imaging, before any drugs or advancement of coronary wire, normal LCA angiography, with small LAD and dominant RCA; asymptomatic state. (**b**) Passing a guidewire into the LCA resulted in critical new narrowing at the proximal LAD (epicardial) and chest pain onset, which was relieved promptly by intracoronary nitroglycerin (100 µg, not shown). (**c**) Three minutes after nitroglycerin, acetylcholine infusion of 50 mcg was followed by chest pain; angiography shows severe LM stenosis, followed by further recurrent stenoses at the LAD (with slow run-off). (**d**) After intracoronary nitroglycerin, the LM and LAD stenoses disappeared and chest pain resolved. This case was interpreted as demonstrating unusual response with coronary spasm, both to mechanical guidewire stimulation and to ACh administration. Calcium antagonists were administered for long-term treatment (clinically successful). See Fig. 8.5 for pressure readings from the same study. *ACH* acetylcholine, *LAD* left anterior descending coronary artery, *LCA* left coronary artery, *LM* left main coronary artery, *RCA* right coronary artery

Unfortunately, at present there are no prospective or controlled studies that compare prognosis in L-ACAOS-IM versus L-ACAOS-IS; however, Eckart and colleagues [7] reported no cases of L-ACAOS-IS in military recruits. As noted, the systolic and diastolic cross-sectional areas differ from each other only in L-ACAOS-IM, whereas L-ACAOS-IS does not result in coronary narrowing other than that induced by superimposed spasm. In ACAOS-IM, disease progression is quite subtle and difficult to quantitate (especially during a limited 1-year follow-up interval [15]). In young athletes, progression of symptoms is mainly related to exercise habits.

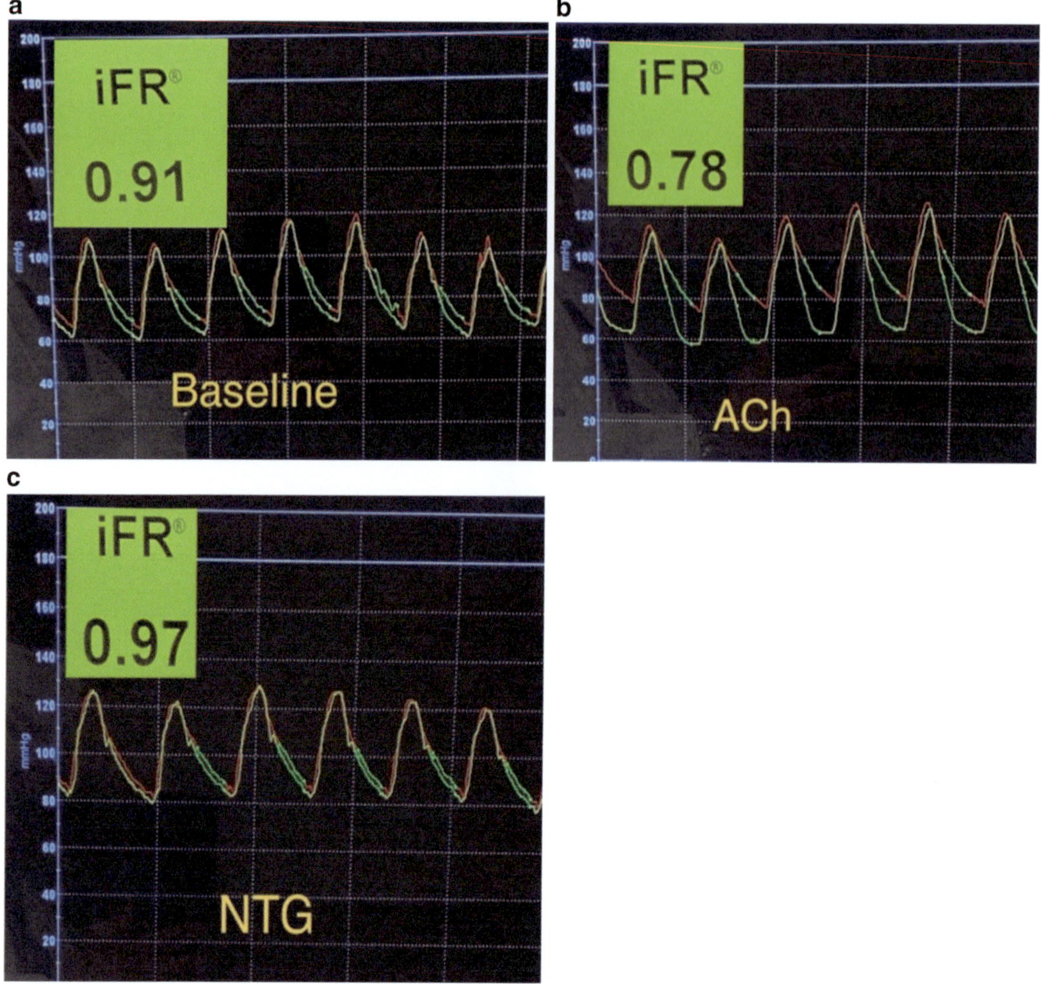

Fig. 8.5 Pressure-wire gradients (iFR) at the distal position to the origin of the left anterior descending coronary artery. The simple passing of the pressure wire created a mild gradient that increased after ACh testing and resolved completely after NTG administration. a Mild initial gradient while passing the wire (corresponding to the angiogram in Fig. 8.4b). (**b**) Gradient at the time of ACh testing, indicating severe stenosis of the left main trunk and left anterior descending coronary artery, which shows slow runoff (corresponding to Fig. 8.4c). (**c**) Gradient after NTG administration, indicating that all stenoses were eliminated; the gradient is absent with the sensor kept distal (corresponding to Fig. 8.4d). *ACh* acetylcholine, *iFR* instantaneous wave-free ratio, *NTG* nitroglycerin

An additional disturbing and objectionable notion has appeared in clinical practice related to ACAOS: the use of the term *interarterial course* (i.e., located in the free space between the aorta and pulmonary artery) that supposedly may or may not have the IM features we described. Besides the fact that the nature of interarterial course has never been clearly defined, this feature would apparently also include the IM variety (an objectionable confusion of 2 different entities).

In reality, especially from our IVUS-based investigative position, the concept that other entities with interarterial course are possible and frequent is not credible; still, 10–15% of patients submitted to surgery "for ACAOS" are not found to have IM course at surgical inspection, and a significant proportion of similar patients (having unroofing or reimplantation of a coronary artery) also have pulmonary translocation [11, 13, 17, 18]. This is difficult to explain, indeed! Clearly, pulmonary artery translocation will not be able to affect IM course inside the aortic wall (the active compressive force is the aortic systolic expansion).

The suspicion is that some clinicians have maintained the early concept of "scissor effect" affecting the ectopic arteries identified as located between the aorta and the pulmonary artery. We do not believe that such stenotic entities exist as an independent entity, and we suggest that much better imaging (especially IVUS) is urgently and routinely needed in all patients recommended for surgery, if doubts persist. The only pass inside the interarterial space is in the proximal IS epicardial course (Fig. 8.1), and neither IM nor IS has any functional result from an interarterial course or a scissor effect. The only relationship that L-ACAOS-IM arteries have with the pulmonary artery is at the level of intramural course, which is inside the aortic wall; the only relationship that L-ACAOS-IS has with the pulmonary artery is by its subpulmonic pass at the right ventricular infundibulum. No scissors can be seen in either of these instances.

References

1. Angelini P, Uribe C. Anatomic spectrum of left coronary artery anomalies and associated mechanisms of coronary insufficiency. Catheter Cardiovasc Interv. 2018;92:313–21. https://doi.org/10.1002/ccd.27656.
2. Maron BJ, Thompson PD, Ackerman MJ, Balady G, Berger S, Cohen D, et al. Recommendations and considerations related to preparticipation screening for cardiovascular abnormalities in competitive athletes: 2007 update: a scientific statement from the american heart association council on nutrition, physical activity, and metabolism: endorsed by the american college of cardiology foundation. Circulation. 2007;115:1643–455. https://doi.org/10.1161/CIRCULATIONAHA.107.181423.
3. Rizzo S, De Gaspari M, Frescura C, Padalino M, Thiene G, Basso C. Sudden death and coronary artery anomalies. Front Cardiovasc Med. 2021;8:636589. https://doi.org/10.3389/fcvm.2021.636589.
4. Angelini P, Muthupillai R, Cheong B, Paisley R. We have plenty of reasons to propose new, updated policies for preventing sudden cardiac death in young athletes. J Am Heart Assoc. 2020;9:e014368. https://doi.org/10.1161/JAHA.119.014368.
5. Angelini P, Cheong BY, Lenge De Rosen VV, Lopez A, Uribe C, Masso AH, et al. High-risk cardiovascular conditions in sports-related sudden death: prevalence in 5,169 schoolchildren screened via cardiac magnetic resonance. Tex Heart Inst J. 2018;45:205–13. https://doi.org/10.14503/THIJ-18-6645.
6. Angelini P, Muthupillai R, Lopez A, Cheong B, Uribe C, Hernandez E, et al. Young athletes: preventing sudden death by adopting a modern screening approach? A critical review and the opening of a debate. Int J Cardiol Heart Vasc. 2021;34:100790. in press.
7. Eckart RE, Scoville SL, Campbell CL, Shry EA, Stajduhar KC, Potter RN, et al. Sudden death in young adults: a 25-year review of autopsies in military recruits. Ann Intern Med. 2004;141:829–34. https://doi.org/10.7326/0003-4819-141-11-200412070-00005.
8. Angelini P, Villason S, Chan AV, Diez JG. Normal and anomalous coronary arteries in humans. In: Angelini P, editor. Coronary artery anomalies: a comprehensive approach. Baltimore MD: Lippincott Williams & Wilkins; 1999. p. 27–150.
9. Cheong BYC, Angelini P. Magnetic resonance imaging of the myocardium, coronary arteries, and anomalous origin of coronary arteries. In: Willerson JT, Holmes Jr DR, editors. Coronary artery disease. London: Springer; 2015. p. 283–337.
10. Angelini P, Uribe C, Monge J, Tobis JM, Elayda MA, Willerson JT. Origin of the right coronary artery from the opposite sinus of valsalva in adults: characterization by intravascular ultrasonography at baseline and after stent angioplasty. Catheter Cardiovasc Interv. 2015;86:199–208. https://doi.org/10.1002/ccd.26069.
11. Doan TT, Zea-Vera R, Agrawal H, Mery CM, Masand P, Reaves-O'Neal DL, et al. Myocardial ischemia in children with anomalous aortic origin of a coronary artery with intraseptal course. Circ Cardiovasc Interv. 2020;13:e008375. https://doi.org/10.1161/CIRCINTERVENTIONS.119.008375.
12. Driesen BW, Warmerdam EG, Sieswerda GT, Schoof PH, Meijboom FJ, Haas F, et al. Anomalous coronary artery originating from the opposite sinus of valsalva (acaos), fractional flow reserve–and intravascular ultrasound-guided management in adult patients. Catheter Cardiovasc Interv. 2018;92:68–75. https://doi.org/10.1002/ccd.27578.
13. Bigler MR, Ashraf A, Seiler C, Praz F, Ueki Y, Windecker S, et al. Hemodynamic relevance of anomalous coronary arteries originating from the opposite sinus of valsalva-in search of the evidence. Front Cardiovasc Med. 2020;7:591326. https://doi.org/10.3389/fcvm.2020.591326.
14. Pijls NH, De Bruyne B, Peels K, Van Der Voort PH, Bonnier HJ, Bartunek JKJJ, et al. Measurement of fractional flow reserve to assess the functional severity of coronary-artery stenoses. N Engl J Med. 1996;334:1703–8. https://doi.org/10.1056/NEJM199606273342604.
15. Tonino PA, De Bruyne B, Pijls NH, Siebert U, Ikeno F, van't Veer M, et al. Fractional flow reserve versus angiography for guiding percutaneous coronary inter-

vention. N Engl J Med. 2009;360:213–24. https://doi.org/10.1056/NEJMoa0807611.

16. Baumann S, Chandra L, Skarga E, Renker M, Borggrefe M, Akin I, et al. Instantaneous wave-free ratio (ifr((r))) to determine hemodynamically significant coronary stenosis: a comprehensive review. World J Cardiol. 2018;10:267–77. https://doi.org/10.4330/wjc.v10.i12.267.

17. Jegatheeswaran A, Devlin PJ, McCrindle BW, Williams WG, Jacobs ML, Blackstone EH, et al. Features associated with myocardial ischemia in anomalous aortic origin of a coronary artery: a congenital heart surgeons' society study. J Thorac Cardiovasc Surg. 2019;158:822–34.e3. https://doi.org/10.1016/j.jtcvs.2019.02.122.

18. Mainwaring RD, Murphy DJ, Rogers IS, Chan FP, Petrossian E, Palmon M, et al. Surgical repair of 115 patients with anomalous aortic origin of a coronary artery from a single institution. World J Pediatr Congenit Heart Surg. 2016;7:353–9. https://doi.org/10.1177/2150135116641892.

Part II

Diagnosis and Risk Stratification

Role of Patient History and Non-invasive Tests in the Workflow of Patients

Julie A. Brothers

Normal coronary artery anatomy consists of one coronary artery arising from the right aortic sinus of Valsalva and one from the left aortic sinus. The left main coronary artery (LMCA) originates from the left aortic sinus and commonly splits into the left anterior descending coronary artery (LAD) and the left circumflex coronary artery. The LAD runs in the anterior interventricular groove, and the left circumflex coronary artery courses in the left atrioventricular groove. The right coronary artery (RCA) arises anteriorly from the right aortic sinus, courses in the right atrioventricular groove, and commonly gives rise to the posterior descending artery (PDA) at its terminus in about 70–80% of the population (right-dominant circulation). The PDA originates from the left circumflex artery in 5–10% of the population (left-dominant) and is supplied by both the left circumflex and right coronary arteries in 10–20% of the population (co-dominant) [1].

The coronary artery ostium is located centrally in the appropriate sinus of Valsalva. Occasionally, the coronary artery may arise close to a valve commissure. As well, one or both coronary ostia may arise from the tubular aorta above the sino-tubular junction, which is commonly a benign condition; however, in some instances, it may be associated with increased risk of myocardial ischemia. This may be clinically important if an aortotomy is necessary for aortic valve replacement; if not recognized, the coronary artery could be transected. Another anomaly is when both coronary arteries arise from the same aortic sinus with either a single ostium or two separate ostia (see Table 9.1). When this occurs, there are different courses the anomalous vessel may take. When the LMCA courses anterior to the aorta (pre-pulmonic), it is believed to be a benign anomaly. When the LMCA courses posterior to the aorta (retro-aortic), this is also usually felt to be benign but there have been case reports of myocardial ischemia, notably when the orifice is slit-like. The anomalous LMCA with an intraconal (intramyocardial/intraseptal/transseptal) course is also generally felt to be a low-risk anomaly but episodes of myocardial ischemia have also been reported [2]. Lastly, a course of either the LMCA or RCA between the aorta and pulmonary artery (interarterial) is clinically significant and may lead to ventricular arrhythmias, myocardial ischemia, and sudden cardiac arrest (SCA)/sudden cardiac death (SCD).

J. A. Brothers (✉)
The Children's Hospital of Philadelphia,
Philadelphia, PA, USA

Perelman School of Medicine at the University of
Pennsylvania, Philadelphia, PA, USA
e-mail: brothersj@email.chop.edu

© Springer Nature Switzerland AG 2023
G. Butera, A. Frigiola (eds.), *Congenital Anomalies of Coronary Arteries*,
https://doi.org/10.1007/978-3-031-36966-7_9

Table 9.1 Anomalous aortic origin of a coronary artery from or above the incorrect sinus of Valsalva, including single coronary artery

1. From right aortic sinus or right coronary artery, left main coronary artery originates and courses:
   (a). Anterior to pulmonary artery (pre-pulmonic)
   (b) Posterior to the aorta (retro-aortic)
   (c) Through interventricular septum (intraseptal)
   (d) Between aorta and pulmonary artery (interarterial)
   (e) Behind mitral and tricuspid valves in the posterior atrioventricular groove (retrocardiac)
2. From right aortic sinus or right coronary artery, left anterior descending coronary artery originates and courses:
   (a) Anterior to pulmonary artery (pre-pulmonic)
   (b) Posterior to the aorta (retro-aortic)
   (c) Through interventricular septum (intraseptal)
3. From right aortic sinus or right coronary artery, circumflex coronary artery originates and courses:
   (a) Posterior to the aorta (retro-aortic)
   (b) Behind mitral and tricuspid valves in the posterior atrioventricular groove (retrocardiac)
4. From left aortic sinus or left main coronary artery, right coronary artery originates and courses:
   (a) Anterior to pulmonary artery (pre-pulmonic)
   (b) Posterior to the aorta (retro-aortic)
   (c) Through interventricular septum (intraseptal/transseptal)
   (d) Between aorta and pulmonary artery (interarterial)
   (e) Behind mitral and tricuspid valves in the posterior atrioventricular groove (retrocardiac)

Anomalous Origin of a Coronary Artery from the Pulmonary Artery

Anomalous origin of a coronary artery from the pulmonary artery is a rare congenital anomaly that is almost always fatal if not diagnosed and treated shortly after diagnosis [3, 4]. Anomalous origin of the LMCA from the pulmonary artery (ALCAPA) is the most common subtype but other coronary arteries may also rarely arise from the pulmonary artery. ALCAPA is otherwise known as the Bland-White-Garland syndrome [5]. The incidence ranges from 1 in 30,000 to 1 in 300,000 people. There is no known genetic predisposition and there is neither racial nor ethnic tendency for the diagnosis. The diagnosis occurs approximately three times as frequently in males as in females. It is the most common cause of myocardial infarction in childhood and should always be included in the differential of a myocardial infarction, even in older children and adolescents. If not diagnosed and treated, the mortality rate approaches 90% by 1 year of age.

Anatomy

In ALCAPA, the LMCA usually arises from the main pulmonary artery (MPA); on occasion, it arises from the right pulmonary artery. It usually originates from the rightward aspect of the posterior (facing) sinus of the MPA, but it may also originate from the leftward aspect of the posterior (facing) and, in rare cases, from the anterior (non-facing) sinus of the MPA (Fig. 9.1).

The development of clinical symptoms will be discussed below but is dependent on the degree of collateral circulation development. The anomalous coronary artery that arises from the pulmonary artery is commonly small, thin-walled, and the coronary arising from the aorta (the RCA in ALCAPA), dilates in compensation. When there is adequate collateralization, the left ventricle (LV) will remain well perfused and the heart will have normal biventricular function. However, more commonly, the collaterals are inadequate and the LV becomes ischemic and dilates. This can imitate that of dilated cardiomyopathy, notably when the fibrosis involves the papillary muscles, leading to incompetence of the mitral valve leaflets. Although ALCAPA usually occurs in isolation, other associated cardiac defects may be present, such as patent ductus arteriosus (PDA), ventricular septal defect (VSD), coarctation of the aorta, and tetralogy of Fallot.

Pathophysiology

Symptoms generally begin in infancy after closure of the ductus arteriosus and the subsequent fall in pulmonary vascular resistance. In fetal life, there is equal pressure in the systemic and pulmonary circulation and myocardial perfusion remains intact due to systemic pulmonary artery pressure. After birth but before ductal closure, the pulmonary artery pressure remains elevated,

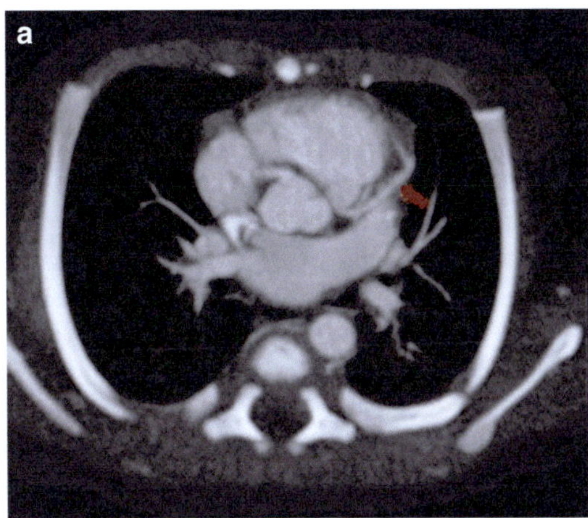

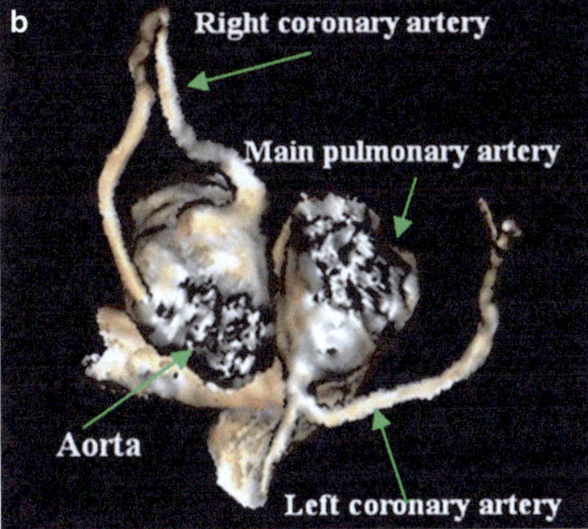

Fig. 9.1 ECG-gated multidetector CT angiography, with oblique axial view (**a**) and 3-D volume-rendered images (**b**), confirmed the diagnosis of ALCAPA (DLP=99 mGy-cm). Reprinted with permission from: Lapierre C, Hugues N. Anomalous origin of the left coronary artery from the pulmonary artery (ALCAPA) in a newborn. Pediatr Radiol. 2010:40:77

allowing for adequate perfusion of the anomalous coronary artery. Due to this, children are rarely diagnosed with ALCAPA during the first few days of life. After ductal closure and with the subsequent decrease in pulmonary vascular resistance, the clinical presentation is dependent on the presence and degree of collateralization from the RCA to the left coronary system. In the event of inadequate collateralization and along with subsystemic pulmonary arterial pressure, the LV will be perfused with poorly saturated blood at a low pressure. This leads to insufficient myocardial perfusion, resulting in LV myocar-

dial ischemia and ventricular dysfunction [6]. At first, myocardial ischemia only occurs at times when there is increased myocardial oxygen demand, such as when the infant is feeding or crying; however, over the next several weeks as the pulmonary vascular resistance continues to fall, reversal of flow into the pulmonary artery from the LMCA in diastole occurs. Ultimately, this causes infarction of the LV free wall, mitral valve papillary dysfunction with mitral valve regurgitation, and subsequent LV volume overload. If there is another cardiac defect, such as a PDA or VSD, the pulmonary artery pressure may remain elevated and the perfusion pressure to the LV may be enough to prevent myocardial ischemia.

With adequate collateralization, the left coronary system remains perfused. When the pulmonary vascular resistance decreases, a left-to-right shunt develops from the RCA to the pulmonary artery, leading to progressive dilation of the RCA and left coronary artery systems. There is a reversal of flow in the left coronary leading to pulmonary-coronary steal. While the shunt is relatively small in relation to cardiac output, it is a significant amount with regard to coronary blood flow. In those with sufficient collateralization who survive past infancy, there is usually progressive left ventricular dysfunction [7]. In a small percentage of cases, the collateral vessels are enough to maintain adequate myocardial perfusion at rest and sometimes even during exertion. These patients may not come to clinical attention until adulthood, usually with exertional symptoms [8].

Clinical Presentation

Infants frequently present between 4 and 6 weeks of age once the pulmonary vascular resistance has dropped [9]. However, many infants may not be diagnosed until 2–3 months of age, when symptoms have increased in severity. A typical presentation is commonly with signs and symptoms of congestive heart failure, including sweating and crying with feeding, tachypnea, poor weight gain, and pallor. The crying with feeds likely represents discomfort from myocardial ischemia. Those who do not present at the typical time may be diagnosed in later infancy due to a loud mitral regurgitation murmur. Older children, adolescents, and adults may remain asymptomatic, while some may come to medical attention after experiencing exertional chest pain, presyncope, or syncope. Other presentations include SCA, respiratory failure, and shock [10].

On physical examination, the infant with ALCAPA typically will show signs of congestive heart failure, including tachypnea, tachycardia, and hepatomegaly. Left ventricular dysfunction caused by ALCAPA can be difficult to distinguish from a dilated cardiomyopathy and is often mistaken for this initially. The left heart is usually enlarged, and the point of maximal impulse may be displaced inferiorly and laterally. If left heart failure has resulted in pulmonary hypertension, then there may also be evidence of right heart enlargement with a close split-second heart sound with a loud P2 component. An S3 gallop rhythm is commonly present. When there is severe mitral regurgitation, a blowing holosystolic murmur will be heard over the apex of the heart. Congestive heart failure is less likely to present in the older presenting patients. However, there may be a continuous murmur auscultated from retrograde blood from the left coronary artery into the pulmonary artery.

Diagnostic Imaging

On chest radiography, infants with ALCAPA may have an enlarged cardiac silhouette from the enlarged left atrium and LV with or without pulmonary venous congestion. When infants present with congestive heart failure, the electrocardiography (ECG) may show an anterolateral infarct pattern with deep Q waves in leads I, aVL, V5, and V6 with poor R wave progression across the precordial leads. There may also be ST segment depression in the inferolateral leads. Although this pattern can be found in other causes of myocardial infarction or cardiomyopathy, if these electrocardiographic abnormalities are seen in an infant with congestive heart failure, ALCAPA

needs to be high on the differential. As well, any infant diagnosed with dilated cardiomyopathy needs to be evaluated for ALCAPA. This diagnosis should also be considered in older children and adolescents with a dilated cardiomyopathy.

Transthoracic echocardiography (TTE) should be performed in all patients presenting with signs and symptoms of congestive heart failure. This usually demonstrates a dilated LV with severe mitral regurgitation, decreased systolic function, and left atrial dilation. The mitral regurgitation seen with ALCAPA is caused by infarction of the posterior leaflet of the mitral valve and subsequent poor movement of the leaflet; fibrosis and fibroelastosis of the papillary muscle also can be present. Imaging of the coronary arteries, including origin and course, has become possible as a result of improved echocardiographic techniques, but it can still be challenging. The short-axis view is the best way to view the coronary arteries. Careful attention should be paid to the origins of both coronary arteries. The LMCA will not be seen arising from the appropriate aortic sinus, but rather from the pulmonary trunk. An enlarged RCA is almost always present and should raise suspicion of this diagnosis. Color Doppler flow interrogation can show retrograde flow from the coronary artery into the pulmonary artery, best seen in diastole (Fig. 9.2). This is pathognomonic for ALCAPA.

Importantly, one needs to distinguish between left main coronary ostial atresia and ALCAPA. Both diseases will show retrograde flow in the LAD coronary artery. Using echocardiography, the two diseases can be distinguished by examining the flow in the left circumflex coronary artery. With ALCAPA, there will be retrograde flow in the left circumflex coronary artery, while with left main coronary ostial atresia, there will be antegrade flow in the left circumflex coronary artery [11].

While echocardiography is an extremely useful imaging modality for evaluation of ALCAPA, underdiagnosis may occur, notably when there are difficulties in identifying the coronary origins and courses. If any question remains about the coronary anatomy and there remains a high clinical suspicion for ALCAPA, then further evaluation is necessary.

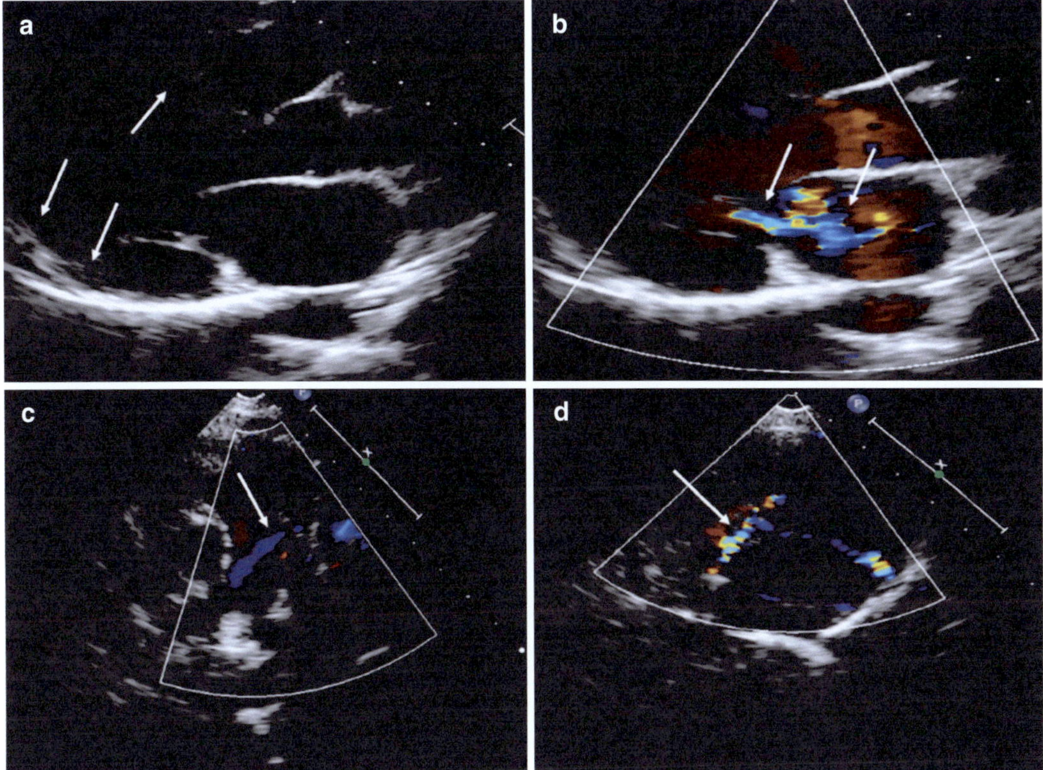

Fig. 9.2 (**a**) 2D on parasternal long axis view. White arrows show the dilated left ventricle (LV). (**b**) Color 2D on parasternal long axis view. White arrows show Mitral regurgitation (MR). (**c**) Color 2D on parasternal short-axis view. White arrow shows the retrograde flow from the left coronary artery (LCA) into the pulmonary artery. (**d**) Color 2D on parasternal short-axis view. White arrow shows the increased flow in the intraventricular collateral vessels from the RCA to the LCA. Reprinted with open access https://creativecommons.org/publicdomain/zero/1.0/, no changes were made. Jinmei Z, Yunfei L, Yue W, Yongjun Q. Anomalous origin of the left coronary artery from the pulmonary artery (ALCAPA) diagnosed in children and adolescents. Journal Cardiothorac Surg. 2020;15:1–6

Magnetic resonance imaging (MRI) is a useful noninvasive diagnostic tool for delineating congenital coronary anomalies [12, 13]. While case reports have been published utilizing MRI to make the diagnosis of ALCAPA, no case series with this anomaly have been reported. Delineation of proximal coronary anatomy by MRI has shown to have similar sensitivity and specificity when compared with coronary angiography and may be especially helpful in delineating the proximal course of anomalous coronary arteries [14]. Computed tomography (CT) has been used extensively for coronary artery delineation in adults and has been used in the diagnosis of ALCAPA in adults [15]. Advantages of CT are the rapid acquisition time and high resolution.

However, the radiation exposure and need for a slower heart rate with ECG gating make its use in infants more challenging.

Cardiac catheterization with angiography remains the gold standard for diagnosing ALCAPA. In infants presenting with ALCAPA, catheterization will commonly demonstrate elevated filling and pulmonary arterial pressures and a low cardiac output. Patients diagnosed at an older age may show only mildly elevated pulmonary arterial pressures but normal filling pressures and cardiac output. There may be a step-up in oxygen saturation in the pulmonary artery if there is significant collateralization leading to a left-to-right shunt. Injection into the aortic root will demonstrate a single, dilated RCA arising normally from the aorta. The origin of the LMCA will not be seen arising from the aortic root. If collaterals are present, aortic root angiography will show the collaterals providing late, retrograde filling of the left coronary artery with a blush of contrast subsequently filling the MPA. An arteriogram in the MPA with distal balloon occlusion will demonstrate the anomalous left coronary artery.

Anomalous Aortic Origin of the Coronary Artery

Anatomy

Anomalous aortic origin of a coronary artery (AAOCA) occurs when one or more coronary arteries do not arise from the usual location within the aortic sinus. AAOCA is the second leading cause of SCD in healthy children and young adults from a cardiac cause and commonly occurs around the time of physical activity. There are different anatomical variants that exist. The description of the anomalous coronary is related to which coronary is anomalous (right, left main, LAD, circumflex), where it originates (which sinus, location in or above the sinus), ostial morphology (round, slit-like or stenotic), and course (pre-pulmonic, retro-aortic, retrocardiac, intraseptal/intraconal, interarterial). The interarterial, intramural course appears to be the highest risk of SCA/SCD, but the challenge remains in determining which patient, given the same coronary anatomy, is at higher risk of LV myocardial ischemia and SCA/SCD.

When there are two separate ostia, either the RCA or the LMCA may arise from the wrong sinus of Valsalva and subsequently course between the great vessels (Fig. 9.3). When the two coronary arteries arise from the same aortic sinus, the anomalous coronary artery ostium is frequently small and slit-like with an acute-angle take-off [16]. When there is a single coronary artery, there can also be an interarterial course. This can occur when there is a single coronary arising from the right aortic sinus and the LMCA or LAD runs between the aorta and pulmonary

artery, or if the single coronary arises from the left aortic sinus and the RCA courses between the great vessels [17–20]. In those with anomalous LMCA (AAOLCA), myocardial ischemia has been found to be associated with an intramural course, a high orifice and a slit-like orifice, and in those with anomalous RCA (AAORCA), risk of ischemia has been associated with a longer intramural course [21].

Pathophysiology

When the anomalous coronary courses in the wall of the aorta (i.e., intramural) there is an increased risk of SCA/SCD [21–30]. The greatest danger is during or just after physical exertion, commonly after an intense effort. Both interarterial, intramural AAOLCA and AAORCA are associated with SCD, but the former carries a much higher risk [21]. Based on autopsy series of patients with AAOLCA, it is hypothesized that SCD occurs from decreased anomalous coronary artery blood flow. This diminished blood flow is likely due to certain anatomical malformations of the anomalous vessel, including a narrowed slit-like orifice that can be elliptical and, in some cases, stenotic. When there is an intramural course, there can be systolic lateral compression of the anomalous vessel from aortic root dilation as it courses in the wall of the aorta. Exercise increases cardiac output, which may lead to ostial obstruction from vessel expansion. As well, vigorous physical exercise leads to tachycardia and shortened diastolic filling time, which could lead to ischemia and/or tachyarrhythmias [31–33].

Clinical Presentation

The true prevalence of AAOCA is unknown, but estimates range from 0.1% to 0.3% of the general population [34, 35]. The challenge with diagnosing these patients is that there are no characteristic patient features or presentation that would be a clue to the diagnosis. Physical examination is nearly always normal. In some children, an innocent murmur may be auscultated and may be the

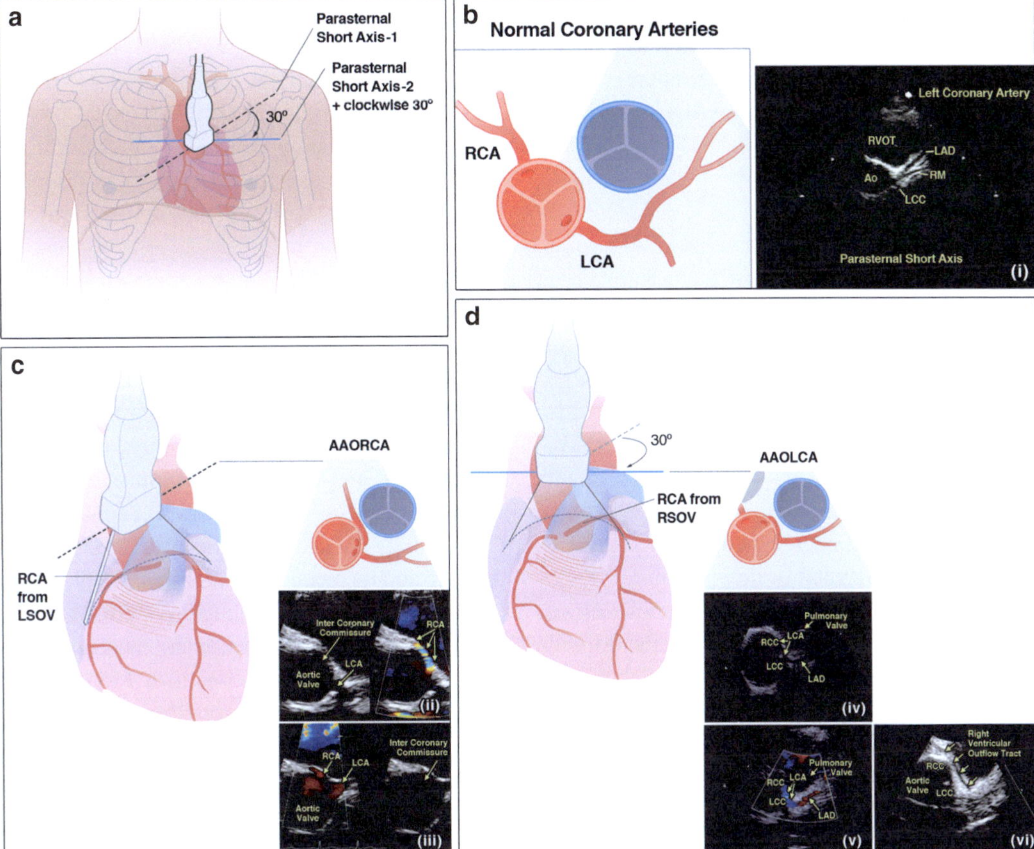

Fig. 9.3 (**a**) Standard PSSAX (1) imaging plane and modified PSSAX (2) with the transducer rotated clockwise and angled to the left shoulder, to a straight right-left axial view. (**b**) Normal origin of coronary arteries. (**c**) PSSAX demonstrating AAORCA. (**d**) PSSAX modified demonstrating AAOLCA. (i) Normal origin of LCA from LSOV with its branched demonstrated on modified PSSAX. (ii) AAORCA in 2D and color PSSAX demonstrating the intramural course of the RCA with **red** color Doppler signal in its lumen as it originates from LSOV and courses within the aortic wall in its proximal course. (iii) AAORCA in 2D and color PSSAX demonstrating a juxtacommissural origin of the RCA from LSOV with a very short versus nonexistent intramural course and absence of color flow hugging the aortic wall. (iv) AAOLCA, intramural proximal course of the LCA after it arises from the RSOV in a modified PSSAX TTE, 2D image. (v) AAOLCA, intramural proximal course of the LCA after it arises from the RSOV in a modified PSSAX TTE, color Doppler image, with **blue** Doppler signal in the proximal coronary lumen. (vi) Modified PSSAX demonstrating the intraconal course of the LCA as it traverses across the conal septum and across the RVOT. AAOLCA = anomalous aortic origin of the left coronary artery; *AAORCA* anomalous aortic origin of the right coronary artery, *Ao* aorta, *LAD* left anterior descending, *LCA* left coronary artery, *LCC* left coronary cusp, *LSOV* left sinus of Valsalva, *PSSAX* parasternal short axis, *RCA* right coronary artery, *RCC* right coronary cusp, *RSOV* right sinus of Valsalva, *RVOT* right ventricular outflow tract, *TTE* transthoracic echocardiography. Reprinted with permission from: Lorber R, Srivastava S, Wilder T, et al. Anomalous aortic origin of coronary arteries in the young: echocardiographic evaluation with surgical correlation. J Am Coll Cardiol Img. 2015;8:1239–49

reason for the initial echocardiogram and subsequent visit with a cardiologist. Many patients with this anomaly are asymptomatic; for some, the first symptom is SCA or SCD [36–38]. When symptoms are present, they commonly are during or just after exertion and include chest pain, palpitations, dizziness, and/or syncope [39–42]. AAOCA should remain in the differential for any young patient with exercise-induced complaints or in those who experience SCA or SCD [43].

Screening first-degree relatives younger than 35 years old with echocardiography is reasonable given that there have been several reports of more than one family member with AAOCA [44].

Diagnostic Imaging

Any young patient with chest pain, palpitations, dizziness, and notably syncope during or just after exertion should be referred to a cardiologist and have a thorough evaluation. A resting ECG should be obtained to evaluate for ventricular hypertrophy, arrhythmias, and evidence of previous myocardial infarction. The majority of patients with AAOCA will have a normal ECG. In patients who present with exertional syncope or SCA/SCD, there may be horizontal or down-sloping ST segment depression in ≥ 2 contiguous leads, suggestive of LV myocardial ischemia. Cardiac troponin levels may also be elevated. Alternately, there may be evidence of ventricular tachycardia or even ventricular fibrillation found when an automated external defibrillator is placed on the chest [45].

A transthoracic echocardiogram should be performed as the initial diagnostic modality for any patient suspected of having a coronary artery anomaly. Echocardiography can be performed in patients without sedation or radiation, is readily available, and is cost-effective. The echocardiogram should ensure normal intracardiac anatomy and evaluate heart function, especially focusing on areas of abnormal wall motion signifying a possible history of ischemia. Close attention should be paid to the proximal coronary anatomy, specifically the coronary artery origins and proximal course (Fig. 9.4). Improvements in two-dimensional echocardiography have made the identification of the origins of both coronary arteries possible in most patients. It is important to also utilize color Doppler flow as two-dimensional imaging alone may be deceptive, notably when there is an intramural course. In these cases, the anomalous vessel may appear to arise normally where it exits the aorta. Color Doppler imaging is helpful in demonstrating the abnormal direction of blood flow within the aortic wall, commonly between the two great vessels.

Other noninvasive techniques, such as cardiac magnetic resonance imaging (MRI) or coronary computed tomographic angiography (CTA), should be used when the coronary artery origins cannot be adequately delineated, to confirm the diagnosis, and to use postoperatively to visualize the neo-coronary ostium and course [46]. In many centers, coronary CTA is utilized for confirmation of a coronary artery anomaly. CTA can provide information about the ostial shape, proximal coronary angulation, and coronary artery course. Given advances in CT technology, current generation scanners can typically obtain the necessary data with high resolution within one breath hold, and sometimes within one to three cardiac cycles [47–49]. However, limitations to CTA include the use of ionizing radiation, motion artifact, and the need for heart rate control, which is more challenging in younger patients. Cardiac MRI is utilized in some centers to determine coronary artery anatomy. Benefits of MRI include no ionizing radiation and the ability to evaluate cardiac function and evidence of fibrosis/scar; however, sedation is needed in younger patients due to the amount of time needed to obtain adequate images. Both CTA and MRI can utilize three-dimensional reconstruction (i.e., virtual angioscopy) to evaluate intraluminal coronary ostial morphology as well as the location of the aortic commissure relative to the anomalous coronary ostium [50]. The decision on which modality, CT or MRI, to use is dependent on the provider and institution and on the availability of the modality. Cardiac catheterization with angiography is rarely utilized for diagnosis of AAOCA in the pediatric population. However, it may be how a coronary anomaly is diagnosed in an adult patient who presents with chest pain and the work-up involves coronary angiography; as well, it may also be utilized in the adult to evaluate for atherosclerotic coronary artery disease before undergoing surgery.

Provocative Testing

Once the diagnosis of AAOCA has been established, a cardiopulmonary exercise test (CPET) is almost always used to evaluate for ischemia and

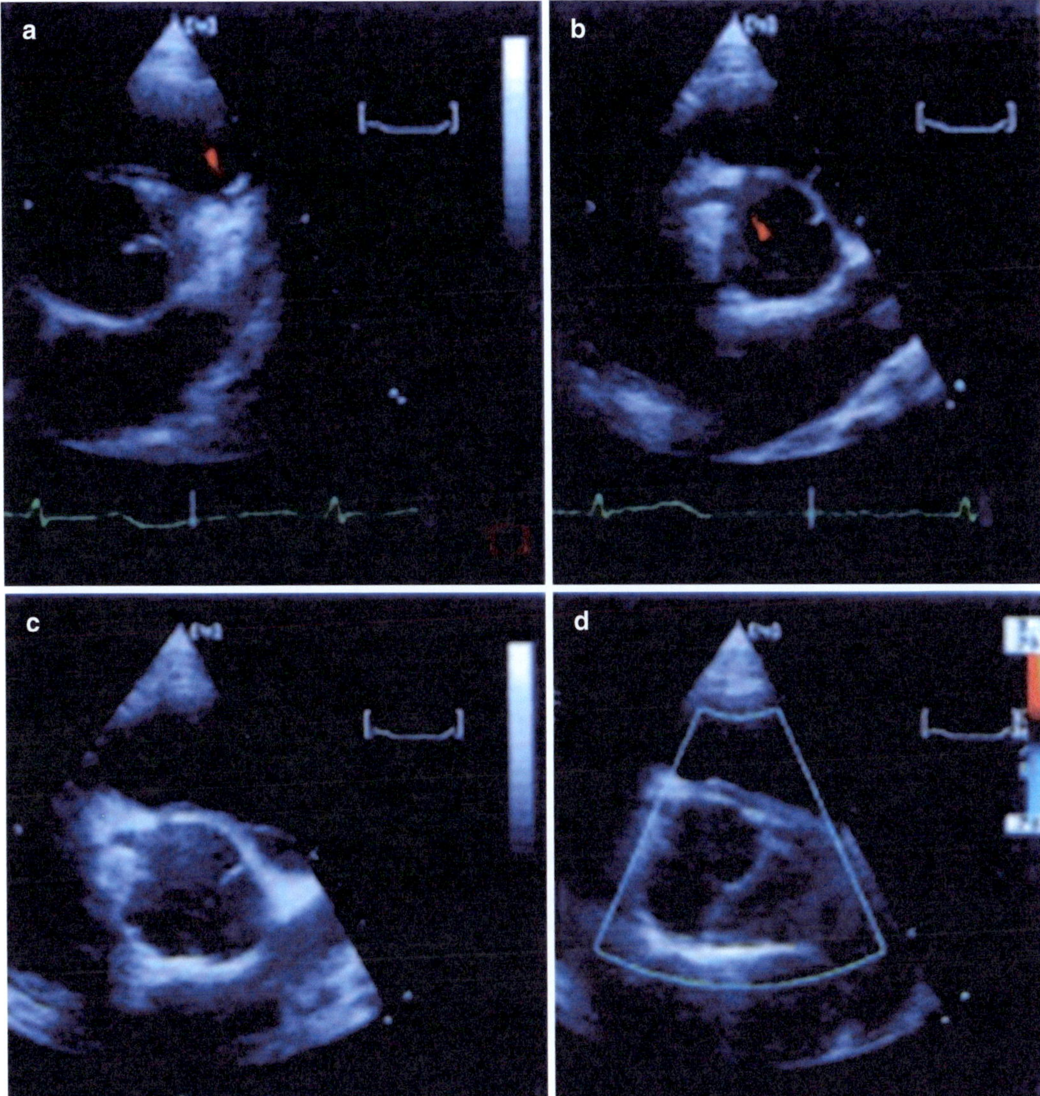

Fig. 9.4 Origin of the LMCA from the right sinus of Valsalva is shown in (**b**) and (**c**). Arrow in (**a**) points to branching of the LMCA into the LAD and LCA. Abnormal direction of blood flow is shown by color Doppler (blue) in (**d**). *LAD* left anterior descending artery, *LCA* left cir-cumflex artery, *LMCA* left main coronary artery. Reprinted with permission from: Davis JA, Cecchin F, Jones TK, Portman MA. Major coronary artery anomalies in a pediatric population: incidence and clinical importance. J Am Coll Cardiol. 2001;37:593–7 [31]

inducible arrhythmias. Those who present with SCA/SCD should not undergo further provocative testing. CPET alone is not a sensitive test in children for myocardial ischemia; it is recommended that an additional imaging modality be used to optimize the sensitivity of stress testing [51]. Commonly, stress echocardiography or a nuclear perfusion study is utilized. Stress imaging studies, such as dobutamine or bicycle MRI or stress PET scan, are additional studies that may be utilized in assessing for myocardial ischemia. CPET is also utilized in the return to sports post-operatively. However, basing treatment decisions on a single CPET may not be reliable, because ischemia is intermittent in patients with AAOCA and the posi-tive predictive value of a positive test in this popu-lation is quite low [52]. For example, in a pediatric study of patients with AAOCA who underwent surgical repair, 9 of 16 who had a preoperative exercise test presented with cardiovascular symptoms, but only one had an abnormal exercise test [52]. Furthermore, normal exercise tests have been reported in patients who subsequently experienced SCD.

Coronary Artery Fistula

A coronary artery fistula occurs when there is an abnormal communication between a coronary artery and a cardiac chamber or one or more of the great vessels [53, 54]. Coronary artery fistulas make up 0.2–0.4% of congenital heart defects and are usually congenital. They make up nearly half of all congenital coronary anomalies. Fistulas are most commonly found in isolation but approximately 20% of the time, they are associated with other congenital heart disease, most commonly tetralogy of Fallot, patent ductus arteriosus, or atrial or ventricular septal defects. Much rarer are acquired fistulas that occur as complications from cardiac surgery, cardiac catheterization, or Kawasaki disease [55].

Anatomy

The right or left coronary artery may give rise to a coronary artery fistula; on occasion, fistulas may arise from more than one coronary artery [56]. Most fistulas arise from a coronary artery with normal distribution. Anatomically, the coronary is usually elongated and dilated in the segment of the coronary proximal to the fistula and the degree of dilation is often proportional to the size of the shunt. Distal to the fistula, the coronary is usually of normal size and caliber. The most common termination sites of coronary fistulas are the right ventricle and right atrium (including the coronary sinus and superior vena cava) and the pulmonary artery [57]. The least common sites of drainage are the left atrium and LV.

Pathophysiology

Coronary fistulas result in a left-to-right or left-to-left shunt. The fistula can cause different pathophysiological consequences due to the resistance to blood flow and differential pressures from where the fistula originates to where the fistula drains. The resistance is affected by the size, length, and tortuosity of the coronary fistula. When the fistula occurs between the coronary and the right side of the heart, the pressure is lower and there is continuous flow during the duration of the cardiac cycle, leading to a left-right shunt [58]. With a large coronary fistula, this could result in coronary steal, where diastolic run-off flows away from the coronary circulation and can lead to myocardial ischemia. Alternately, a left-left shunt is established when the coronary fistula drains into a left-sided structure, such as the left atrium, LV, or pulmonary vein, and may act like aortic valve regurgitation. Depending on the size of the shunt, it may ultimately lead to volume overload.

When there is a chronically high flow state in the coronary artery fistula, this can lead to dilation and aneurysm formation. Valvar regurgitation secondary to papillary muscle dysfunction may be present. Other complications from coronary artery fistulas may include atherosclerosis, mural thrombus, calcification, and rupture. However, when a coronary fistula drains to the right ventricle, there may be a chance for spontaneous closure in the younger child [59].

Clinical Presentation

Children with coronary artery fistulas are commonly asymptomatic. The diagnosis is often made due to an echocardiogram performed for a different reason, such as an innocent heart murmur evaluation. When symptoms are present, the most common complaints are exertional dyspnea and fatigue. Angina is rare in children, even when coronary steal may be present. While ventricular dysfunction and congestive heart failure are occasionally seen in childhood in the presence of a large fistula, these are found more commonly in the adult. In the adult patient, atrial fibrillation may be found from right atrial enlargement when a coronary artery fistula drains to the right atrium. While rare, adults may also present with exertional symptoms due to ischemia in the myocardial territory distal to the origin of the fistula caused by increased myocardial oxygen demand during exercise.

Physical examination of a patient with a coronary artery fistula may reveal a continuous murmur. Most commonly, the murmur is a crescendo-decrescendo type, but should be louder during diastole. The location of the loudest intensity of the murmur can give a clue to the drainage site of the fistula. When a fistula drains into the right atrium, the murmur should be loudest along the sternal border; drainage into the pulmonary artery the murmur should be loudest at the second intercostal space just to the left of the sternum; and drainage into the LV, the murmur should be loudest near the apex. A PDA should be on the differential, but fistulas are generally heard lower down on the chest than the patent ductus arteriosus. In older patients with coronary artery fistulas, most commonly the fistula was present early in life and gradually increased in size over several years. Although there may be progressive enlargement, it is rare for rupture to occur. When rupture does occur, it is usually from aneurysm formation with the weakening of the coronary wall, either from a congenital defect or due to atherosclerosis. Bacterial endocarditis has been reported believed to be due to turbulence in the fistula.

Diagnostic Imaging

In most cases of coronary artery fistula, the ECG is normal. However, in older patients or those with large fistulas, there may be evidence of volume overload, atrial fibrillation, or myocardial ischemia, if there is coronary steal present. As previously noted, atrial fibrillation is most commonly found in the adult with a fistula connection to the right atrium. Chest radiographs are almost always normal but, in some cases, may show cardiomegaly or evidence of congestive heart failure. If giant aneurysms are present, they may be seen on the chest X-ray.

Two-dimensional echocardiography should be the initial diagnostic test performed. It can demonstrate the origin of the fistula, the size of the coronary artery, the chamber or vessel into which it drains, and any cardiac chamber enlargement or hypertrophy. It can also assess biventricular function and any evidence of wall motion abnormalities due to myocardial ischemia. Color Doppler flow will help demonstrate the fistula and will also be useful to determine the amount of shunting and if there is turbulence present. Echocardiography is also useful after surgical or transcatheter intervention to evaluate the coronary and the LV function. If surgical closure is recommended, transesophageal echocardiography (TEE) can give a clearer view of the fistula anatomy, including the origin, course and termination as well as the amount of blood flow through the fistula.

Echocardiography alone should be enough for evaluation in patients with tiny or small fistulas. However, in those that are medium or large or when the extent of the fistula cannot be adequately evaluated, then multidetector CT or MRI should be used. CT allows for very good delineation of the coronary artery fistula. Contrast opacification can help demonstrate where the fistula enters the drainage chamber or vessel. The cardiac MRI is an additional non-invasive imaging technique to diagnose the coronary artery fistula, examine the fistula origin and drainage site, delineate the coronary anatomy both proximal and distal to the fistula, and help determine the extent of shunting. Limitations for both CT and MRI are like those described above for AAOCA. Coronary catheterization with selective coronary angiography remains the gold standard in defining the coronary anatomy and the hemodynamic significance of the fistula. In fistulas that require closure, an experienced interventional cardiologist can successfully coil embolize the fistula without incurring the morbidity associated with cardiopulmonary bypass and sternotomy [60]. In the more recent era, transcatheter closure is a first-line therapy in certain patients instead of surgical repair.

In patients with moderate or large coronary artery fistulas, exercise testing with either myocardial perfusion scan or stress echocardiogram may be helpful in assessing for symptoms and signs of myocardial ischemia in the territory of the coronary fistula. If there is evidence of inducible ischemia or concerning symptoms, there should be a discussion with the patient about transcatheter or surgical closure versus medical management. As well, anyone who is asymptomatic and has a moderate or large fistula may be considered for elective repair. Children with small fistulas usually do not require closure but they should be followed for potential enlargement as the child grows [61].

Congenital Ostial Atresia of the Left Main Coronary Artery

Congenital atresia of the LMCA is very rare, with no more than solitary cases reported thus far [11, 62]. In this disease, there is no left main coronary from the aortic root (Fig. 9.5). The LAD and left circumflex coronary arteries are in their anatomically "typical" location but they end blindly; blood flow to the left side occurs retrograde from the RCA, usually through collateral vessels. Because these collaterals are generally inadequate to perfuse the left side of the heart, patients are typically symptomatic on presentation. This lesion may be confused with a single RCA; however, with a single RCA, that gives rise to all three major coronary arteries, the flow is antegrade (not retrograde) and patients are generally asymptomatic. While this lesion usually occurs in isolation, other associated congenital anomalies may include supravalvar aortic stenosis, VSD with pulmonic stenosis, and PDA [11, 62].

Pathophysiology

The pathophysiology of congenital LMCA ostial atresia is due to perfusion of the left coronary system by collateral vessels. Because the collateral vessels are typically smaller than the left-sided coronary arteries, blood flow through these vessels is typically not adequate to meet myocardial oxygen demand. This results in left ventricular myocardial ischemia, and the potential for SCD.

Clinical Presentation

There is a wide range of clinical presentations from infancy into adulthood, but patients are almost always symptomatic at the time of presentation. The difference in age at presentation is likely related to the degree and adequacy of the collateral circulation. The youngest patients generally come to medical attention due to signs and symptoms of congestive heart failure, like those with ALCAPA or dilated cardiomyopathy [11, 64]. Parents may report failure to thrive, feeding difficulties, sweating with feeds, fatigue, and dyspnea. The younger patients are also more likely to have associated congenital heart disease. It is possible that a concomitant congenital heart lesion may cause increased myocardial oxygen demand, and therefore, these patients come to clinical attention at a younger age. Older children, adolescents, and adults commonly present with symptoms of chest pain, dyspnea, and syncope with exertion as well as ventricular arrhythmias. SCD may be the first presentation, even at a young age. Physical examination may reveal a holosystolic murmur of mitral regurgitation from infarcted papillary muscles.

Diagnostic Testing

Accurate diagnostic imaging is essential because symptoms are nonspecific and can be potentially attributed to other causes. In infants and children who present with congestive heart failure, the chest X-ray may show cardiomegaly with pulmonary edema; in older patients, the chest X-ray may be normal. A 12-lead ECG may show ischemia with anterolateral Q waves and lateral T wave inversion; right bundle branch block or ventricular ectopy, including ventricular tachycardia, may also be present.

The initial imaging procedure should be a transthoracic echocardiogram. In infants and young children, this is likely to show a dilated LV with poor function and mitral regurgitation, two findings that are also found in ALCAPA and dilated cardiomyopathy. Like with ALCAPA,

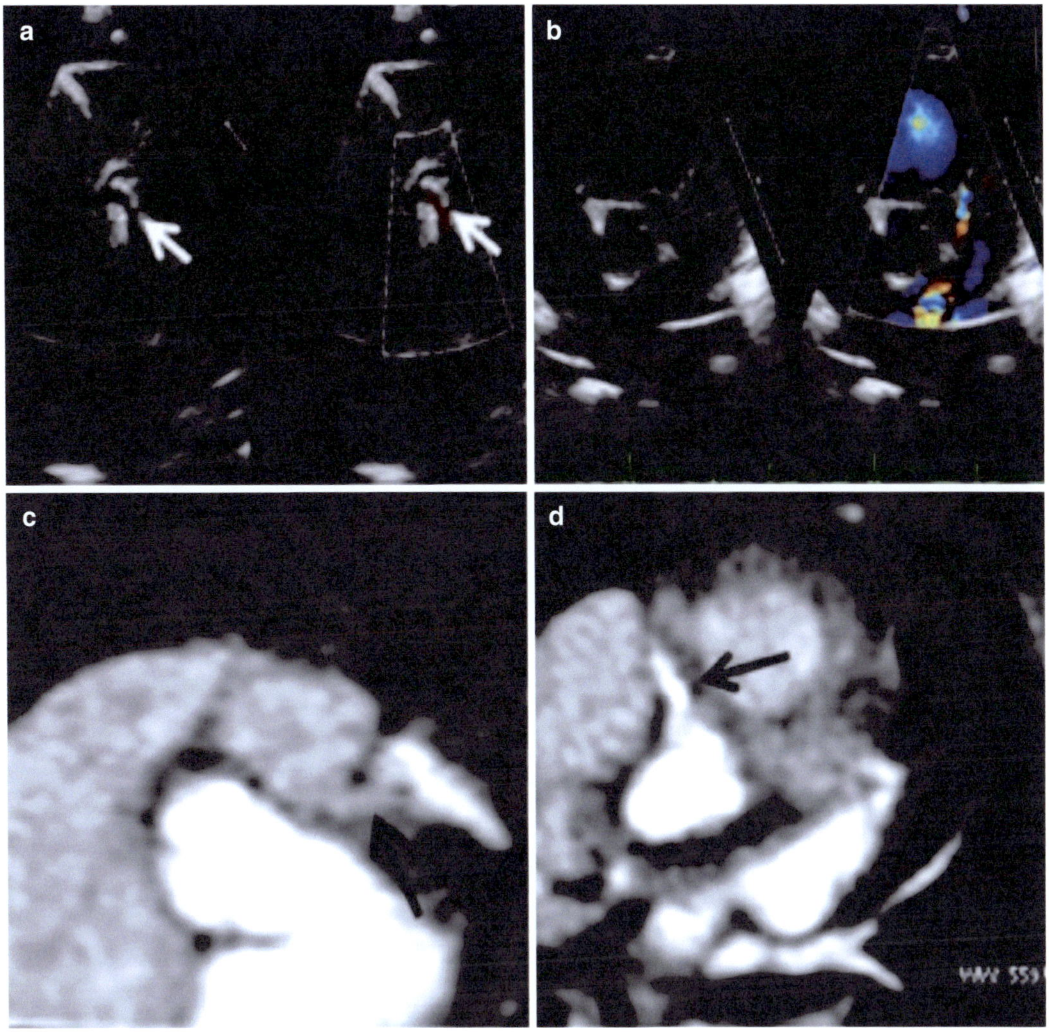

Fig. 9.5 (**a**) Prominent RCA with normal ostial origin and antegrade flow with a prominent branch arising anteriorly. (**b**) Antegrade flow seen in the usual location of the LAD; however, ostial origin of the LMCA from the aorta is not seen. (**c**) LCA stump arising from the mid-part of the left posterior facing sinus of the pulmonary artery (arrow). The gray contrast of the LCA stump is clearly different from the bright contrast of the RCA-fed portion of the left coronary system. D, RCA arising normally from the right aortic sinus is bright in contrast and mildly dilated (arrow). *LAD* left anterior descending artery, *LMCA* left main coronary artery, *RCA* right coronary artery. Reprinted with open access https://creativecommons.org/publicdomain/zero/1.0/, no changes were made: Alsalehi M, Jeewa A, Wan A, et al. A case series of left main coronary artery ostial atresia and a review of the literature. Congenit Heart Dis 2019;14:901–23 [63]

delineating the coronary anatomy is essential. Doppler color flow may be used to show retrograde flow from the RCA to the left coronary system without filling in the pulmonary trunk, as would be seen with ALCAPA. Notably, an orifice for the LMCA will not be clearly demonstrated. Another way to help differentiate LMCA ostial atresia from ALCAPA is to fully evaluate and interrogate with Doppler color flow the left circumflex coronary artery. In ALCAPA, retrograde flow will be demonstrated in the left circumflex coronary artery whereas in LMCA ostial atresia, antegrade flow will be demonstrated in the left circumflex coronary artery [11, 65]. Although echocardiographic techniques have improved over the past several years, delineating coronary anatomy and blood flow can be difficult in some cases. Therefore, cardiac catheterization with coronary angiography remains the gold standard for diagnosis. The direction of flow from the RCA to the left coronary system and whether the PA is filled retrograde should be delineated. If any question remains regarding the diagnosis, selective RCA angiography should be performed.

References

1. Shriki JE, Shinbane JS, Rashid MA, et al. Identifying, characterizing, and classifying congenital anomalies of the coronary arteries. Radiographics. 2012;32:453–68.
2. Doan TT, Zea-Vera R, Agrawal H, et al. Myocardial ischemia in children with anomalous aortic origin of a coronary artery with intraseptal course. Circ Cardiovasc Interv. 2020;13:e008375.
3. Brooks HSJ. Two cases of an abnormal coronary artery of the heart, arising from the pulmonary artery; with some remarks upon the effect of this anomaly in producing cirsoid dilatation of the vessels. J Anat Physiol. 1885;20:26–9.
4. Smith A, Arnold R, Anderson RH, et al. Anomalous origin of the left coronary artery from the pulmonary trunk. J Thorac Cardiovasc Surg. 1989;98:16–24.
5. Bland EF, White PD, Garland J. Congenital anomalies of the coronary arteries: report of an unusual case associated with cardiac hypertrophy. Am Heart J. 1933;8:787–801.
6. Berdjis F, Takahashi M, Wells WJ, et al. Anomalous left coronary artery from the pulmonary artery. Significance of intercoronary collaterals. J Thorac Cardiovasc Surg. 1994;108:17–20.
7. Shivalkar B, Borgers M, Daenen W, et al. ALCAPA syndrome: an example of chronic myocardial hypoperfusion. J Am Coll Cardiol. 1994;23:772–8.
8. Schwerzmann M, Salehian O, Elliot T, et al. Anomalous origin of the left coronary artery from the main pulmonary artery in adults: coronary collateralization at its best. Circulation. 2004;110:e511–3.
9. Wesselhoeft H, Fawcett JS, Johnson AL. Anomalous origin of the left coronary artery from the pulmonary trunk. Its clinical spectrum, pathology, and pathophysiology, based on a review of 140 cases with seven further cases. Circulation. 1968;68:403–25.
10. Kwiatkowski DM, Mastropietro CW, Cashen K, et al. Characteristics and surgical outcomes of patients with late presentation of anomalous left coronary artery from the pulmonary artery: a multicenter study. Semin Thorac Cardiovasc Surg. 2021;33:141–50.
11. Weigand JD, Gowda S, Lorber R, Madan N. Echocardiographic diagnosis of left main coronary artery atresia. World J Pediatr Congenit Heart Surg. 2017;8:101–2.
12. Douard H, Barat JL, Laurent F, et al. Magnetic resonance imaging of an anomalous origin of the left coronary artery from the pulmonary artery. Eur Heart J. 1988;9:1356–60.
13. Molinari G, Balbi M, Bertero G, et al. Magnetic resonance imaging in Bland-White-Garland syndrome. Am Heart J. 1995;129:1040–2.
14. Danias PG, Roussakis A, Ioannidis JP. Diagnostic performance of coronary magnetic resonance angiography as compared against conventional X-ray angiography: a meta-analysis. J Am Coll Cardiol. 2004;44:1867–76.
15. Takemoto K, Hirata K, Tanimoto T, et al. Combined non-invasive Doppler echocardiography and coronary computed tomography lead to diagnosis of anomalous left coronary artery from the pulmonary artery (ALCAPA) syndrome. Circ J. 2015;79:1136–8.
16. Virmani R, Chun PKC, Goldstein RE, et al. Acute takeoffs of the coronary arteries along the aortic wall and congenital coronary ostial valve-like ridges: association with sudden death. J Am Coll Cardiol. 1984;3:766–71.
17. Roberts WC. Major anomalies of coronary arterial origin seen in adulthood. Am Heart J. 1986;111:941–63.
18. Roberts WC, Shirani J. The four subtypes of anomalous origin of the left main coronary artery from the right aortic sinus (or from the right coronary artery). Am J Cardiol. 1992;70:119–21.
19. Roynard JL, Cattan S, Artigou JY, et al. Anomalous course of the left anterior descending coronary artery between the aorta and pulmonary trunk: a rare cause of myocardial ischaemia at rest. Br Heart J. 1994;72:397–9.
20. Shirani K, Roberts WC. Solitary coronary ostium in the aorta in the absence of other major congenital cardiovascular anomalies. J Am Coll Cardiol. 1993;21:137–43.
21. Jegatheeswaran A, Devlin PJ, McCrindle BW, et al. Features associated with myocardial ischemia in anomalous aortic origin of a coronary artery: a congenital heart Surgeons' Society study. J Thorac Cardiovasc Surg. 2019;158:822–34.
22. Basso C, Maron BJ, Corrado D, et al. Clinical profile of congenital coronary artery anomalies with origin from the wrong aortic sinus leading to sudden death in young competitive athletes. J Am Coll Cardiol. 2000;35:1493–501.
23. Cheitlin MD, DeCastro CM, McAllister HA. Sudden death as a complication of anomalous left coronary origin from the anterior sinus of Valsalva: a not-so-minor congenital anomaly. Circulation. 1974;50:780–7.
24. Liberthson RR, Dinsmore RE, Fallon JT. Aberrant coronary artery origin from the aorta: report of 18 patients, review of literature and delineation of natural history and management. Circulation. 1979;59:748–54.
25. Maron BJ, Shirani J, Poliac LC, et al. Sudden death in young competitive athletes: clinical, demographic and pathological profiles. JAMA. 1996;276:199–204.
26. Mustafa I, Gula G, Radley-Smith R, et al. Anomalous origin of the left coronary artery from the anterior aor-

tic sinus: a potential cause of sudden death. J Thorac Cardiovasc Surg. 1981;82:297–300.

27. Taylor AJ, Rogan KM, Virmani R. Sudden cardiac death associated with isolated congenital coronary artery anomalies. J Am Coll Cardiol. 1992;20:640–7.

28. Frescura C, Basso C, Thiene G, et al. Anomalous origin of coronary arteries and risk of sudden death: a study based on an autopsy population of congenital heart disease. Hum Pathol. 1998;29:689–95.

29. Kragel AH, Roberts WC. Anomalous origin of either the right or left main coronary artery from the aorta with subsequent coursing between aorta and pulmonary trunk: analysis of 32 necropsy cases. Am J Cardiol. 1988;62:771–9.

30. Roberts WC, Kragel AH. Anomalous origin of either the right or left main coronary artery from the aorta without coursing of the anomalously arising artery between aorta and pulmonary trunk: analysis of 32 necropsy cases. Am J Cardiol. 1988;62:1263–7.

31. Davis JA, Cecchin F, Jones TK, Portman MA. Major coronary artery anomalies in a pediatric population: incidence and clinical importance. J Am Coll Cardiol. 2001;37:593–7.

32. Zeppilli P, dello Russo A, Santini C, et al. In vivo detection of coronary artery anomalies in asymptomatic athletes by echocardiographic screening. Chest. 1998;114:89–93.

33. Brothers JA, McBride MG, Seliem MA, et al. Evaluation of myocardial ischemia following surgical repair of anomalous aortic origin of a coronary artery in a series of pediatric patients. J Am Coll Cardiol. 2007;50:2078–82.

34. Brothers JA, Stephens P, Gaynor JW, et al. Anomalous aortic origin of a coronary artery with an interarterial course: should family screening be routine? J Am Coll Cardiol. 2008;51:2062–4.

35. Frommelt PC, Frommelt MA, Tweddell JS, et al. Prospective echocardiographic diagnosis and surgical repair of anomalous origin of a coronary artery from the opposite sinus with an interarterial course. J Am Coll Cardiol. 2003;42:148–54.

36. Romp RL, Herlong R, Landolfo CK, et al. Outcome of unroofing procedure for repair of anomalous aortic origin of left or right coronary artery. Ann Thorac Surg. 2003;76:589–96.

37. Towbin JA. Myocardial infarction in childhood. In: Garson A, Bricker JT, DG MN, editors. The science and practice of pediatric cardiology. hiladelphia: Lea & Febiger; 1990. p. 1684.

38. Frommelt PC, Berger S, Pelech AN, et al. Prospective identification of anomalous origin of left coronary artery from the right sinus of Valsalva using transthoracic echocardiography: importance of color Doppler flow mapping. Pediatr Cardiol. 2001;22:327–32.

39. Post JC, van Rossum AC, Bonzwaer JGF, et al. Magnetic resonance angiography of anomalous coronary arteries. A new gold standard for delineating the proximal course? Circulation. 1995;92:3163–71.

40. Taylor AM, Thorne SA, Rubens P, et al. Coronary artery imaging in grown up congenital heart disease: complementary role of magnetic resonance and X-ray coronary angiography. Circulation. 2000;101:1670–8.

41. Brothers JA, Stephens P, Gaynor JW, Lorber R, Vricella LA, Paridon SM. Anomalous aortic origin of a coronary artery with an interarterial course: should family screening be routine? J Am Coll Cardiol. 2008;51:2062–4.

42. Greet B, Quinones A, Srichai M, Bangalore S, Roswell RO. Anomalous right coronary artery and sudden cardiac death. Circ Arrhythm Electrophysiol. 2012;5:e111–2.

43. Brothers JA, Frommelt MA, Jaquiss RDB, Myerburg RJ, Fraser CD Jr, Tweddell JS. Expert consensus guidelines: anomalous aortic origin of a coronary artery. J Thorac Cardiovasc Surg. 2017;153:1440–57.

44. Tresoldi S, Mezzanzanica M, Campari A, Salerno Uriarte D, Cornalba G. Role of computed tomography coronary angiography in the management of coronary anomalies. J Card Surg. 2013;28:33–6.

45. Attili A, Hensley AK, Jones FD, Grabham J, DiSessa TG. Echocardiography and coronary CT angiography imaging of variations in coronary anatomy and coronary abnormalities in athletic children: detection of coronary abnormalities that create a risk for sudden death. Echocardiography. 2013;30:225–33.

46. Baird CW. Intraluminal 3-D CT identifies coronary osteal and commissural relationships in anomalous aortic origin of coronary arteries. Ann Thorac Surg. 2010;89:1341. Author reply 1341-2.

47. Brothers JA, Whitehead KK, Keller MS, et al. Cardiac MRI and CT: differentiation of normal ostium and intraseptal course from slitlike ostium and interarterial course in anomalous left coronary artery in children. Am J Roentgenol. 2015;204:W104–9.

48. Brothers J, Carter C, McBride M, et al. Anomalous left coronary artery origin from the opposite sinus of Valsalva: evidence of intermittent ischemia. J Thorac Cardiovasc Surg. 2010;140:e27–9.

49. Brothers JA, McBride MG, Seliem MA, et al. Evaluation of myocardial ischemia after surgical repair of anomalous aortic origin of a coronary artery in a series of pediatric patients. J Am Coll Cardiol. 2007;50:2078–82.

50. Liberthson RR, Sagar K, Berkoben JP, et al. Congenital coronary arteriovenous fistula. Report of 13 patients, review of the literature and delineation of management. Circulation. 1979;59:849–54.

51. McNamara JJ, Gross RE. Congenital coronary artery fistula. Surgery. 1969;65:59–69.

52. Koenig PR, Kimball TR, Schwartz DC. Coronary artery fistula complicating the evaluation of Kawasaki disease. Pediatr Cardiol. 1993;14:179–80.

53. Davis JT, Allen HD, Wheller JJ, et al. Coronary artery fistula in the pediatric age group: a 19-year institutional experience. Ann Thorac Surg. 1994;58:760–3.

54. Fernandes ED, Kadivar H, Hallman GL, et al. Congenital malformations of the coronary arteries: the Texas heart institute experience. Ann Thorac Surg. 1992;54:732–40.

55. Gowda RM, Vasavada BC, Khan IA. Coronary artery fistulas: clinical and therapeutic considerations. Int J Cardiol. 2006;107:7–10.
56. Santoro G, Formigari R, Di Carlo D, Ballerini L. Chiusura spontanea delle fistole coronariche: possibile ruolo prognostico della sede di comunicazione [Spontaneous closure of coronary fistulas: a possible prognostic role of the site of drainage]. G Ital Cardiol. 1994;24:1223–6.
57. Reidy JF, Anjos RT, Qureshi SA, et al. Transcatheter embolization in the treatment of coronary artery fistulas. J Am Coll Cardiol. 1991;18:187–92.
58. Farooki ZQ, Nowlen T, Hakimi M, et al. Congenital coronary artery fistulae: a review of 18 cases with special emphasis on spontaneous closure. Pediatr Cardiol. 1993;14:208–13.
59. Musiani A, Cernigliaro C, Sansa M, et al. Left main coronary artery atresia: literature review and therapeutical considerations. Eur J Cardiothorac Surg. 1997;11:505–14.
60. Chou HH, Chan CH, Tsai KT, et al. Congenital atresia of the left main coronary artery associated with patent ductus arteriosus and aortic regurgitation. Circ J. 2009;73:1163–6.
61. Kaczorowski DJ, Sathanandam S, Ravishankar C, et al. Coronary ostioplasty for congenital atresia of the left main coronary artery ostium. Ann Thorac Surg. 2012;94:1307–10.
62. Lorber R, Srivastava S, Wilder T, et al. Anomalous aortic origin of coronary arteries in the young: echocardiographic evaluation with surgical correlation. J Am Coll Cardiol Img. 2015;8:1239–49.
63. Alsalehi M, Jeewa A, Wan A, et al. A case series of left main coronary artery ostial atresia and a review of the literature. Congenit Heart Dis. 2019;14:901–23.
64. Jinmei Z, Yunfei L, Yue W, Yongjun Q. Anomalous origin of the left coronary artery from the pulmonary artery (ALCAPA) diagnosed in children and adolescents. J Cardiothorac Surg. 2020;15:1–6.
65. Lapierre C, Hugues N. Anomalous origin of the left coronary artery from the pulmonary artery (ALCAPA) in a newborn. Pediatr Radiol. 2010;40:77.

Advanced Imaging in Congenital Abnormalities of Coronary Arteries in Children

Jan Marek, Kristian Mortensen, and Claudio Capelli

Introduction

Improved cardiac imaging over the last two decades resulted in qualitative changes in diagnostic morphological and functional protocols in children suspected of having congenital or acquired heart conditions. Incorporating coronary artery views (origins and proximal branches) into comprehensive echocardiographic segmental sequential scans [1] in all children referred for cardiology review in most cardiac centres worldwide has resulted in increased detection rate of congenital coronary abnormalities in asymptomatic children, including abnormalities with uncertain haemodynamic implication such as anomalous aortic origin from opposite sinus (AAOCA). High-volume centres such as Great Ormond Street Hospital for Children, identify accidentally up to 15–30 patients with AAOCA every year, resulting in significantly increased demands for further detailed advanced multimodal imaging [2] at rest and on exertion to enable correct risk stratification and further management and treatment.

In this chapter, we aim to offer a brief review of current multimodal imaging of coronary arteries in paediatric population such as 3D modelling, virtual reality and stress tests, offering diagnostic strategies and pathways, and share our experience with diagnostic imaging in children from prenatal period of time, through early infancy and childhood, until young adulthood.

Echocardiography

2D Transthoracic Echocardiography

In children, transthoracic echocardiography (TTE) with high-frequency probes (6–12Mhz) permits rapid visualisation of coronary ostia and proximal branches, typically examined from parasternal short axis views [1, 3, 4]. Apart from parasternal short axis views, the left main coronary artery (LMCA) origin can be visualised from apical or subcostal five-chamber (anteriorly tilted 4-CH) view to allow accurately image coronary origin from the sinus, sino-tubular junction, or proximal ascending aorta (AO). The right coronary artery (RCA) origin can be seen from a parasternal long-axis view with slight rightward tilt of the transducer allowing identification of the coronary origin similar to LMCA. The left anterior descendent (LAD) coursing alongside the anterior interventricular groove can visualised in a high parasternal short axis with the transducer

J. Marek (✉) · K. Mortensen · C. Capelli
Great Ormond Street Hospital for Children and Institute of Cardiovascular Imaging, University College London, London, UK
e-mail: Jan.Marek@gosh.nhs.uk;
Kristian.mortensen@gosh.nhs.uk;
C.capelli@ucl.ac.uk

tilted more leftward laterally or in the long axis view with leftward anterior tilt as the imaging plane sweeps between aortic root and pulmonary trunk (PA).

Visualising LMCA from PA in anomalous origin of coronary artery from pulmonary trunk (ALCAPA) may be challenging particularly in cases with LMCA in close proximity to aortic wall or with the take-off from lateral aspect of PA adhering to left pleural space. All views including modified parasternal and subcostal modified views should be attempted to visualised origins of RCA and LMCA in non-perpendicular way to the ultrasound beam aiming to visualise flow pattern at the level of entering ostia from aortic sinuses on colour flow mapping (CFM). Optimised CFM modality with low Nyquist limit (20–40 cm/s), 2D, and colour gain optimisation should be applied to correctly image flow within coronary arteries. Default coronary CFM pre-set is routinely used to enhance CFM coronary flow imaging at the cost of suppressed quality of 2D imaging. Although parasternal short axis views are recommended to visualise the proximal branches on 2D imaging, these views however may not allow to image flow within on CFM as ultrasound beam is transmitted often perpendicularly to coronary course (RCA aortic origin at 9 o'clock, LMCA at 3 o'clock).

Interestingly, and according to our experience, well-visualised coronary colour flow may suspect ALCAPA or AAOCA more reliably than 2D image as the coronary arteries with acute angle in AAOCA are running more parallel with ultrasound beam such as in RCA originating from left aortic sinus (AAORCA, Fig. 10.1). The intramural segment in AAOCA is longer and usually running certain distance through the aortic wall before exiting the aortic wall from the opposite sinus. Intramural segment with the anomalous coronary ostium arising adjacent to the commissure between the right and left coronary cusps. CFM should always be used to document the flow from aortic sinus into coronary ostium in all variants of congenital coronary abnormalities. Reversal diastolic flow on CFM within the LAD suggestive of coronary steal from RCA territory is highly suspicious of ALCAPA even if coronary artery is convincingly connected to the AO on 2D

image. Careful assessment of left ventricle (LV) and mitral valve function remains imperative for all patients suspicious of coronary-induced ischaemia. Myocardial fibrosis of papillary muscles with regional wall motion abnormalities on conventional echocardiography and on tissue deformation imaging are sensitive diagnostic features in any coronary abnormalities causing myocardial hypoperfusion at rest or on exercise [5]. However, in contrast to adults, babies and small children tend to develop coronary collateral vessels from RCA resulting in well-maintained LV function on conventional echocardiograms. In these cases, the proximal RCA is usually dilated with multiple small collateral vessels connected to the LMCA territory, and is usually well visualised in multiple parasternal and subcostal views.

Although the echocardiographic diagnostic correlations between institutional and expert echocardiography compared with surgical findings were reported rather poor [6], improvement in diagnostic accuracy of congenital coronary abnormalities can be documented by significantly increasing numbers of echocardiographically diagnosed AAOCA incidentally identified in asymptomatic children.

Prenatal 2D Transabdominal Echocardiography

Although prenatal imaging of coronary arteries is not amongst the requirements for antenatal cardiac screening in second trimester, current ultrasound technology enables to image coronary arteries in a variety of conditions mainly causing coronary artery dilatation such as isolated coronary fistulae [7] or as a part of the spectrum of more severe conditions such as in pulmonary atresia with intact ventricular septum [8]. Moreover, foetal coronary Doppler flow patterns can also be assessed, and increased velocities were identified in foetuses suffering from anaemia [9]. With current ultrasound technology, it is however not surprising that isolated coronary abnormality such as anomalous origin of right coronary artery from left aortic sinus (AAORCA) can be reliably identified as early as in 22nd week of gestation [10]. In late trimester, proximal

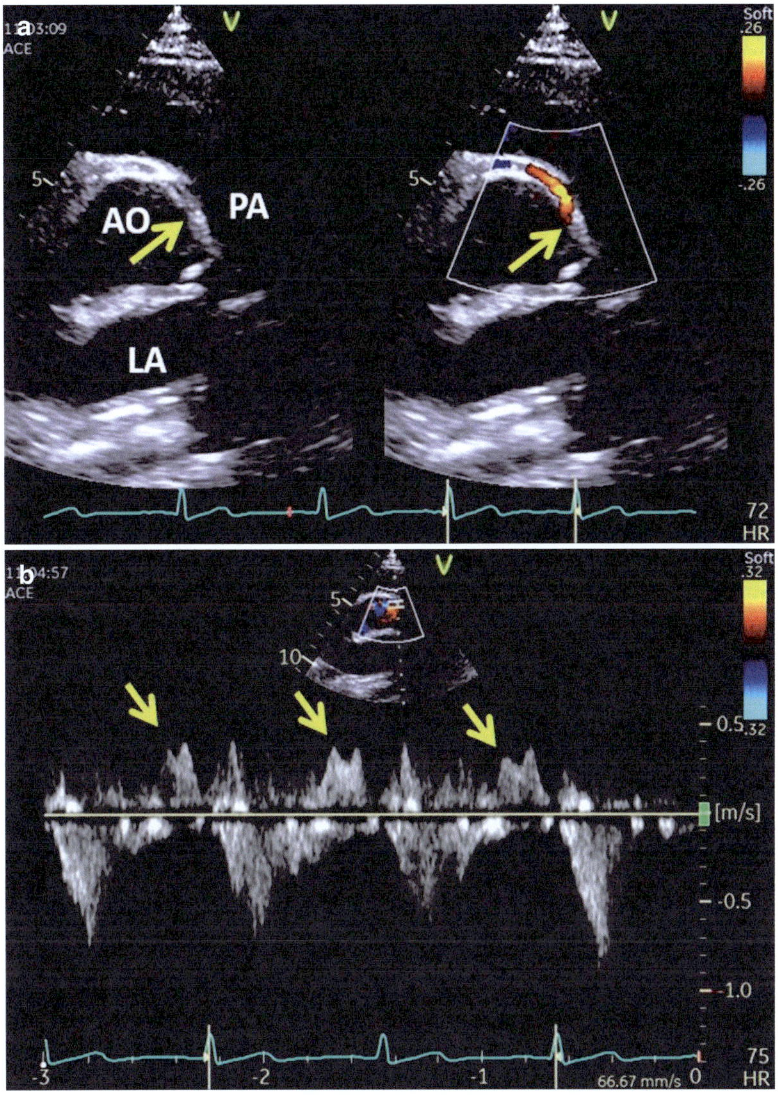

Fig. 10.1 12 years old competitive swimmer with AAORCA. 2D transthoracic echocardiography with colour flow mapping in parasternal short axis view and (**a**) shows take-off of right coronary artery (arrow) from opposite sinus with interarterial course between AO and PA. Puled Doppler tracing (**b**) demonstrated normal diastolic flow (arrows)

coronary branches can be occasionally identified (Fig. 10.2), and assessing coronary arrangement in transposition of the great arteries could be considered although data on accuracy are not available.

3D Transthoracic and Transoesophageal Echocardiography (3DE)

The 3DE visualisation of coronary arteries and the detection of coronary artery abnormalities are generally possible in children; however, high-resolution 2D echocardiography remains superior

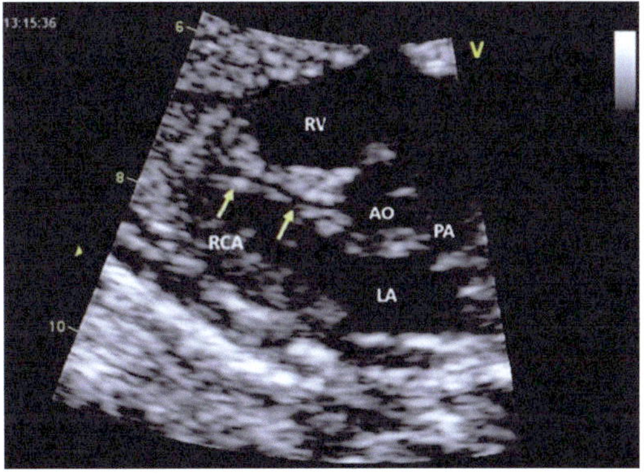

Fig. 10.2 Right coronary artery (RCA, arrows) imaged in 28-week-old foetus. *RV* right ventricle, *PA* pulmonary artery, *AO* aorta, *LA* left atrium

to 3DE. Higher sensitivity and specificity values were obtained by 2D than by 3D echocardiography when tested in adults [11]. The desired end-face views to assess ostial shape are possible to obtain in patients with very good acoustic windows or by transoesophageal approach; however, image quality remains far inferior to those obtained by high-resolution computed-tomographic (CT) angiography.

Transoesophageal Echocardiography

Transoesophageal echocardiography (TEE) is not routinely used as primary diagnostic modality for children with coronary abnormalities. TEE has been, however, routinely used in children to identify coronary problems mainly as additional imaging modality during general anaesthetics required for cross-section imaging or as a part of perioperative pre- and post-bypass assessment.

Multiplane TEE probe views from mid-oesophageal window in short axis angulated around 30–40° can image coronary artery just above the aortic valve (Fig. 10.3.). In this view CFM can usually indicate entry into ostium. The RCA is best seen at 90–120°. CFM of both coronary arteries is important to evaluate the direction, velocity, and timing of flow. In selective patients, TEE may improve visualisation of proximal coronary arteries and their relation to surrounding structures such as aortic and pulmonary commissures and may offer better visualisation of ostia and it's course through aortic wall in patients suspected of AAOCA. In addition, pharmacological (dobutamine) Stress TEE can be considered in children to assess dynamic change in coronary ostial shape and flow dynamics

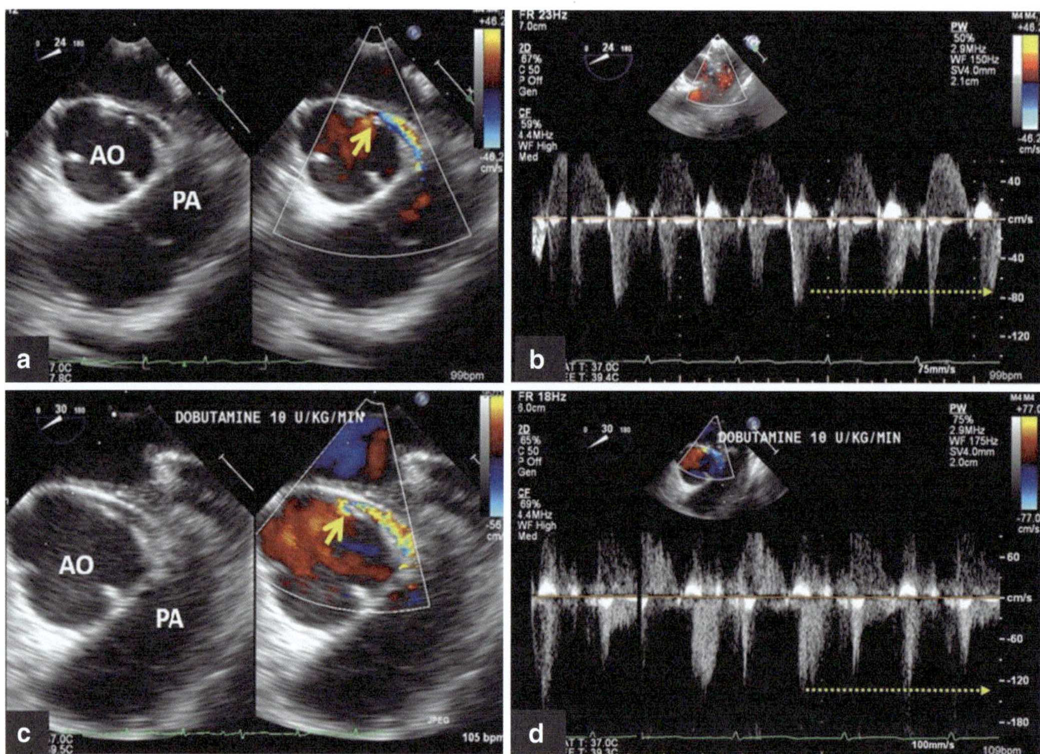

Fig. 10.3 Transoesophageal dobutamine stress echocardiography in a 7-year-old boy with incidental finding of single coronary artery from non-coronary sinus with intramural course of LMCA and interarterial and intramural course of the RCA. 2D echocardiography with colour flow mapping (**a**) demonstrated juxtacommisural take-off of LMCA (**b**) with Vmax on PDE around 0.7 m/s (**b**). Low-dose dobutamine stress echocardiogram confirmed narrow LMCA ostium with turbulent flow on colour flow mapping (**c**) with Vmax up to 1.2 m/s (**d**)

together with global and regional ventricular function to better understand physiology in patients with AAOCA [12].

Epicardial Echocardiography

Similar to transoesophageal echocardiography, epicardial echocardiography is indispensable intraoperative imaging modality mainly reserved for babies and small children referred for heart operation involving interventions on coronary arteries such as for arterial switch for transposition of the great arteries [13, 14]. Focused two-dimensional, colour, and spectral Doppler imaging of the coronary arteries using 9–12 MHz probe is performed during operation requiring coronary re-implantation or manipulation, particularly in those with unexpected ventricular dysfunction or ST changes on ECG monitor suggestive of myocardial ischaemia (Fig. 10.4). Imaging of the coronary arteries should include ostial areas and proximal branches to assess any calibre change, kinking, angulation, narrowing and relationship with surrounding structures potentially causing extrinsic compression.

Epicardial echocardiography is rather under-utilised due to variable skills of surgeons performing epicardial echocardiograms, limited experience and time demands for cardiologists, as well as absence of national and international guidelines [15].

Intravascular Ultrasound

Intravascular ultrasound (IVUS) imaging of coronary arteries has become a routine procedure in most adult cardiac catheterisation laboratories. Clinical application of IVUS in children is rather limited [16–19] and mainly refers to complications following heart transplantation [20, 21]. In our institution, IVUS is reserved for assessing adverse effects in patients undergoing heart transplantation. In congenital coronary abnormalities in adults, IVUS has been used as integrated imaging modality in comprehensive assessment in AAOCA involving selective coronary angiograms, IVUS, and fractional flow reserve measurements with provocative testing using adenosine and/or dobutamine infusions. Fractional flow reserve and IVUS is offered as a standard work-up for adult patients with AAOCA and proposed as a flowchart to aid in decision-making although the data should be interpreted with caution, as the validity of fractional flow reserve findings in this population has not been established [22]. Only anecdotal reports are referring to clinical application of IVUS in children with congenital or acquired coronary abnormalities such as AAOCA and Kawasaki disease [23].

Stress Echocardiography

Stress echocardiography is well recognised and probably currently underused functional imaging modality for routine screening and monitoring of children with coronary abnormalities (native or post-procedural) providing real-time cardiac imaging [24]. Ergometric stress echocardiography is the preferred technique over the pharmacological (Dobutamine) test for its dynamic nature; however, the methodology requires significant modifications as compared to adults due to the rapid decline in heart rate. Semi-supine bicycle ergometric stress echocardiography has been accepted as standard method with little risk for children and can be safely and accurately performed in children from 7–8 years of age (body height > 135 cm) using commercially available devices. It is a test that is relatively simple to conduct. In our institution, dynamic SE has been included in diagnostic follow-up protocol for all patients with asymptomatic AAOCA as well as for all patients after surgical treatment [25]. Scarce data exist on risk stratification of AAOCA using SE, one study confirmed regional wall motion abnormalities in some patients on subjective assessment as well as on tissue deformation imaging in older children using treadmill exercise testing rather than real-time semi-supine stress echocardiography [26]. It is however important to mention that any stress tests are, at best, incompletely reassuring. They are most

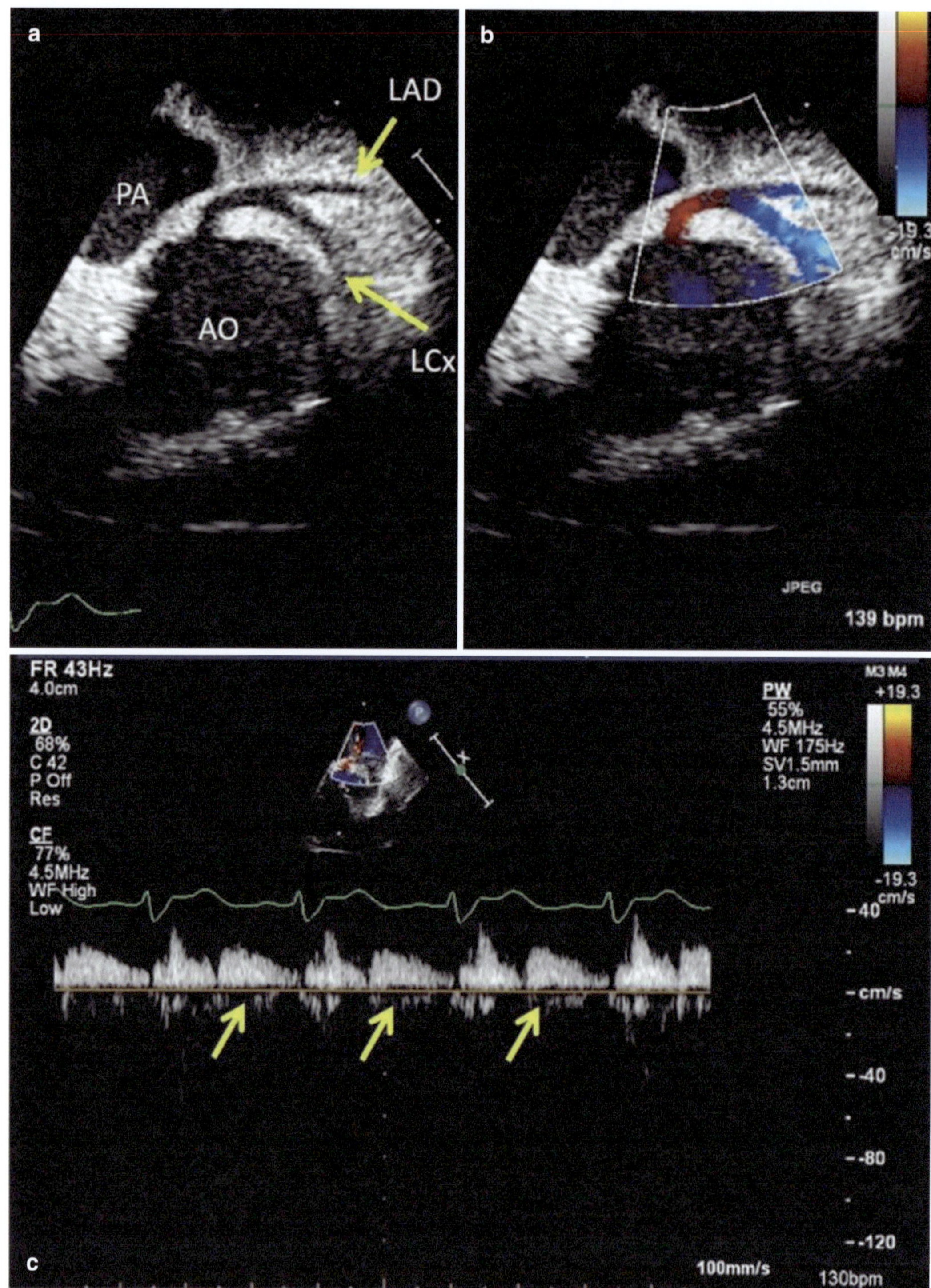

Fig. 10.4 Epicardial echocardiogram performed in 18-day-old boy after arterial switch for transposition and ventricular septal defect. Left main stem, anterior descendent (LAD), and left circumflex imaged from epicardial short axis view (**a**), laminar flow demonstrated by colour flow mapping (**b**) and on pulsed Doppler interrogation (**c**). *PA* pulmonary artery after Lecompt manoeuvre, *AO* aorta

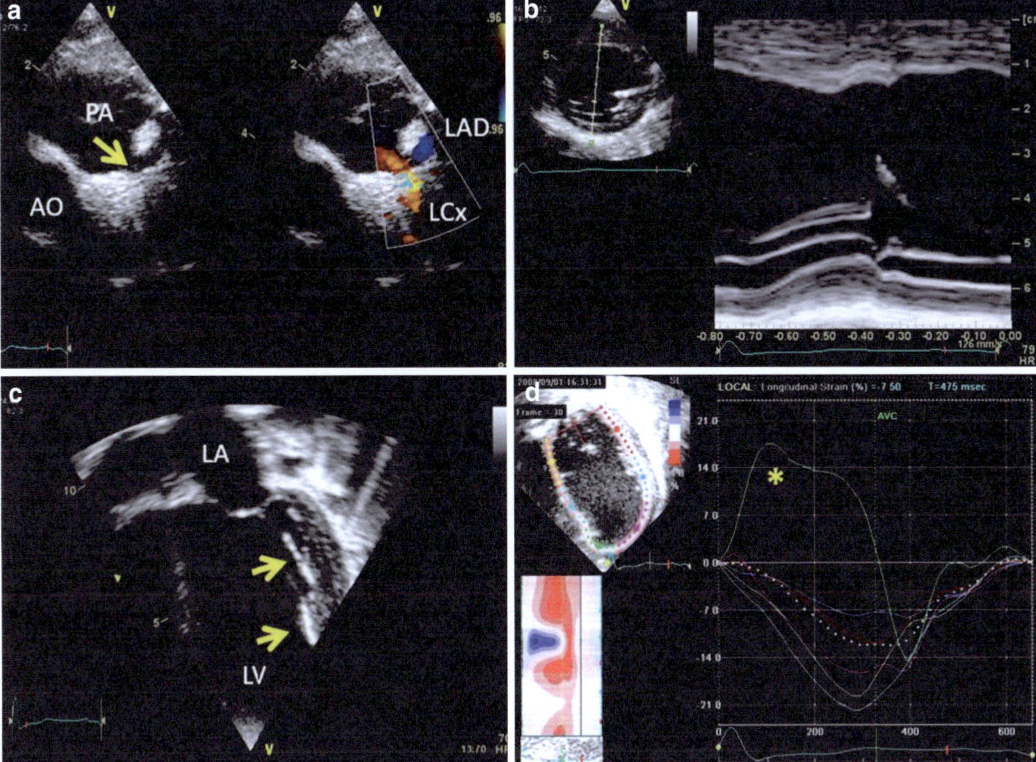

Fig. 10.5 3-months old infant with ALCAPA. LMCA with both branches originated from posterior sinus of pulmonary trunk with typical retrograde diastolic flow on colour flow mapping (**a**). Conventional M-mode suggested good contractility of anterior myocardial septal and posterior wall segments (**b**). Bright echogenicity of papillary muscles was consistent with coronary-induced ischaemia (**c**). 2D Strain imaging confirmed myocardial dyskinesia of apical segment and reduced contractility of lateral segments (**d**). *AO* aorta, *PA* pulmonary trunk, *LAD* left anterior descendance, *LCx* left circumflex, *LA* left atrium, *LV* left ventricle

helpful if they are positive as most of the published data and our experience confirmed a low negative predictive value.

Functional assessment of all children with congenital or acquired coronary abnormalities should include conventional as well as advanced echocardiographic techniques. Tissue deformation imaging (2D or 3D speckle tracking) may identify areas of myocardial ischaemic injury better than conventional 2D or M-mode imaging (Fig. 10.5.). Our study [5] suggested that children presenting with ALCAPA with preserved global LV systolic function on conventional echocardiography did have impaired longitudinal and radial strain, when compared with controls. Surgical treatment led to improvement in deformation indices, although post repair evidence of abnormal deformation in LV segments supplied by the anomalous left coronary artery remains.

Cross-sectional Imaging

Both computer tomography coronary angiography (CTCA) and cardiac magnetic resonance (CMR) are vital components in the non-invasive multimodality imaging approach to congenital coronary arterial abnormalities in children, owing to their ability to provide non-invasive, isotropic 3D imaging of the entire coronary arterial system [2, 27]. CTCA and CMR avoid limitations by acoustic windows and imaging planes, and also eliminate risks associated with invasive techniques that also require general anaesthesia in the majority of children. Technological advances have improved spatial and temporal resolution and heightened speed of acquisition and, in the case of CTCA, decreased radiation doses thus facilitating widespread use in children [28, 29]. However, imaging of the coronary arteries in children remains challenging due to the small size of the coronary arteries, high heart rates, and a propensity for motion artefacts from respiration and general body movement.

Cardiovascular Magnetic Resonance Imaging

CMR documents coronary arterial take-off and course mainly by mode of a non-contrast-enhanced, isotropic, ECG-triggered 3D 'whole heart' angiography acquired during free breathing that covers the entire heart to the ascending AO in one isotropic volume [30]. This sequence avoids the use of contrast medium and ionising radiation, and therefore is potentially advantageous in children [2]. However, CMR is often challenging in children due to the small patient size with resultantly small vascular structures, high heart rates, and relatively lengthy acquisition times [31–33]. In addition, 'whole heart' imaging is often inadequate for coronary arterial imaging beyond the proximal artery. An alternative to the 'whole heart' is volume-targeted imaging by CMR, but this sequence faces similar challenges in children and does not generally provide comprehensive coronary assessment either. [1] Various 2D CMR sequences have very limited roles in children, because this approach necessitates breath-holding, and precise positioning can be challenging in small vessels. Taking into consideration these limitations along with the need for general anaesthesia in the younger child, CMR may be the preferred modality for radiation-free screening for an anatomical coronary arterial abnormality, especially in larger children with larger coronary arteries and lower heart rates who cooperate wholly during image acquisition. In these con-

texts, when CMR with contrast medium is performed then the 'whole heart' will have better contrast if performed after administration of contrast medium.

Computed Tomographic Imaging

CTCA provides high spatial resolution, and comprehensive imaging of the entire coronary arterial system in children, akin to adults, even though specific considerations are required due to the smaller arteries, elevated heart rates, and often limited cooperation during image acquisition [34]. Despite the potential of both CTCA and CMR to provide isotropic 3D coronary arterial imaging, CTCA has become the preferred choice for conclusive, non-invasive coronary arterial anatomical imaging in children by means of rapid 3D data acquisition with submillimetre spatial resolution [31]. Detailed coronary arterial assessment requires ECG-gating for elimination of cardiac motion artefact (Fig. 10.6), although the origins and course of the proximal coronary arteries may be apparent even on non-ECG-gated, high-pitch scans used in the ultra-rapid and low-dose assessment of complex congenital heart disease [35, 36]. Anomalous coronary arteries are common in 'non-coronary' congenital heart disease, and unequivocal mapping is important since these associated abnormalities may be clinically unimportant in isolation but they will often determine the possible surgical repair technique [37]. Resultingly, CTCA has a role both in the isolated, outcome determining coronary arterial abnormalities and before repair of congenital heart disease [38, 39]. The mode of ECG-gating is guided by heart rate, similar to adults, and heart rate reduction is sought using comparable drugs to facilitate scanning with the lowest possible radiation dose [40, 41]. Image quality may, despite lowering heart rates, still be adversely impacted by a propensity to sinus arrhythmia in children (Fig. 10.7); early breath-holding helps alleviate this by allowing the heart rate to settle before image acquisition. In addition, careful information is important in older children when

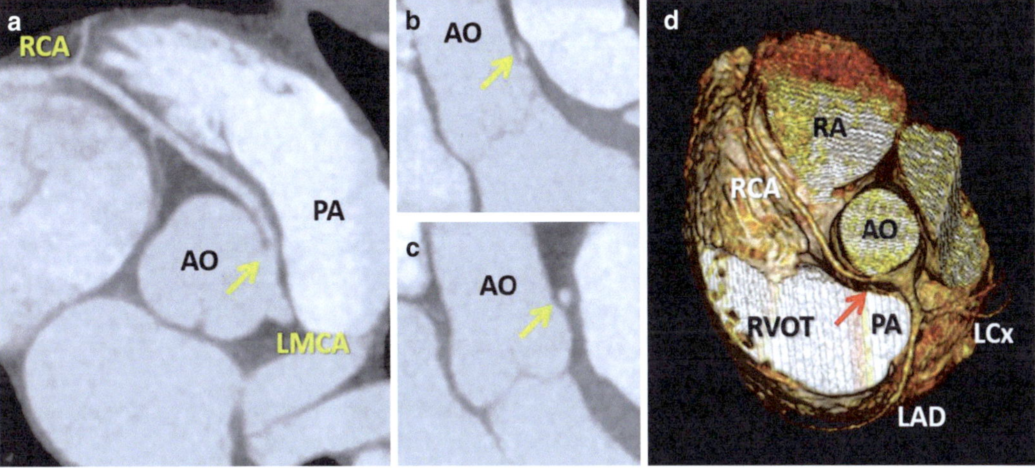

Fig. 10.6 16-year-old girl with ALCAPA and presenting with out-of-hospital cardiac arrest imaged using a retrospectively ECG-gated CT coronary angiogram. The select 2D images from multiplanar reformats show anomalous take-off of the left coronary artery from the pulmonary artery and (**a**) left-sided system adapting a usual epicardial position in the distal course (**b, c**), and a 3D volume-rendered reformat also shows the course of the dilated coronary arteries in relation to the cardiac structures (**c**). *AO* aorta, *PA* pulmonary trunk, *LMCA* left main coronary artery, *LAD* left anterior descending coronary artery, *RCA* right coronary artery

Fig. 10.7 11-year-old asymptomatic boy with AAORCA and a family history of sudden cardiac death in a brother due to AAORCA is imaged using a retrospectively ECG-gated CT coronary angiogram was performed during an average heart rate of 63 beats per minute on beta-blocker treatment with marked RR interval variability (53–76 beats per minute) due to sinus arrhythmia. A juxta-commissural, slit-like origin of the RCA from the left coronary sinus adjacent to and separate from the left main stem is shown on 2D (**a**) and 3D volume-rendered images (**d**) with end-on 2D images showing the proximal interarterial and intramural course with narrowing and oval shape (**b**) and the more distal interarterial but not intramural RCA with a round shape and of good calibre (**c**). *AO* aorta, *PA* pulmonary trunk, *RA* Right atrium, *RVOT* right ventricular outflow tract; *LMCA* left main coronary artery, *LAD* left anterior descending coronary artery; *LCx* left circumflex coronary artery, *RCA* right coronary artery

scanning without sedation or general anaesthesia in order to minimise anxiety that may cause marked reflex heart rate increments, poor breath-holding, or even body movement during contrast administration.

Even following pharmaceutical heart rate modification, heart rates often remain high in children and the lowest dose, ECG-triggered 'single heart beat' acquisitions tend to be inadequate for comprehensive assessment of the coronary arterial system in this situation [42]. This

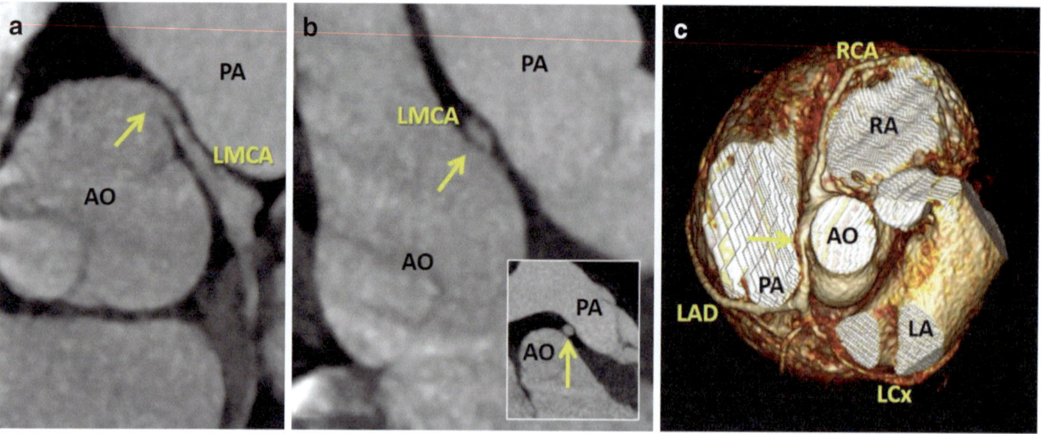

Fig. 10.8 13-year-old boy with AAOLCA and presenting with exercise-induced syncope imaged using a retrospectively ECG-gated CT coronary angiogram performed with a heart rate of 81 beats per minute flowing beta-blocker treatment. The select 2D images from multiplanar reformats show an interatrial left main stem originating from a slit-like orifice in the right coronary cusp with a narrowed and oval shape proximally, consistent with an intramural course in the wall of the right coronary sinus (**a, c**). The left main stem later becomes extramural and of good calibre as evident with the round shape adjacent to the left coronary sinus (**b**). *AO* aorta, *PA* pulmonary trunk, *LMCA* left main coronary artery, *LAD* left anterior descending coronary artery, *LCx* left circumflex coronary artery, *RCA* right coronary artery

ultra-rapid and low radiation dose scan may, however, be adequate for visualisation of the very proximal coronary arteries in the uncooperative child when general anaesthesia or sedation is contraindicated and rapid acquisition is crucial [43]. The more radiation-heavy, ECG-triggered prospective 'sequential step-and-shoot' scanning is possible in a larger proportion of children. The prospective mode is often utilised in children at higher heart rates than would often be the case in adults. For these ECG-trigged scans (including 'single heart beat' scans), a diastolic phase (around 70% of RR interval) increases the likelihood of imaging free of cardiac motion at relatively lower heart rates, whereas a systolic phase (around 40% of RR interval) may provide a motion free visualisation at relatively higher heart rates [44, 45]—although the systolic phase mainly is reliable for origin and course because limited luminal information is often obtained for the distal coronary arterial system. Padding around the selected acquisition phase (not possible for 'single heart beat' scanning), with for instance 5–10% of the RR interval before and after the desired phase, increases the likelihood of a diagnostic study in irregular RR intervals by increasing the number of cardiac phases available, but this will be at the cost of higher radiation dose. The most radiation-heavy, retrospectively ECG-gated multiphase acquisition may be preferred in children with very high heart rates or irregular RR intervals (Fig. 10.8). Here, data acquisition should be as narrow as possible in the RR interval and a minimal dose exposure approach should be applied outside this interval. A multiphase acquisition may also be preferred where high-resolution, anatomical assessment of a dynamic nature is required such as for ostial changes or myocardial bridges across the cardiac cycle [46].

Radiation doses have decreased for CTCA owing to significant technological advances and CTCA has emerged as a pivotal modality in the non-invasive multimodality approach for suspected, outcome-determining coronary arterial abnormalities also in children [29]. Inventions such as iterative reconstruction have dramatically altered the dose landscape, and automatic dose-reduction strategies maintain the lowest radiation dose tailored to the individual child, be it through automated exposure control or weight-based tube current and voltage settings [46]. Still, careful tailoring on a case-by-case basis of the chosen protocol against the clinical question remains pivotal in order to achieve the lowest possible radiation exposure [29, 47]. An understanding of the in-built, automated scanner settings is also essential in order to keep radiation exposure as low as possible; adaptive settings may for instance in the context of variations in the RR interval automatically expand the exposure beyond the predefined parts of the RR interval in ECG-triggered and ECG-gated sequences, increasing the likelihood of diagnostic data in the face of arrhythmia. The necessity of these features should be carefully assessed at the time of each scan, overriding any unwanted and excessive adaptation and padding. In addition, operators should ensure that the z-axis (craniocaudal direction) coverage is sufficient to fully capture any anomalous anatomy but avoid unnecessary z-axis scanning.

Lowering the heart rate enables lower dose scanning modes that are characterised by rapid acquisition and shorter breath holds. Longer acquisitions are nonetheless often required in children with elevated heart rates or arrhythmia, necessitating longer breath holds due with 'step and shoot' approach or with the lower pitch and table movement speed in continuous retrospective ECG-gating. Older children may be able to comply with breath-holding instructions, often from 8–10 years of age depending on maturity and helped by distractions from videos or parents. Younger children need sedation or general anaesthesia in order to reduce the risk of a non-diagnostic radiation exposure due to breathing or general body motion. In the smallest children, gentle swaddling can be a low-risk alternative to general anaesthesia and a feed, a pacifier or an oral glucose solution work well as further calming measures [40]. This is important as multiple anaesthetics in children have been proposed linked to learning disabilities [48]. Planning should therefore factor in the child's maturity, risks of drugs administered, and the likelihood of a diagnostic study with the various approaches.

Contrast administration is generally performed using a biphasic protocol and a chaser consisting of 20% contrast and 80% saline solution can help reduce artefacts. When coronary arterial anomalies are associated with other congenital cardiovascular anomalies it can be better to deploy a triphasic injection protocol, ensuring visualisation of all anatomical features in the same scan [47]. Children weighing <40 kg are given 1–3 mL/kg (typically 2 mL/kg) of a non-ionic low-osmolar iodinated contrast agent, with adult contrast doses utilised in children weighing >40 kg [40]. Injection rates are adjusted according to the child's body weight, often extrapolating from adults and using a large range—typically from 0.5 to 6 mL/s. A low total contrast dose should be considered for newborns due to an, at least theoretically, increased risk of contrast-induced nephropathy [49]. A careful balance must be sought, when a low total contrast dose is available, between the total contract dose, injection rate, and timing of data acquisition to avoid non-diagnostic imaging.

Timing of the CTCA acquisition relative to the contrast injection is similar to adults with data acquired during peak opacification of the coronary arteries. Different approaches to setting this time can be taken according to operator preference, including: (1) standard delay from the start or end of an injection, (2) delay according to a test bolus, (3) automated bolus triggering, or (4) visual triggering [50]. Each approach has its strengths and disadvantages. It can be important, especially in smaller children, to avoid a test bolus that uses part of the contrast dose and, of course, to take an approach that minimises total radiation exposure by limiting the need for planning scans [40]. Automated triggering can be challenging in small children with small vessels and potential for movement, and standard delays can be difficult to predict in complex congenital heart disease especially when ventricular function is poor or shunts are present [46]. When timing the study based on maximum contrast enhancement in the aortic root, there is limited evidence for optimal delays for best coronary arterial enhancement, but 2–8 s can be deployed depending on patient size, length of the contrast bolus, injection rate, scan range, and any need for non-coronary visualisation [47]. Large central shunts often result in widespread early opacification and a saline chaser (with risk of poor visualisation) may thus also reach the coronary arteries at an early time point. Visual triggering is, therefore, often chosen using the lowest possible dose of monitoring scans along with the latest possible start and frequency of these scans. The triggering time point must consider the duration of the scan plus any delay until the scan starts [40, 46]. Contrast medium is mainly administered via an upper limb cannula, but in small children streak artefact from contrast in the superior caval vein (SVC) may degrade the image quality of the coronary arteries and aortic root. This is minimizable by acquisition during a low contrast level chaser in the central veins, by use of a foot cannula for contrast medium injection, or with higher tube voltage (at the cost of radiation exposure) [40].

Functional Imaging by Cross-sectional Imaging

Whereas CTCA takes centre stage due to its ability to rapidly provide comprehensive 3D coronary arterial imaging in suspected coronary arterial abnormalities in children, CMR is the gold standard for non-invasive assessment of associated features, including ventricular function and volumes, myocardial wall motion, myocardial perfusion at rest and stress [51], and myocardial fibrosis and scar in children with anomalous coronary arteries [2, 52–54]. The approach to CMR mirrors that in adults with a good safety profile also during pharmacological stress in congenital coronary arterial abnormalities [55, 56]. The currently used gadolinium-based contrast agents are considered safe when applied to children with normal renal function, but the impact of deposition with repeated administrations is unresolved so the use should always be critically appraised [57]. Compared with CT, children more often require general anaesthesia for diagnostic image quality due to intolerance to lying in the scanner bore combined with the longer duration of image acquisition. However, accelerated CMR sequences are increasing the age range where CMR can be performed without sedation or general anaesthesia by increasing the speed of scanning and minimising the need for breath-holding [58–60]. A more pragmatic approach is often taken to the deployment of CMR than CT, attempting an awake CMR study in younger children because a failed CMR study mainly involves a waste of resources compared to a non-diagnostic radiation exposure when a non-diagnostic CTCA is performed.

Modelling and Simulations in AAOCA

Biomechanical engineering using patient-specific modelling and precision medicine approaches has offered novel insights into studying cardiovascular problems. Recently, such tools have been applied also to AAOCA by focusing on the physio-pathology, trying to unveil mechanisms leading to sudden cardiac death, and tailoring surgical interventions. In particular, computational fluid dynamics (CFD) and structural simulations based on finite element (FE) methods have been applied to investigate the complex biomechanics of AAOCA.

With the improvement of imaging and numerical techniques, the creation of highly realistic AAOCA models can be very useful to represent both anatomical and physiological patients' characteristics. Patient-specific models are created by segmenting raw imaging data. Overall, reconstructing coronary arteries can be complex because of the size, the motion of the heart, and, in case of AAOCA, the identification of intramural segments (Fig. 10.9). Both computed tomography angiography and cardiac magnetic resonance imaging (CMRI) should offer high-resolution data to generate such models. 3D models of AAOCA per se allow precise morphometrical analysis. It has been reported, for example, that intramural segments consistently present features of noncircular coronary compression. These characteristics are immediately visible in patient-specific models making the use of 3D models in AAOCA both feasible and informative (Fig. 10.10).

Computational models and simulations of AAOCA cases require precise boundary condi-

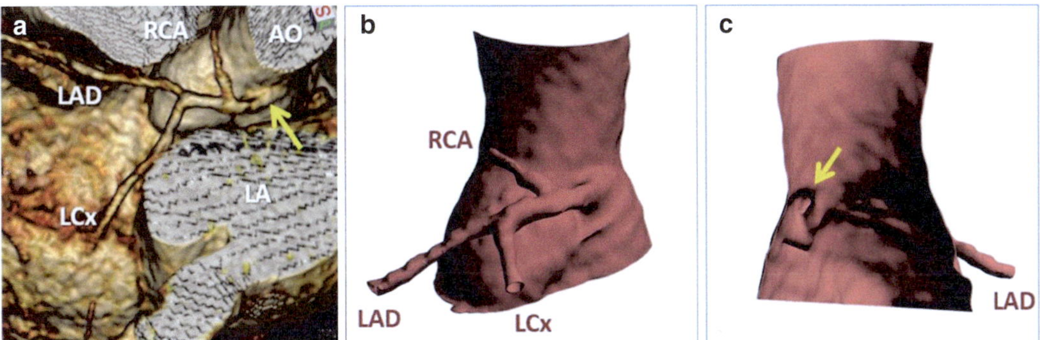

Fig. 10.9 7-year-old boy with incidental finding of single coronary artery from non-coronary sinus with intramural course of LMCA and interarterial and intramural course of the RCA. 3D rendered CT angio (**a**) with single coronary ostium (arrow). External 3D model (**b**) and intralu- menal view (**c**) documenting slit coronary ostium (arrow). *AO* aorta, *LA* left atrium, *LAD* left anterior descendent, *LCx* left circumflex, *RCA* right coronary artery

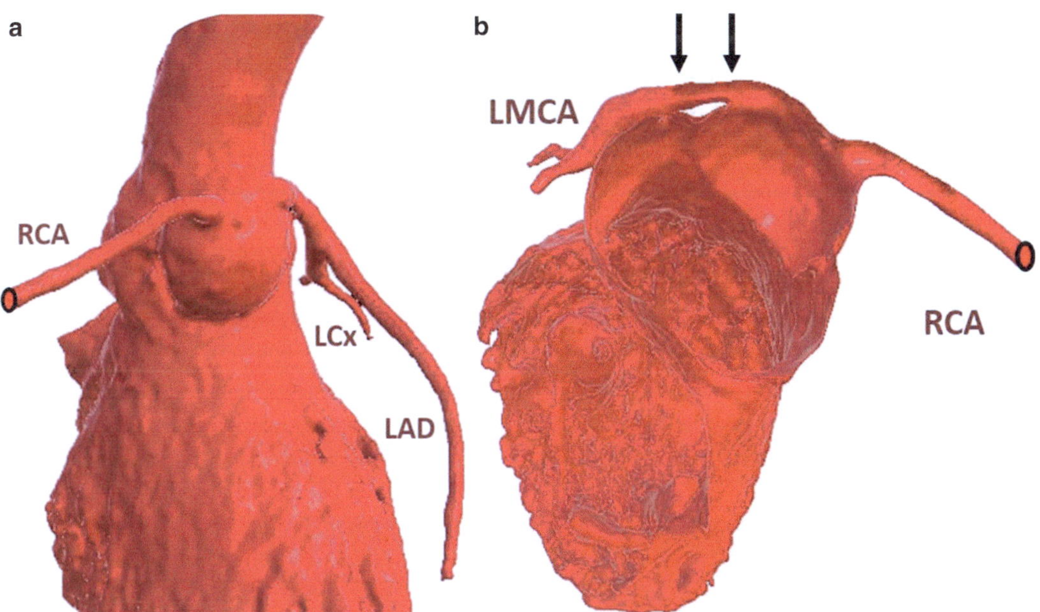

Fig. 10.10 11-year-old boy with a family history of sudden cardiac death in older brother with AAORCA and interarterial and intramural course (two younger brothers have same RCA morphology). 3D model from retrospective ECG-gated CT angiogram. External blood pool view (**a**) and intraluminal view (**b**) documenting proximal narrowing of left main coronary artery (LMCA, arrows). *LAD* left anterior descendent, *LCx* left circumflex, *RCA* right coronary artery

tions, which take into account the behaviour of the system downstream and upstream of the 3D model. Selection of accurate BCs is critical in patient-specific cardiovascular modelling as they can significantly affect local haemodynamics. Modelling the working conditions of AAOCA can be particularly complex as a comprehensive model may also include valve dynamics and arterial deformations to ensure the highest level of realism of the simulations. In addition, resistance of the small arteries and arterioles of the coronary micro-vasculature affects changes in blood pressure in larger arteries. Modellers have been used in various strategies to reduce the complexity of this system. The most advanced approach [61] is setting up a lumped parameter network (LPN) to consider the effects and the changes of the downstream vasculature by representing it as a collection of electrical elements.

Modelling patient-specific AAOCA is very complex and, only over the past few years, this has been reported only in studies which show a successful integration of highly specialised clinical and bioengineering knowledges.

The haemodynamics of the anomalous origin of the right coronary artery from the left coronary artery sinus has been recently studied by Cong et al. 2021 [62]. In these patients, the RCA is usually characterised by an acute take-off angle. The authors modelled two relatively groups of patients respectively with a normal RCA and with AAORCA from the left coronary sinus and correlated fluid-dynamics parameters with morphological assessment. The acute take-off angle of AAORCA was measured as 20–40°, with the starting angle of a normal RCA between 45° and 90°. The study measured a lower pressure and higher wall shear stresses (WSS) in patients with an anomalous origin of the RCA from the left coronary artery sinus. In particular, patients with an acute take-off angle were shown to have significantly lower pressure in systole which may be the cause of clinical symptoms such as dizziness and chest tightness.

The biomechanical outcomes of unroofing procedure were analyzed by Razavi et al. 2020 [63]. CFD modelling from CMR data acquired from a group of eight patients with intramural AAOCA was performed to analyze and compare coronary haemodynamics before and after intervention. Results showed how surgical intervention reduces and normalises time-averaged wall shear stress (TAWSS). These findings suggest that acute angle of origin of the coronary may create abnormal coronary flow patterns and haemodynamics that could leave patients more susceptible to the early onset and progression of atherosclerosis. Despite the small sample size, this study shows how the characterisation of haemodynamics in patient-specific models can be useful to explain myocardial morbidity associated with intramural AAOCA.

The importance of intramural segment in AAOCA was investigated also by Formato et al. 2018 [64] and Hatoum et al. 2020 [65]. The first study focused on the mechanisms underlying the coronary occlusions and quantified how the expansion of the anomalous coronaries is impaired especially at the ostium. The acute take-off angles can in fact cause elongated coronary ostia, with an eccentricity increasing with aortic expansion. The latter study showed how to use patient-specific 3D-printed models of AAOCA to identify a drop in fractional flow reserve in the intramural segment and decreasing coronary flow with increasing aortic pressure in an ischemic model of AAORCA.

Although in its infancy, modelling AAOCA can represent an important step in our understanding of haemodynamics in AAOCA [66]. These studies show the development and the potentials of using patient-specific modelling and simulations to investigate the physio-pathology and the effects of treatments in patients with AAOCA (Fig. 10.11). Technological developments in computer modelling allow to explore also such a complex and rare condition. Hence, in the near future, more studies are expected which include a larger number of cases and scenarios simulated. This will contribute to strengthening the statistical inference and the mapping of haemodynamic indices with patient conditions and outcomes. AAOCA modelling will be able to answer how different anatomical properties impact coronary pressure and flow variations in patients with AAOCA. This in turn may allow clinicians to better risk-stratify AAOCA patients and decide which operation may be more appropriate for a particular patient. After all, simulation is a process of knowledge creation and a better understanding of the pathophysiology of AAOCA

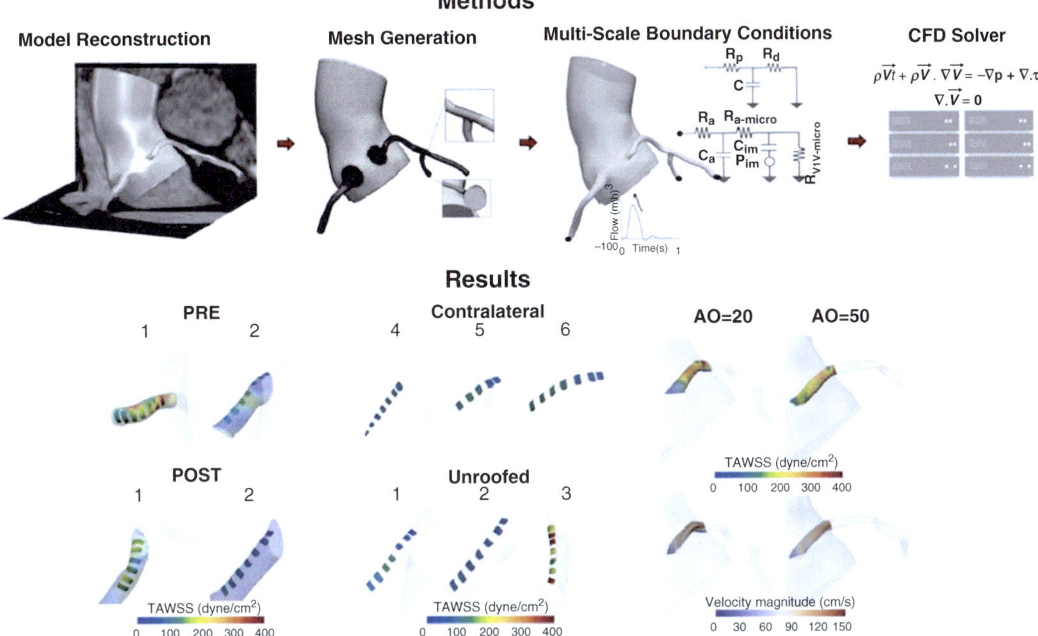

Fig. 10.11 Summary of the steps conducted for patient-specific computational analysis of AACOA in the current investigation included model reconstruction from cardiac magnetic resonance imaging (CMR) data, mesh generation with local refinements on the ostial region and left main coronary artery (LMCA) bifurcation, assigning multiscale boundary conditions, and postprocessing of resulting haemodynamics to visualise and quantify changes in coronary artery velocity and indices of wall shear stress (WSS). Results showed that: [1] time-averaged wall shear stress (TAWSS) was higher preoperatively due to more skewed velocity profiles along the length of the angulated anomalous arteries, [2] unroofing may normalise WSS, [3] changes in AO led to significant alterations in the local flow patterns and haemodynamics. "Adapted from [63] with permission"

will allow us to move from anecdote-based to data-based clinical decision-making.

References

1. Lai WW, Geva T, Shirali GS, Frommelt PC, Humes RA, Brook MM, et al. Guidelines and standards for performance of a pediatric echocardiogram: a report from the Task Force of the Pediatric Council of the Journal of the American Society of Echocardiography Volume 33 Number 3 Frommelt et al 289American Society of Echocardiography. J Am Soc Echocardiogr. 2006;19:1413–30.
2. Frommelt P, Lopez L, Dimas VV, Eidem B, Han BK, Ko HH, Lorber R, Nii M, Printz B, Srivastava B, Valente AV, Cohen MS. Recommendations for multimodality assessment of congenital coronary anomalies: a guide from the American Society of Echocardiography: developed in collaboration with the Society for Cardiovascular Angiography and Interventions, Japanese Society of Echocardiography, and Society for Cardiovascular Magnetic Resonance. J Am Soc Echocardiogr. 2020;33(3):259–94.
3. Brown LM, Duffy CE, Mitchell C, Young L. A practical guide to pediatric coronary artery imaging with echocardiography. J Am Soc Echocardiogr. 2015;28(4):379–91.
4. Fuse S, Kobayashi T, Arakaki Y, Ogawa S, Katoh H, Sakamoto N, Hamaoka K, Saji T. Standard method for ultrasound imaging of coronary artery in children. Pediatr Int. 2010;52(6):876–82.
5. Naqvi N, Babu-Narayan SV, Krupickova S, Muthialu N, Maiya S, Chandershekar P, Cheang MH, Kostolny M, Tsang V, Marek J. myocardial function following repair of anomalous origin of left coronary artery from the pulmonary artery in children. J Am Soc Echocardiogr. 2020;33(5):622–30.
6. Lorber R, Srivastava S, Wilder TJ, McIntyre S, DeCampli WM, Williams WG, Frommelt PC, Parness IA, Blackstone EH, Jacobs ML, Mertens L, Brothers JA. Herlong JR; AAOCA working Group of the Congenital Heart Surgeons Society. Anomalous aortic origin of coronary arteries in

the Young: echocardiographic evaluation with surgical correlation. JACC Cardiovasc Imaging. 2015;8(11):1239–49.

7. Sharland GK, Konta L, Qureshi SA. Prenatal diagnosis of isolated coronary artery fistulas: progression and outcome in five cases. Cardiol Young. 2016;26(5):915–20.

8. Liu L, Wang H, Cui C, Li Y, Liu Y, Wang Y, Fan T, Peng B. Prenatal echocardiographic classification and prognostic evaluation strategy in fetal pulmonary atresia with intact ventricular septum. Medicine (Baltimore). 2019;98(42):e17492.

9. Baschat AA, Muench MV, Gembruch U. Coronary artery blood flow velocities in various fetal conditions. Ultrasound Obstet Gynecol. 2003;21(5):426–9.

10. Vargas LA, Dyar DA, Davis CK, Dummer KB. Prenatal detection of anomalous right coronary artery with an interarterial course. CASE (Phila). 2019;4(2):63–5.

11. Stoebe S, Lange K, Pfeiffer D, Hagendorff A. Feasibility of proximal right coronary artery imaging by 2D and 3D echocardiography in comparison to coronary angiography. Echo Res Pract. 2015;2(3):73–9.

12. Bonello B, Bo I, Mortensen K, Banks RL, Mc Leod IW, Kaski JP, Hsia TY, Marek J. Value of Stress transesophageal echocardiography in an asymptomatic patient with single coronary artery from noncoronary sinus, intramural course, and ostial stenosis. Circ Cardiovasc Imaging. 2019;12(1):e008560.

13. Dragulescu A, Golding F, Van Arsdell G, Caldarone C, Mertens L, Al-Radi O, Lee KJ. The impact of additional epicardial imaging to transesophageal echocardiography on intraoperative detection of residual lesions in congenital heart surgery. Cardiovasc Surg. 2012;143(2):361–7.

14. Nield LE, Dragulescu A, MacColl C, Manlhiot C, Brun H, McCrindle BW, Kuipers B, Caldarone CA, Miner SES, Mertens L. Coronary artery Doppler patterns are associated with clinical outcomes post-arterial switch operation for transposition of the great arteries. Eur Heart J Cardiovasc Imaging. 2018;19(4):461–8.

15. Awasthy N, Girotra S, Dutta N, Azad S, Radhakrishnan S, Iyer KS. A systematic approach to epicardial echocardiography in pediatric cardiac surgery: an important but underutilized intraoperative tool. Ann Pediatr Cardiol. 2021;14(2):192–200.

16. Sang CJ 3rd, Prejean S, Von Mering G, Ahmed M, Law MA. Intravascular ultrasound use for stent optimization during percutanous coronary intervention in a toddler with post-surgical stenosis after coronary reimplantation for ALCAPA. J Cardiol Cases. 2020;22(2):77–80.

17. Agrawal H, Molossi S, Alam M, Sexson-Tejtel SK, Mery CM, McKenzie ED, Fraser CD Jr, Qureshi AM. Anomalous coronary arteries and myocardial bridges: risk stratification in children using novel cardiac catheterization techniques. Pediatr Cardiol. 2017;38(3):624–30. https://doi.org/10.1007/s00246-016-1559-4.

18. McElhinney DB. Direct physiologic assessment of anomalous aortic origin of a coronary artery: Enhanced diagnostics or illusion of insight? Catheter Cardiovasc Interv. 2018;92(1):76–7.

19. Angelini P, Velasco JA, Ott D, Khoshnevis GR. Anomalous coronary artery arising from the opposite sinus: descriptive features and pathophysiologic mechanisms, as documented by intravascular ultrasound. J Invasive Cardiol. 2003;15:207–14.

20. Costello JM, Wax DF, Binns HJ, Backer CL, Mavroudis C, Pahl E. A comparison of intravascular ultrasound with coronary angiography for evaluation of transplant coronary disease in pediatric heart transplant recipients. J Heart Lung Transplant. 2003;22(1):44–9.

21. Auerbach SR, Fenton MJ, Grutter G, Albert DC, Di-Filippo S, Burch M, Kuhn MA. The complication rate of intravascular ultrasound (IVUS) in a multi-center pediatric heart transplant population: A study of the international pediatric IVUS consortium. Clin Transpl. 2020;34(9):e13981.

22. Driesen BW, Warmerdam EG, Sieswerda GT, Schoof PH, Meijboom FJ, Haas F, Stella PR, Kraaijeveld AO, Evens FCM, Doevendans PAFM, Krings GJ, van Dijk APJ, Voskuil M. Anomalous coronary artery originating from the opposite sinus of Valsalva (ACAOS), fractional flow reserve- and intravascular ultrasound-guided management in adult patients. Catheter Cardiovasc Interv. 2018;92(1):68–75.

23. Watanabe M, Fukazawa R, Ogawa S, Ohkubo T, Abe M, Hashimoto K, Hashimoto Y, Itoh Y. Virtual histology intravascular ultrasound evaluation of coronary artery lesions within 1 year and more than 10 years after the onset of Kawasaki disease. J Cardiol. 2020;75(2):171–6.

24. Cifra B, Dragulescu A, Border WL, Mertens L. Stress echocardiography in paediatric cardiology. Eur Heart J Cardiovasc Imaging. 2015;16(10):1051–9.

25. Ciliberti P, McLeod I, Cairello F, Kaski JP, Fenton M, Giardini A, Marek J. Semi-supine exercise stress echocardiography in children and adolescents: feasibility and safety. Pediatr Cardiol. 2015;36(3):633–9.

26. Binka E, Zhao N, Wood S, Zimmerman SL, Thompson WR. Exercise-induced abnormalities of regional myocardial deformation in anomalous aortic origin of the right coronary artery. World J Pediatr Congenit Heart Surg. 2020;11(6):712–9.

27. Warnes CA, Williams RG, Bashore TM, Child JS, Connolly HM, Dearani JA, del Nido P, Fasules JW, Graham TP Jr, Hijazi ZM, Hunt SA, King ME, Landzberg MJ, Miner PD, Radford MJ, Walsh EP, Webb GD, Smith SC Jr, Jacobs AK, Adams CD, Anderson JL, Antman EM, Buller CE, Creager MA, Ettinger SM, Halperin JL, Hunt SA, Krumholz HM, Kushner FG, Lytle BW, Nishimura RA, Page RL, Riegel B, Tarkington LG, Yancy CW. ACC/AHA 2008 guidelines for the management of adults with congenital heart disease: a report of the American College

of Cardiology/American Heart Association Task Force on Practice Guidelines (Writing Committee to Develop Guidelines on the Management of Adults With Congenital Heart Disease). Developed in collaboration with the American Society of Echocardiography, Heart Rhythm Society, International Society for Adult Congenital Heart Disease, Society for Cardiovascular Angiography and Interventions, and Society of Thoracic Surgeons. J Am Coll Cardiol. 2008;52:e143–263.

28. Cheng Z, Wang X, Duan Y, Wu L, Wu D, Chao B, Liu C, Xu Z, Li H, Liang F, Xu J, Chen J. Low-dose prospective ECG-triggering dual-source CT angiography in infants and children with complex congenital heart disease: first experience. Eur Radiol. 2010;20:2503–11.

29. Han BK, Lindberg J, Overman D, Schwartz RS, Grant K, Lesser JR. Safety and accuracy of dual-source coronary computed tomography angiography in the pediatric population. J Cardiovasc Comput Tomogr. 2012;6:252–9.

30. Beerbaum P, Sarikouch S, Laser KT, Greil G, Burchert W, Körperich H. Coronary anomalies assessed by whole-heart isotropic 3D magnetic resonance imaging for cardiac morphology in congenital heart disease. J Magnetic Resonance Imaging. 2009;29:320–7.

31. Goo HW. Coronary artery imaging in children. Korean J Radiol. 2015;16:239–50.

32. Tangcharoen T, Bell A, Hegde S, Hussain T, Beerbaum P, Schaeffter T, Razavi R, Botnar RM, Greil GF. Detection of coronary artery anomalies in infants and young children with congenital heart disease by using MR imaging. Radiology. 2011;259:240–7.

33. Rajiah P, Setser RM, Desai MY, Flamm SD, Arruda JL. Utility of free-breathing, whole-heart, three-dimensional magnetic resonance imaging in the assessment of coronary anatomy for congenital heart disease. Pediatr Cardiol. 2011;32:418–25.

34. Tada A, Sato S, Kanie Y, Tanaka T, Inai R, Akagi N, Morimitsu Y, Kanazawa S. Image quality of coronary computed tomography angiography with 320-row area detector computed tomography in children with congenital heart disease. Pediatr Cardiol. 2016;37:497–503.

35. Kanie Y, Sato S, Tada A, Kanazawa S. Image quality of coronary arteries on non-electrocardiography-gated high-pitch dual-source computed tomography in children with congenital heart disease. Pediatr Cardiol. 2017;38:1393–9.

36. Nie P, Wang X, Cheng Z, Ji X, Duan Y, Chen J. Accuracy, image quality and radiation dose comparison of high-pitch spiral and sequential acquisition on 128-slice dual-source CT angiography in children with congenital heart disease. Eur Radiol. 2012;22:2057–66.

37. Yu FF, Lu B, Gao Y, Hou ZH, Schoepf UJ, Spearman JV, Cao HL, Sun ML, Jiang SL. Congenital anomalies of coronary arteries in complex congenital heart disease: diagnosis and analysis with dual-source CT. J Cardiovasc Comput Tomogr. 2013;7:383–90.

38. Goo HW. Identification of coronary artery anatomy on dual-source cardiac computed tomography before arterial switch operation in newborns and young infants: comparison with transthoracic echocardiography. Pediatr Radiol. 2018;48:176–85.

39. Han BK, Rigsby CK, Hlavacek A, Leipsic J, Nicol ED, Siegel MJ, Bardo D, Abbara S, Ghoshhajra B, Lesser JR, Raman S, Crean AM. Computed tomography imaging in patients with congenital heart disease part I: rationale and utility. An expert consensus document of the Society of Cardiovascular Computed Tomography (SCCT): endorsed by the Society of Pediatric Radiology (SPR) and the north American Society of Cardiac Imaging (NASCI). J Cardiovasc Comput Tomogr. 2015;9:475–92.

40. Mortensen KH, Tann O. Computed tomography in paediatric heart disease. Br J Radiol. 2018;91:20180201.

41. Rigsby CK, deFreitas RA, Nicholas AC, Leidecker C, Johanek AJ, Anley P, Wang D, Uejima T. Safety and efficacy of a drug regimen to control heart rate during 64-slice ECG-gated coronary CTA in children. Pediatr Radiol. 2010;40:1880–9.

42. Chen B, Zhao S, Gao Y, Cheng Z, Duan Y, Das P, Wang X. Image quality and radiation dose of two prospective ECG-triggered protocols using 128-slice dual-source CT angiography in infants with congenital heart disease. Int J Card Imaging. 2019;35:937–45.

43. Han BK, Overman DM, Grant K, Rosenthal K, Rutten-Ramos S, Cook D, Lesser JR. Non-sedated, free breathing cardiac CT for evaluation of complex congenital heart disease in neonates. J Cardiovasc Comput Tomogr. 2013;7:354–60.

44. Zhang W, Bogale S, Golriz F, Krishnamurthy R. Relationship between heart rate and quiescent interval of the cardiac cycle in children using MRI. Pediatr Radiol. 2017;47:1588–93.

45. Araoz PA, Kirsch J, Primak AN, Braun NN, Saba O, Williamson EE, Harmsen WS, Mandrekar JN, McCollough CH. Optimal image reconstruction phase at low and high heart rates in dual-source CT coronary angiography. Int J Card Imaging. 2009;25:837–45.

46. Secinaro A, Curione D, Mortensen KH, Santangelo TP, Ciancarella P, Napolitano C, Del Pasqua A, Taylor AM, Ciliberti P. Dual-source computed tomography coronary artery imaging in children. Pediatr Radiol. 2019;49:1823–39.

47. Rigsby CK, McKenney SE, Hill KD, Chelliah A, Einstein AJ, Han BK, Robinson JD, Sammet CL, Slesnick TC, Frush DP. Radiation dose management for pediatric cardiac computed tomography: a report from the image gently 'Have-A-Heart' campaign. Pediatr Radiol. 2018;48:5–20.

48. Wilder RT, Flick RP, Sprung J, Katusic SK, Barbaresi WJ, Mickelson C, Gleich SJ, Schroeder DR, Weaver AL, Warner DO. Early exposure to anesthesia and learning disabilities in a population-based birth cohort. Anesthesiology. 2009;110:796–804.

49. Krishnamurthy R. Neonatal cardiac imaging. Pediatr Radiol. 2010;40:518–27.

50. Duan Y, Chen L, Wu D, Chao B, Cheng Z, Yan X, Zhao S, Chen B, Xu M, Wang X, Lu G. Image quality and radiation dose of different scanning protocols in DSCT cardiothoracic angiography for children with tetralogy of fallot. Int J Card Imaging. 2020;36:1791–9.

51. Agrawal H, Wilkinson JC, Noel CV, Qureshi AM, Masand PM, Mery CM, Sexson-Tejtel SK, Molossi S. Impaired myocardial perfusion on stress CMR correlates with invasive FFR in children with coronary anomalies. J Invasive Cardiol. 2021;33:E45–e51.

52. Secinaro A, Ntsinjana H, Tann O, Schuler PK, Muthurangu V, Hughes M, Tsang V, Taylor AM. Cardiovascular magnetic resonance findings in repaired anomalous left coronary artery to pulmonary artery connection (ALCAPA). J Cardiovasc Magn Reson. 2011;13:27.

53. Latus H, Gummel K, Rupp S, Mueller M, Jux C, Kerst G, Akintuerk H, Bauer J, Schranz D, Apitz C. Cardiovascular magnetic resonance assessment of ventricular function and myocardial scarring before and early after repair of anomalous left coronary artery from the pulmonary artery. J Cardiovasc Magn Reson. 2014;16:3.

54. Browne LP, Kearney D, Taylor MD, Chung T, Slesnick TC, Nutting AC, Krishnamurthy R. ALCAPA: the role of myocardial viability studies in determining prognosis. Pediatr Radiol. 2010;40:163–7.

55. Doan TT, Molossi S, Sachdeva S, Wilkinson JC, Loar RW, Weigand JD, Schlingmann TR, Reaves-O'Neal DL, Pednekar AS, Masand P, Noel CV. Dobutamine stress cardiac MRI is safe and feasible in pediatric patients with anomalous aortic origin of a coronary artery (AAOCA). Int J Cardiol. 2021;334:42.

56. Wilkinson JC, Doan TT, Loar RW, Pednekar AS, Trivedi PM, Masand PM, Noel CV. Myocardial stress perfusion MRI using Regadenoson: a weight-based approach in infants and Young children. Radiol Cardiothoracic Imaging. 2019;1:e190061.

57. McDonald RJ, McDonald JS, Kallmes DF, Jentoft ME, Murray DL, Thielen KR, Williamson EE, Eckel LJ. Intracranial gadolinium deposition after contrast-enhanced MR imaging. Radiology. 2015;275:772–82.

58. Olivieri L, Cross R, O'Brien KJ, Xue H, Kellman P, Hansen MS. Free-breathing motion-corrected late-gadolinium-enhancement imaging improves image quality in children. Pediatr Radiol. 2016;46:983–90.

59. Steeden JA, Kowalik GT, Tann O, Hughes M, Mortensen KH, Muthurangu V. Real-time assessment of right and left ventricular volumes and function in children using high spatiotemporal resolution spiral bSSFP with compressed sensing. J Cardiovasc Magn Reson. 2018;20:79.

60. Steeden JA, Quail M, Gotschy A, Mortensen KH, Hauptmann A, Arridge S, Jones R, Muthurangu V. Rapid whole-heart CMR with single volume super-resolution. J Cardiovasc Magn Reson. 2020;22:56.

61. Razavi A, Sachdeva S, Frommelt PC, LaDisa JF Jr. Selection of patient-specific boundary conditions with application to anomalous aortic origin of a coronary artery under resting and stress conditions. Bimed Sci Instrument. 2019;55:388–98.

62. Cong M, Zhao H, Dai S, Chen C, Xu X, Qiu J, Qin S. Transient numerical simulation of the right coronary artery originating from the left sinus and the effect of its acute take-off angle on hemodynamics. Quant Imaging Med Surg. 2021;11(5):2062.

63. Razavi A, Sachdeva S, Frommelt PC, LaDisa Jr JF. Patient-specific numerical analysis of coronary flow in children with intramural anomalous aortic origin of coronary arteries. In Seminars in thoracic and cardiovascular surgery 2021 (Vol. 33, 1, pp. 155-167). WB Saunders.

64. Formato GM, Lo Rito M, Auricchio F, Frigiola A, Conti M. Aortic expansion induces lumen narrowing in anomalous coronary arteries: a parametric structural finite element analysis. J Biomech Eng. 2018;140(11):111008.

65. Hatoum H, Krishnamurthy R, Parthasarathy J, Flemister DC, Krull CM, Walter BA, Mery CM, Molossi S, Dasi LP. Flow Dynamics in Anomalous Aortic Origin of a Coronary Artery in Children: Importance of the Intramural Segment. In: Seminars in thoracic and cardiovascular surgery. WB Saunders; 2020.

66. Hatoum H, Dasi LP, Krishnamurthy R, Molossi S, Mery CM. Commentary: Computational fluid dynamics in anomalous coronaries: moving from anecdote-based to data-based clinical decision-making. In: Seminars in thoracic and cardiovascular surgery. Elsevier; 2020.

Role of Invasive and Provocative Tests

11

Mauro Agnifili, Luca Arzuffi, Omar Alessandro Oliva, Miriam Deamici, and Francesco Bedogni

Introduction

Ostium of an anomalous origin of coronary arteries is usually in atypical position and also the pathway of the coronary itself may represent a great challenge for the invasive cardiologist. In this setting, a prior Computed tomographic study is highly warranted in order to both identify the major characteristics of the coronary arteries and guide the invasive study and treatments.

Coronary Artery Anomalies

Absent Left Trunk

This anomaly occurs in 0.41% of the general population and is characterized by the separate origin of the left anterior descending artery (LAD) and left circumflex coronary artery (LCx). Usually, a Left Judkins coronary artery catheter with a 4.0 curve is used to enter the LCx while for the LAD the same catheter is chosen but with a 3.5 curve (Fig. 11.1).

The original version of the chapter has been revised. A correction to this chapter can be found at https://doi.org/10.1007/978-3-031-36966-7_23

M. Agnifili · L. Arzuffi · O. A. Oliva · M. Deamici
IRCCS Policlinico San Donato, San Donato
Milanese, Milan, Italy
e-mail: miriam.deamici@grupposandonato.it

F. Bedogni (✉)
Policlinico, San Donato, University Hospital,
San Donato Milanese, Milan, Italy
e-mail: Francesco.Bedogni@grupposandonato.it

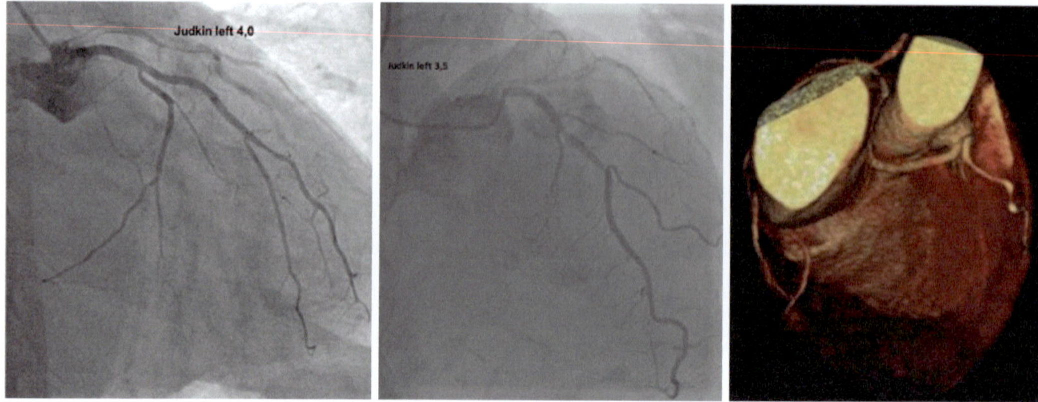

Fig. 11.1 Separate Ostia of Left Anterior Descending Coronary Artery and Left Circumflex Coronary Artery. Computed tomographic angiographic imaging of absent left trunk variant with separate ostia of left anterior descending coronary artery (LAD) and left circumflex coronary artery (LCx): angiographic image with Judkins left 4.0 engagement for LCx and Judkins left 3.5 for LAD

Anomalous Origin of the Right Coronary Artery

The right coronary artery can have different anomalous origins as clearly depicted in Fig. 11.2.

An anomalous right coronary artery (RCA) can arise from different locations. The Central Illustration summarizes these different locations: (A) RCA ostium contiguous to left main (LM) coronary artery ostium; (B) RCA ostium inferior to LM ostium; (C) RCA ostium near the commissure of the right and left cusps; (D) ostium above the sino-tubular junction; (E) ostium from right cusp superior and adjacent the left cusp; and (F) usual origin.

Location A

This location is the most common and it is characterized by an RCA ostium contiguous to the LM coronary artery ostium. Usually, there is a "slit-like" ostium and there is an intramural course of the proximal segment which is significantly angulated. Selective angiography can be challenging and there is a risk of dissection during catheter manipulations. The preferred catheter for such anatomy is usually a 7 Fr Leya catheter left coronary Amplatz 45 or 90° (Cordis Cardinal Health, Dublin, Ohio). Figure 11.3 shows CT scan imaging with significant lateral compression of the proximal

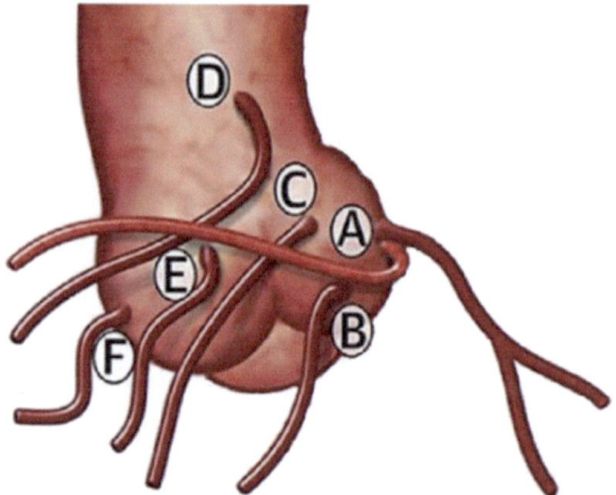

Fig. 11.2 Representative Diagram of Anomalous Origin of Right Coronary Artery From Left Sinus of Valsalva Ben-Dor, I. et al. J Am Coll Cardiol Intv. 2021;14(9):995–1008. (A) Origin adjusted to the ostium of the left main coronary artery; (B) inferior to left main coronary artery ostium; (C) toward the commissure of the right and left cusps; (D) origin from the aorta above the sino-tubular plane; (E) origin from right cusp superior and toward the left cusp; (F) usual origin. Catheter suggested for cannulation: (A) Leya catheter, Amplatz 45/90°; R-ACAOS, Launcher; (B) Amplatz left 1,2, 3; (C) Amplatz left 1,2,3; Amplatz right 1,2,3; (D) Judkins right; Multi-purpose; Kockey stick; (E) Sherpa NX Balances; Amplatz left 0.75, 1, 2, 3; Amplatz right 1,2,3; 3DRC; (F) Judkins right

segment of the RCA. Angiography from the same patient is shown in the middle. Finally, on the right is the picture of the catheter used in these anomalies.

Alternatively, a 6 Fr Launcher coronary guide catheter (Medtronic, Minneapolis, Minnesota) can be used (Fig. 11.4).

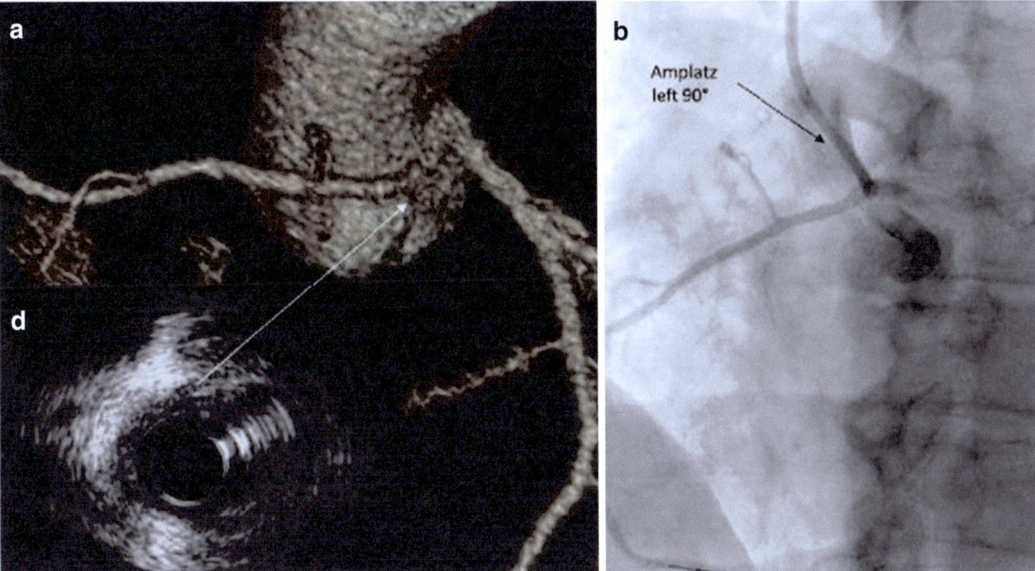

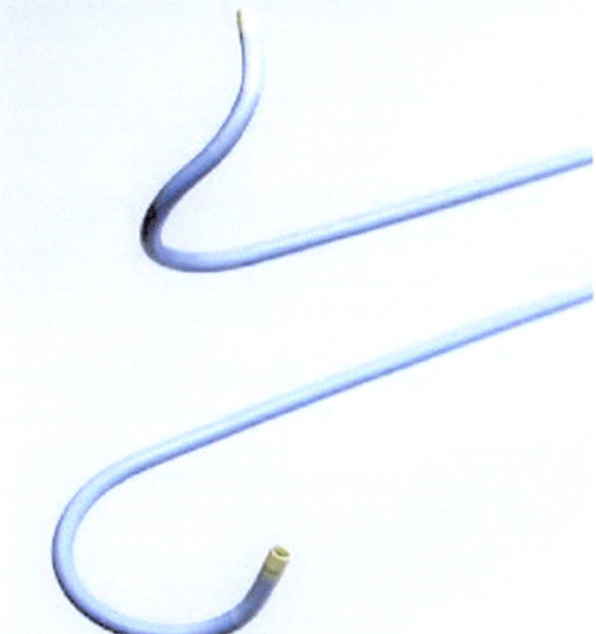

Fig. 11.3 Anomalous Right Coronary Artery from the Left Cusp Engaged With Leya Catheter; Ref [1]. (**a**) Computed tomographic angiographic imaging of the intramural course of the right coronary artery (RCA) from the left sinus. (**b**) Anomalous RCA adjusted to the left main coronary artery engaged with Leya catheter: Amplatz left 90. (**c**) Leya catheter: Amplatz left 45 and 90. (**d**) Intravascular ultrasound pullback shows severe lateral compression of the proximal anomalous RCA, which increases during systole

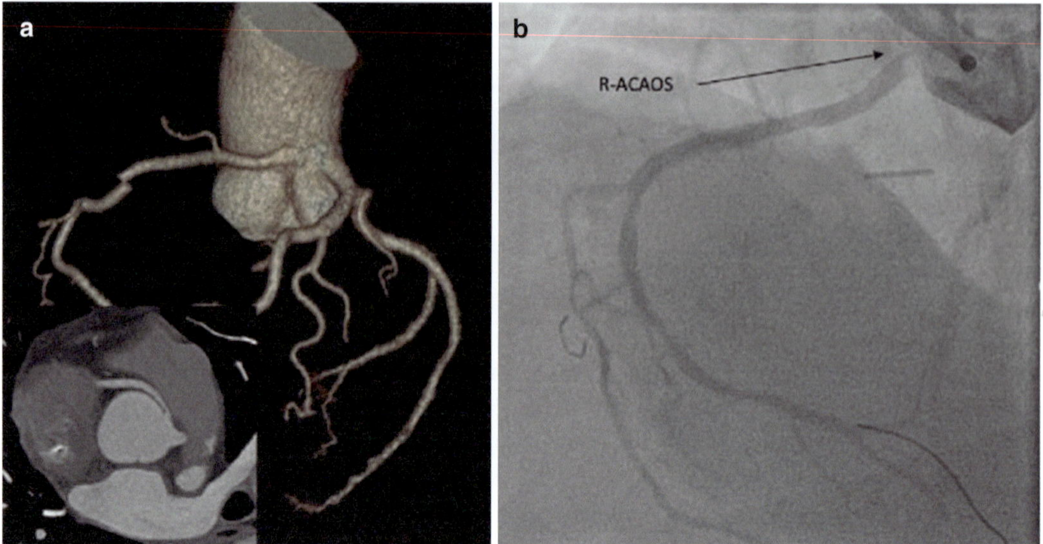

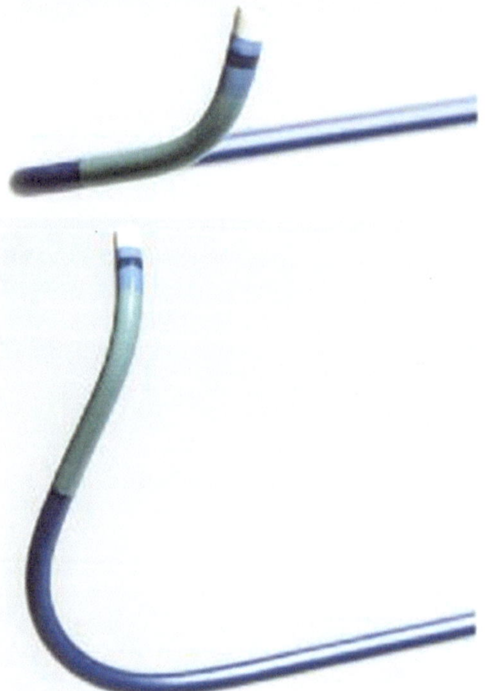

Fig. 11.4 Anomalous Right Coronary Artery From the Left Cusp Engaged With R-ACAOS Catheter Ref [1]. (**a**) Computed tomographic angiographic imaging of the intramural course of the right coronary artery (RCA) from the left sinus. (**b**) Anomalous RCA adjusted to the left main coronary artery engaged with R-ACAOS catheter. (**c**) R-ACAOS catheter

Locations B and C

Location B is characterized by the ostium of the RCA just inferior to the LM ostium. In location C the ostium of the RCA is near the commissure of the right and left cusps; In these situations, usually a coronary artery catheter Amplatz Left or right with curves 1,2, or 3 is used according to aortic root size.

Location D

Location D is characterized by the RCA ostium right above the sino-tubular junction. This anatomy is similar to that of a saphenous venous graft, therefore the preferred catheters used are the multipurpose Amplatz right or left, Hockey stick, or a Judkins right catheter curve 4 (Fig. 11.5).

Location E

This anatomy is characterized by the RCA ostium arising from right cusp superior and close to the left cusp. This is another challenging anatomy to be engaged in. Usually, an Amplatz left or right catheter can be used successfully or a 3DRC (Fig. 11.6). Sometimes when support is needed, the Sherpa NX Balanced (Medtronic) is used (Fig. 11.7).

Finally, sometimes selective engagement cannot be obtained. In these situations, a useful trick can be used. A guiding catheter is approached to the ostium, then a hydrophilic coronary guidewire can be advanced inside the coronary artery. The following step is to advance a microcatheter over the hydrophilic guidewire. Eventually, in order to gain more support, the hydrophilic guidewire can be exchanged for a supportive non-hydrophilic coronary guidewire.

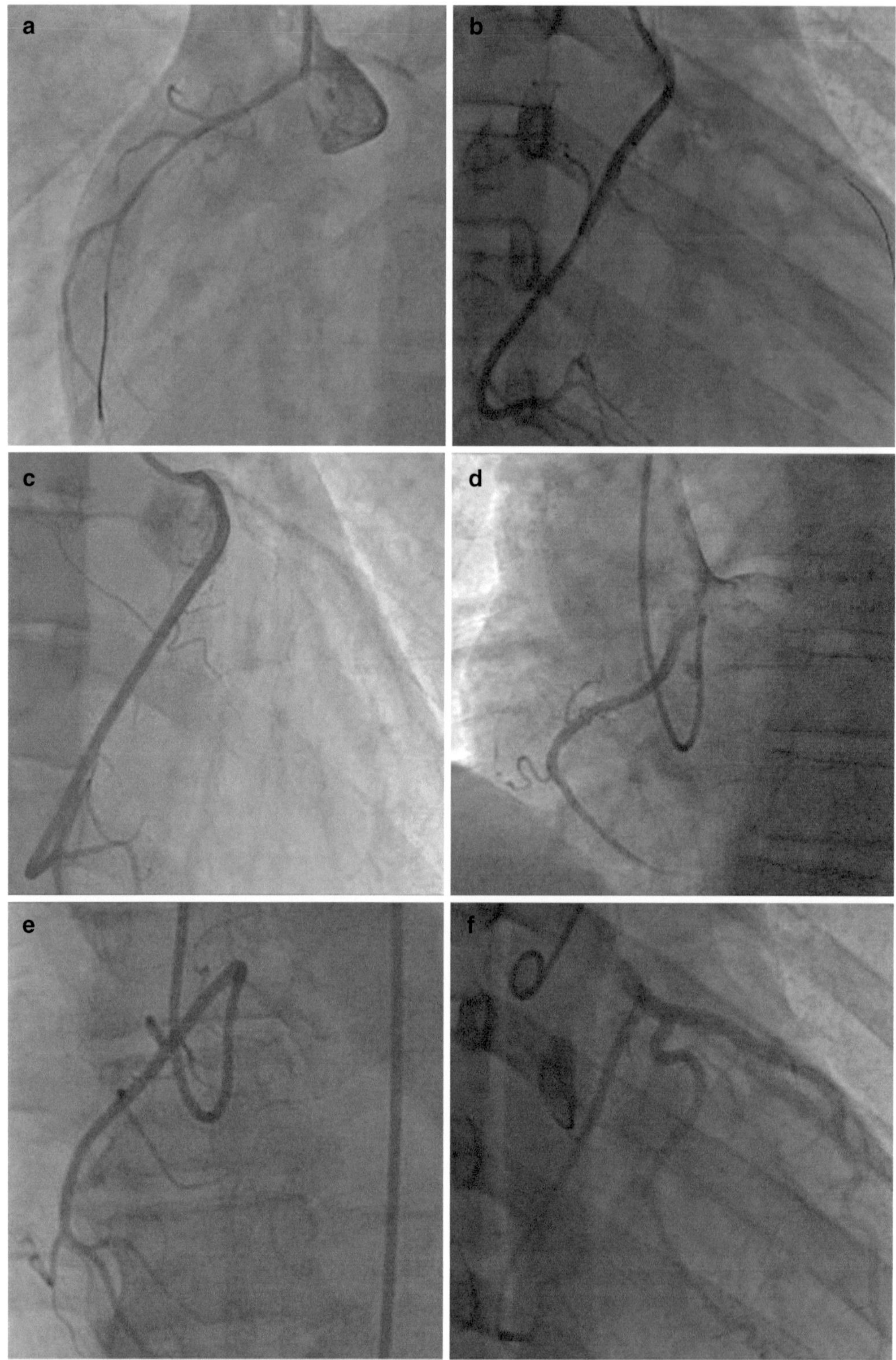

Fig. 11.5 Anomalous Right Coronary Artery in Various Locations Engaged With Different Catheters; Anomalous right coronary artery not adjusted to the left main coronary artery, engaged with (**a**) Hockey stick. (**b**) Multipurpose catheter. (**c**) Judkins right 4 (**d**) AL1 (**e**) AL2. (**f**) Pigtail catheter

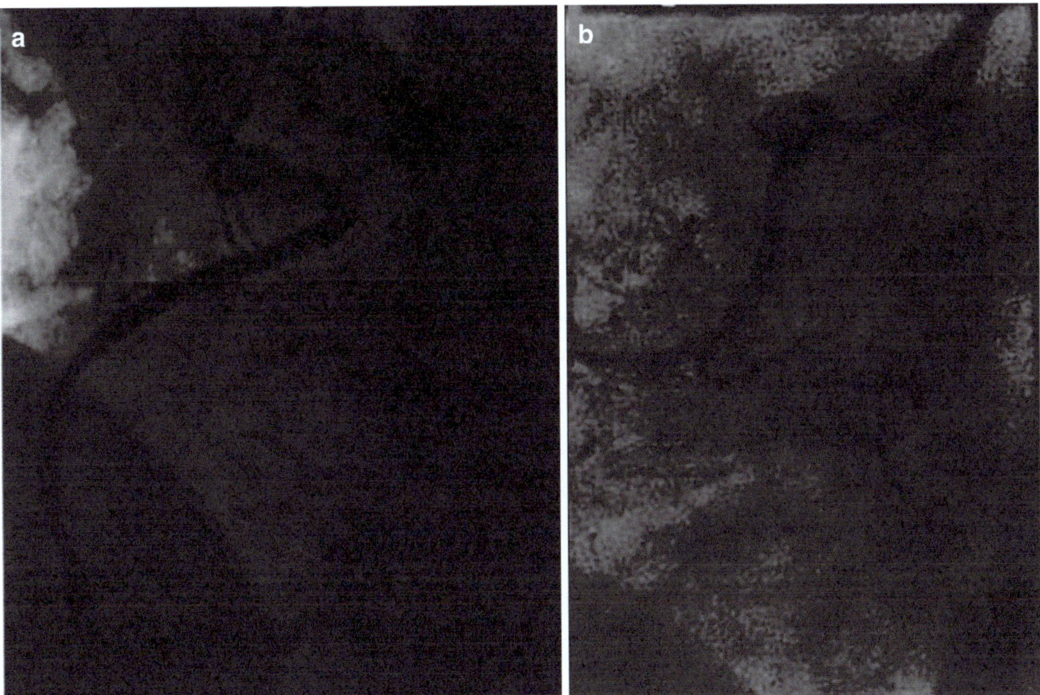

Fig. 11.6 Anomalous Right Coronary Artery From Right Cusp Engaged With Amplatz Right and 3DRC Guide Ref [1]. Anomalous right coronary artery from right cusp superior or toward the left cusp engaged with (**a**) Amplatz right and (**b**) 3DRC guide

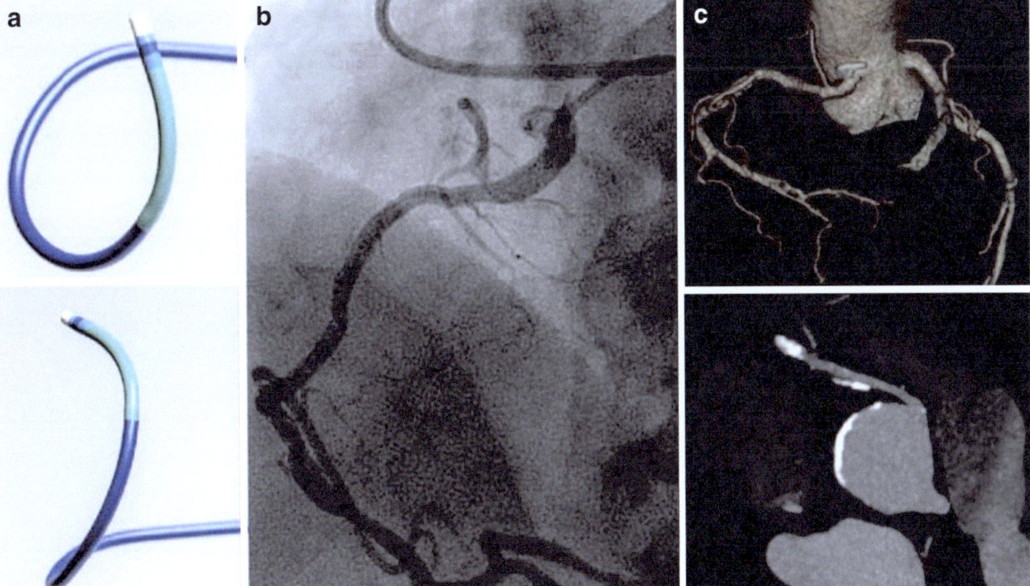

Fig. 11.7 Anomalous RCA from right cusp engaged with Sherpa NX Balanced guide Ref [1]. (**a**) Sherpa NX Balanced guide. (**b**) Anomalous RCA from right cusp superior and toward the left cusp engaged with Sherpa NX Balanced guide. (**c**) Computed tomographic images of anomalous right coronary artery from right cusp superior and toward the left cusp

Anomalous LCx from the Right Cusp

Anomalous LCx from the right coronary sinus associated with a retro-aortic course has a prevalence of 0.3% and is usually considered as a benign anomaly. However, in case of aortic valve replacement surgery, it may make the surgical procedure more difficult since it can be complicated with closure of the LCx. This anomaly may also have an impact on TAVI procedures, since there is a risk of compression due to the TAVI valve. In this scenario, a balloon angioplasty of the aortic valve may precede TAVI in order to screen for that risk. In the latter case, a self-expanding valve is the first choice over a balloon expandable valve. An alternative strategy is to have a guidewire placed into the coronary artery and have a bail-out stent available.

The preferred projection to show this anomaly is the right anterior oblique (RAO) 30° view. The ideal catheter to show the anomaly is the Amplatz left or right catheter, Judkins 4 right, and hockey stick. A major detail to be kept in mind is that if the catheter is too deep into the RCA then the anomaly cannot be demonstrated. Therefore, it is useful to place a guidewire in the distal RCA and then play with a second guidewire in order to get access to the difficult position of the LCx (Figs. 11.8, 11.9, and 11.10).

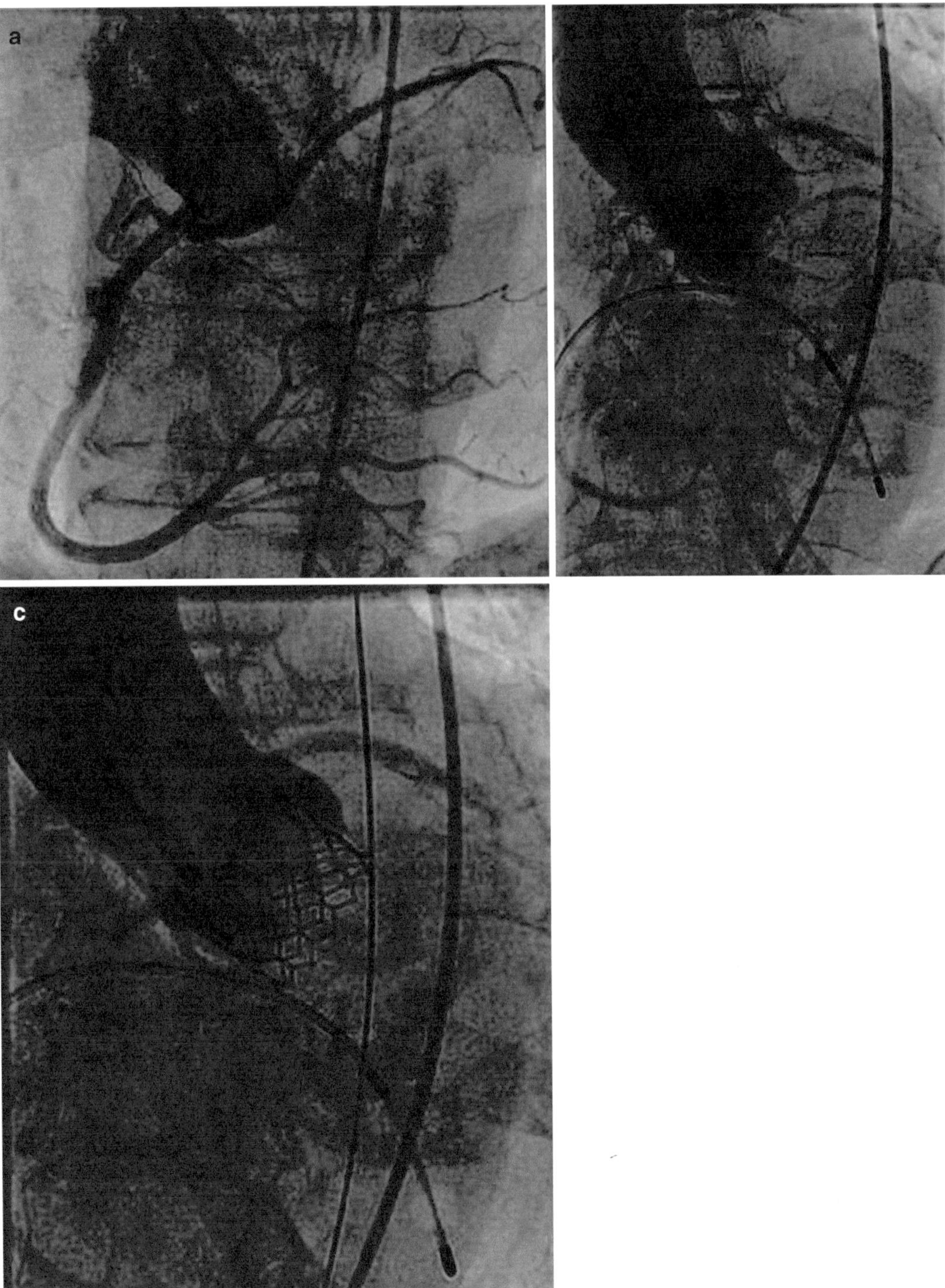

Fig. 11.8 Transcatheter aortic valve in a patient with anomalous left circumflex coronary artery from right coronary artery Ref [1]. (**a**) Anomalous circumflex from right cusp retro aortic course engaged with Judkins right catheter. (**b**) Aortogram pre-transcatheter aortic valve replacement. (**c**) Aortogram post-transcatheter aortic valve replacement (Sapien S3) demonstrating risk for compression of the anomalous artery by a prosthetic valve

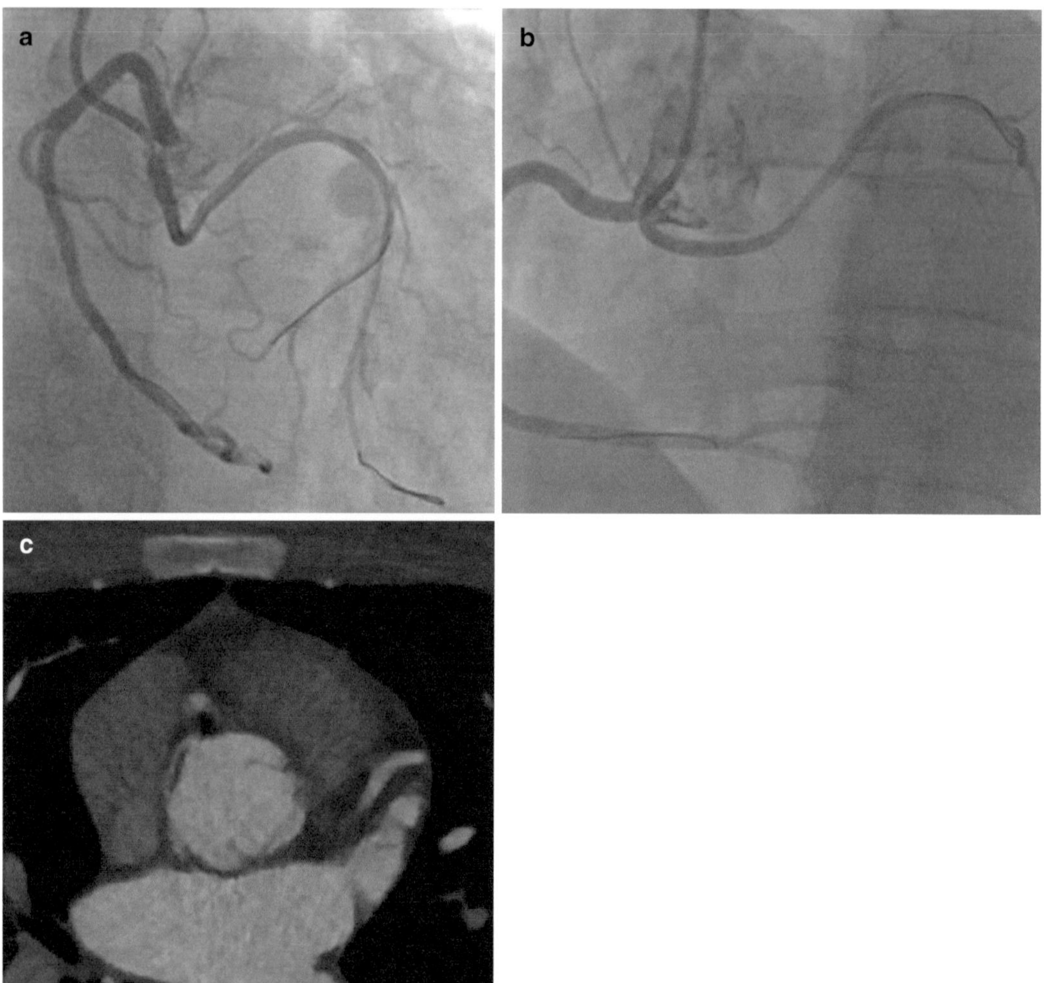

Fig. 11.9 Anomalous left circumflex coronary artery (LCx) from right cusp engaged with (**a**) Amplatz right catheter. (**b**) Multipurpose catheter. (**c**) Computed tomographic imaging of anomalous LCx for right cusp with retro-aortic course

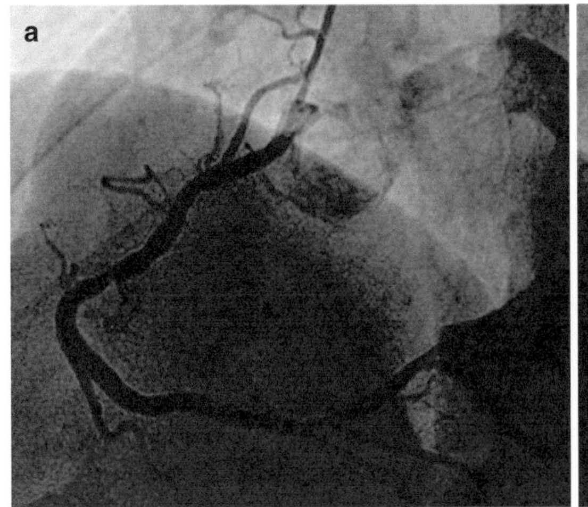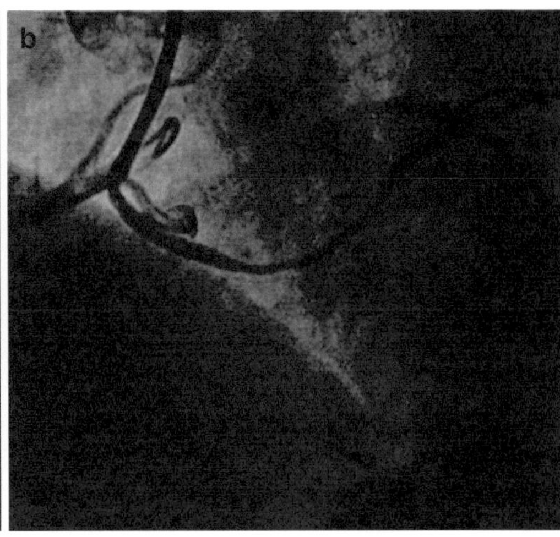

Fig. 11.10 Catheterization technique of how to engage anomalous circumplex artery from right coronary artery Ref [1]. (**a**) Image of the right coronary artery (RCA) with Judkins right seated deep, missing the ostium of anomalous left circumflex coronary artery (LCx). (**b**) Using hockey stick guide and coronary wire in distal RCA to stabilize the guide and pulling back the guide close to the ostium, and a second guidewire used to direct the wire to an anomalous LCx with a selective image

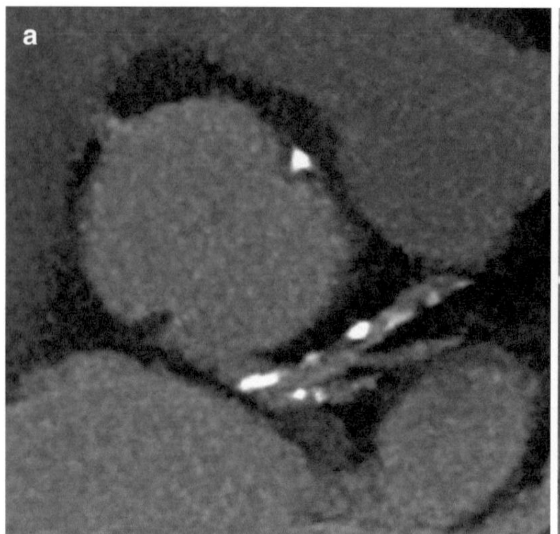 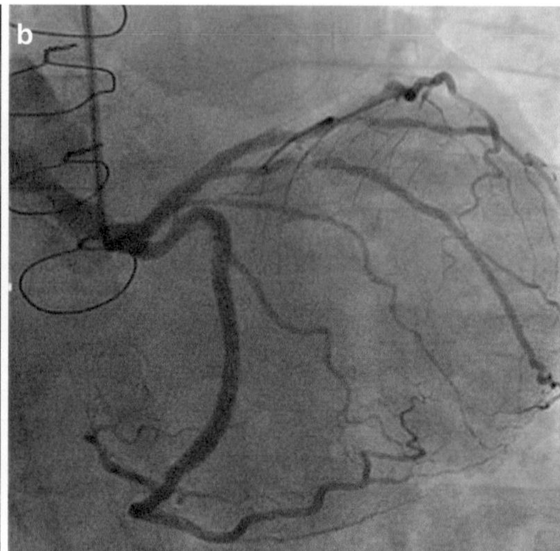

Fig. 11.11 Left main coronary artery origin at the posterior of the left cusp Ref [1]. (**a**) Computed tomographic image. (**b**) Angiographic view engaged with Judkins right catheter. *L* left coronary cusp, *NC* noncoronary cusp, *R* right coronary cusp

Posterior Origin of the Left Main from the Left Cusp or Noncoronary Cusp

This anatomy is rare but can be difficult to selectivate. The ideal is to use guiding catheters as EBU or CLS (Figs. 11.11 and 11.12).

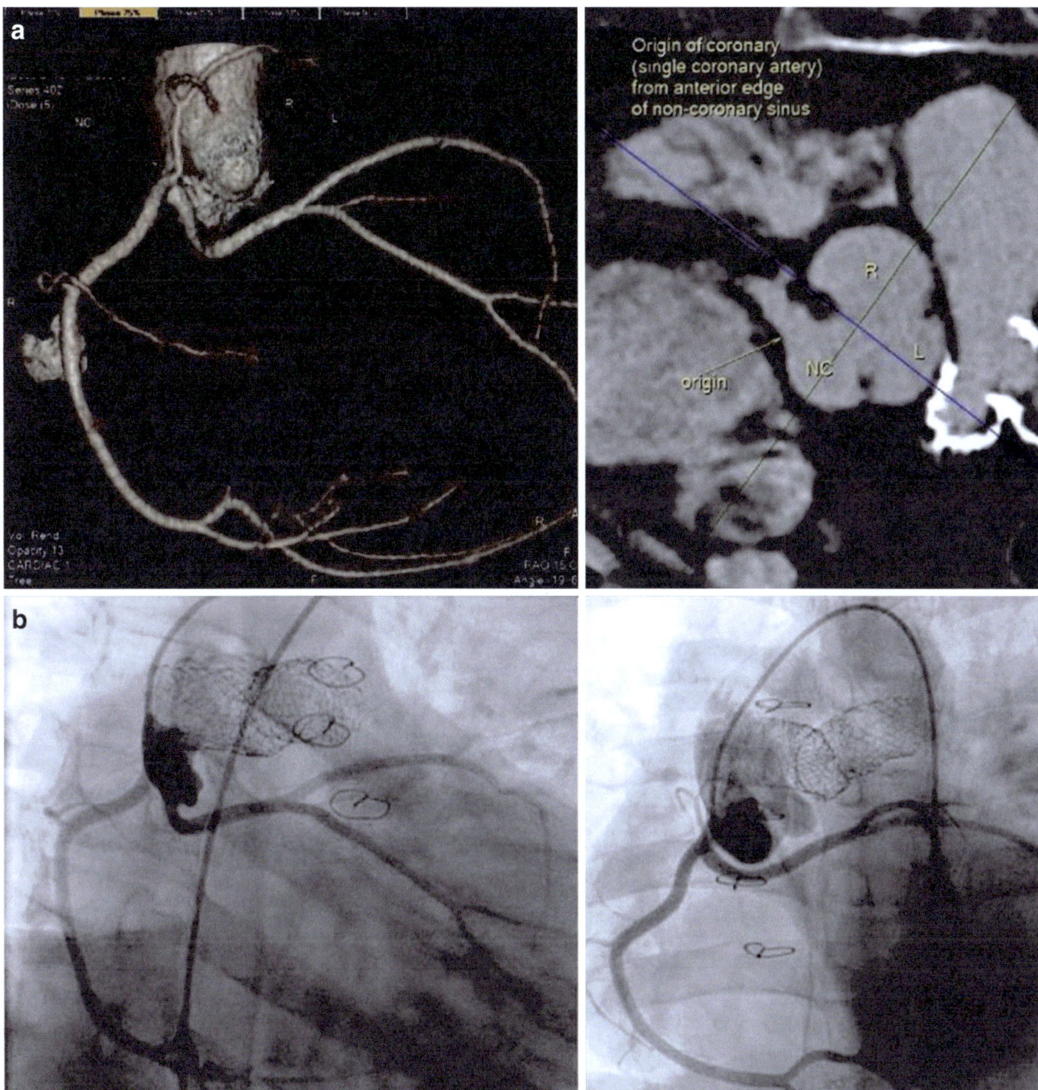

Fig. 11.12 Left main coronary artery origin from non-coronary cusp. Ref [1]. (**a**) Computed tomographic image. (**b**) Angiographic view engaged with Judkins right cathe-ter. *L* left coronary cusp, *NC* noncoronary cusp, *R* right coronary cusp

Anomalous Left Main Coronary Artery from the Right Cusp

This anomaly occurs in up to 0.7% of the population and can have inter-arterial, septal (subpulmonic), retro-aortic, or anterior-pulmonic course.

A selective angiography is performed by using a hockey stick or a right Judkins coronary catheter curve 4. The ideal angiographic projection is the RAO with caudal angulation view. Sometimes placing a Swan-Ganz catheter in the main pulmonary artery may help locate the position and course of the coronary artery in relationship to the pulmonary artery and the aorta (Figs. 11.13, 11.14, 11.15, 11.16, and 11.17).

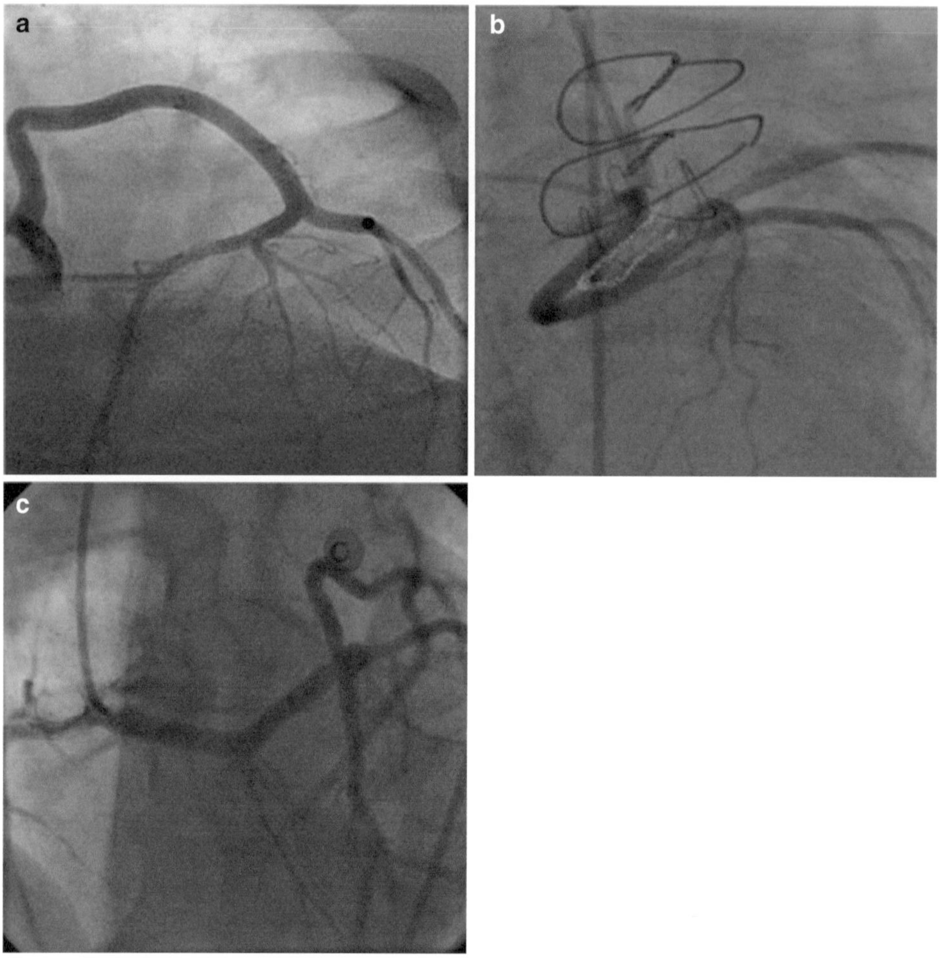

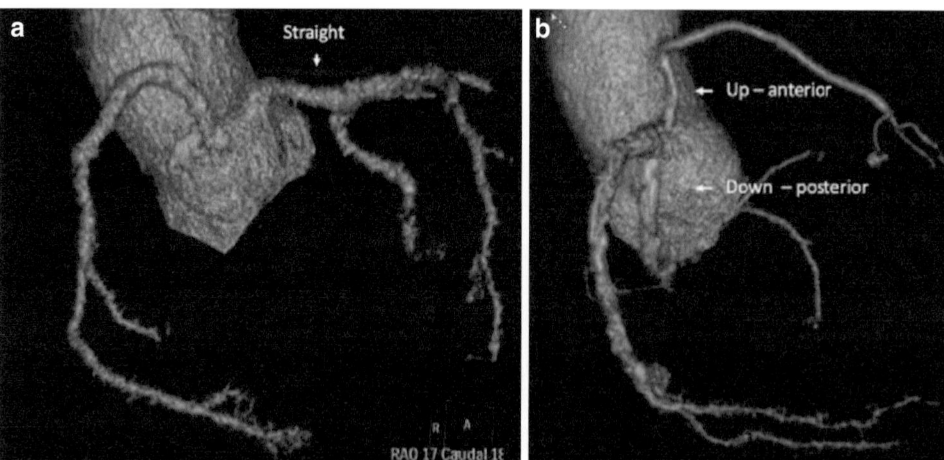

Fig. 11.13 Angiographic views to identify left main course from the right cusp Ref [1]. Right anterior oblique caudal views of (**a**) left main coronary artery going up ante- rior to pulmonary artery, (**b**) left main coronary artery down posterior to pulmonary artery, and (**c**) left main coronary artery straight in between the aorta and pulmonary artery

Fig. 11.14 Computed tomographic images Ref [1]. (**a**) Caudal view left main coronary artery straight between the aorta and pulmonary artery and (**b**) left anterior descending coronary artery going up anterior to pulmo- nary artery, left circumflex coronary artery down posterior to aorta. RAO 1/4 right anterior oblique

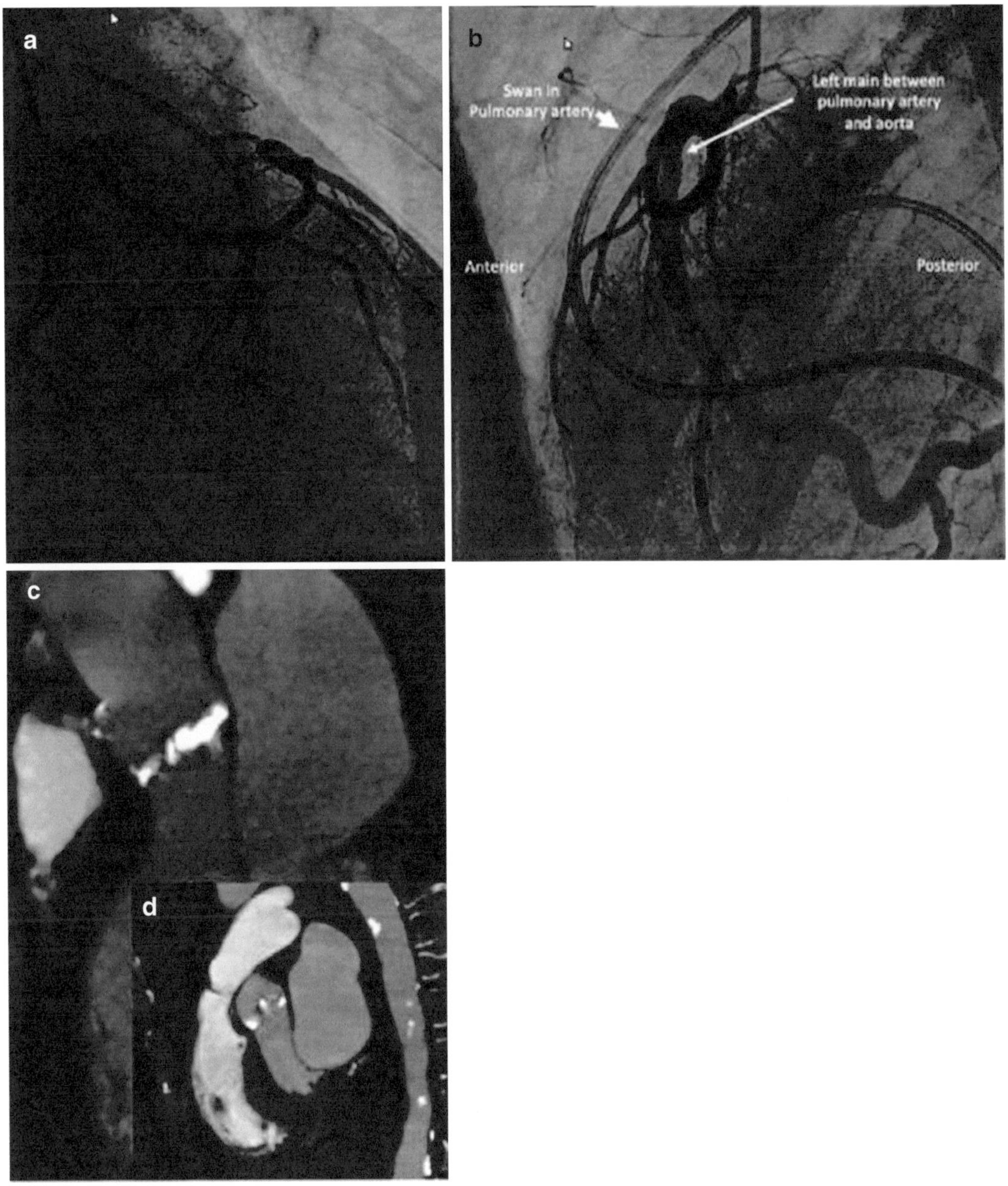

Fig. 11.15 Identify left main course with pulmonary artery catheter in place Ref [1]. (**a**) Caudal view showing left main coronary artery and Swan-Ganz but unable to tell if in between pulmonary artery and aorta. (**b**) Lateral view 90 with Swan-Ganz in the pulmonary artery showing left main coronary artery in between aorta and pulmonary artery. (**c**) CT image showing left main coronary artery in between aorta and pulmonary artery diving down with intraseptal course. (**d**) Computed tomographic lateral view 90, same projection as angiography in (**b**)

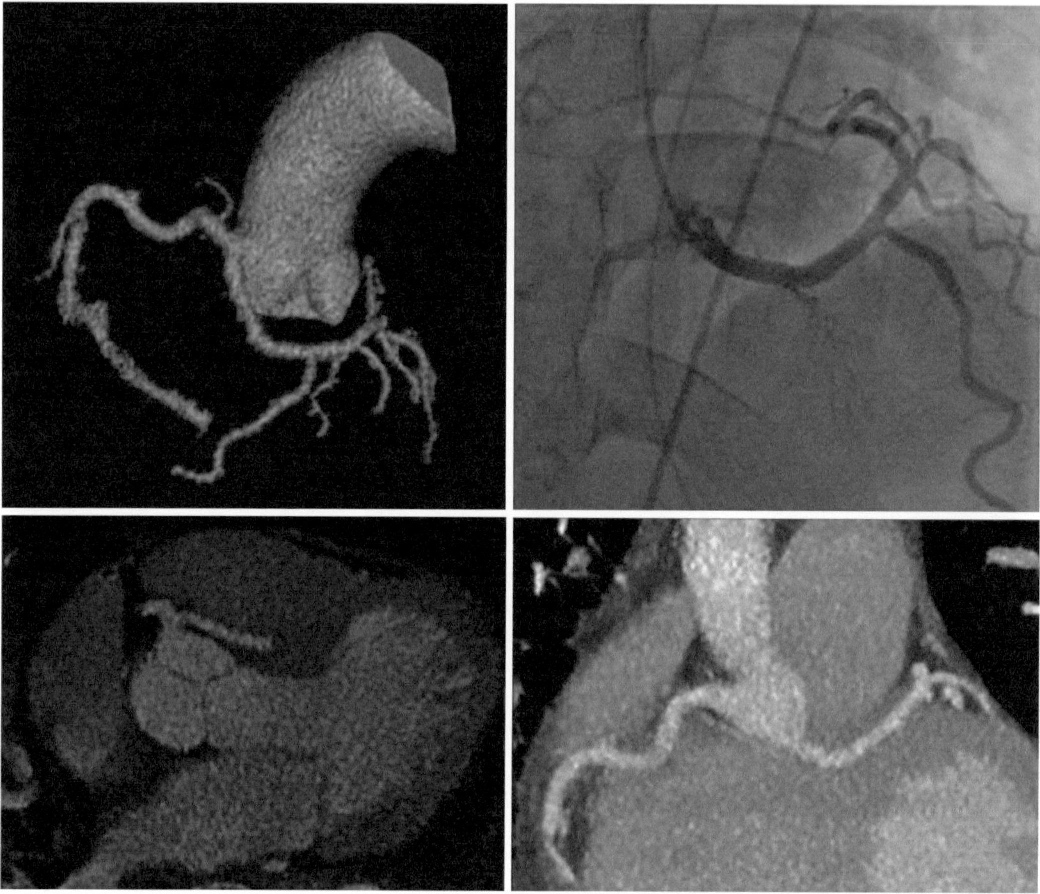

Fig. 11.16 Computed tomography and angiography of left main coronary artery between the pulmonary artery and aorta diving down through the crista supraventricular is (within the ventricular septum beneath the right ventricular infundibulum) Ref [1]

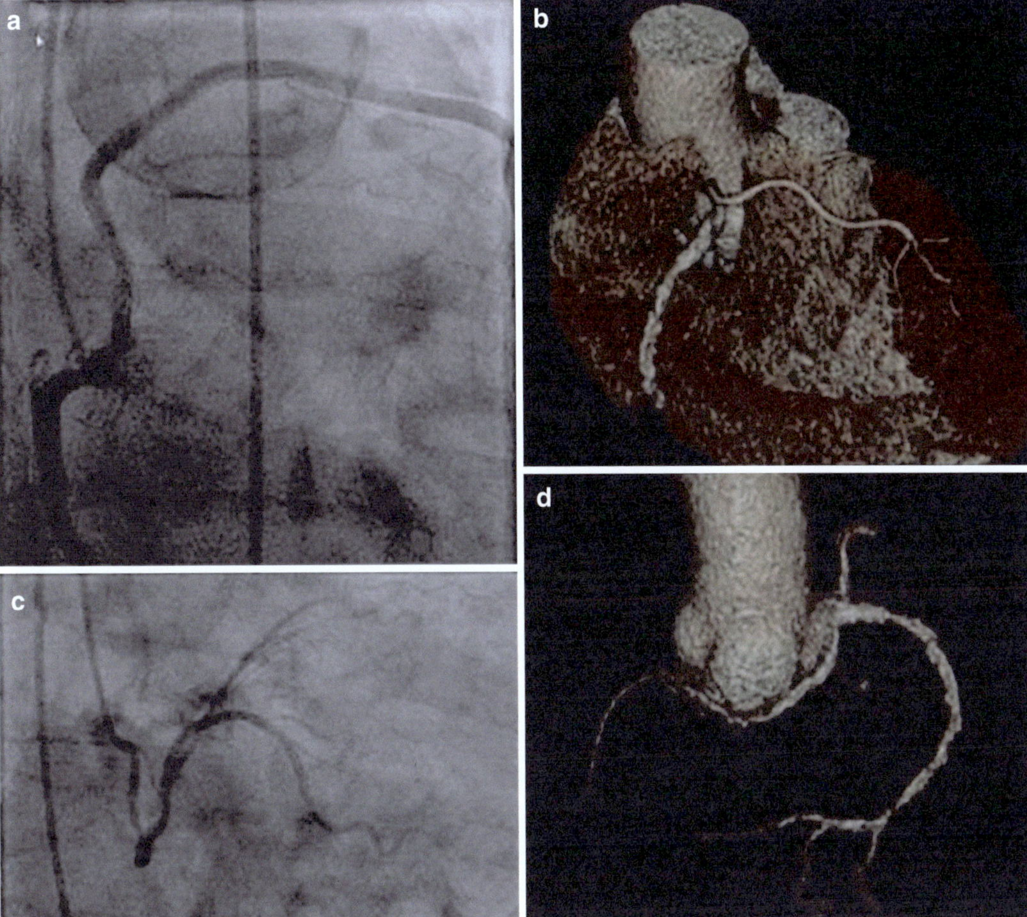

Fig. 11.17 Anomalous left main coronary artery from the right cusp Ref [1]. (**a**) Angiography shows left anterior descending coronary artery (LAD) anterior to pulmonary artery. (**b**) Computed tomography (CT) shows LAD ante- rior to pulmonary artery. (**c**) Angiography shows left cir- cumflex coronary artery (LCx) retro-aortic. (**d**) CT shows LCx retro-aortic

Anomalous Coronary Arteries Originating from the Opposite Sinus of Valsalva (ACAOS)

ACAOS are quite rare occurring in 0.26% of the general population (03% for left coronary ACAOS: L-ACAOS, 0.23% for right coronary ACAOS: R-ACAOS) [2, 3]. There are several risk factors associated to ischemic events in these anomalies: they include a) slit-like ostium; b) acute take-off angle; c) an intramural course; d) inter-arterial course (Fig. 11.18),

(a) *Slit-like ostium* at the anomalous ostium is defined as $a \geq 50\%$ reduction of the minimal lumen diameter compared to the normal dis- tal reference diameter [5] [<50% = oval ostium [5]].

(b) Acute *take-off angle* (below 45°), defined as an axial course of the proximal segment tan- gential to the great vessel circumference [6, 7], In this anatomical situation, exercise leads to expansion of the aortic root, which may decrease the acute take-off angle and consequently increased narrowing at the

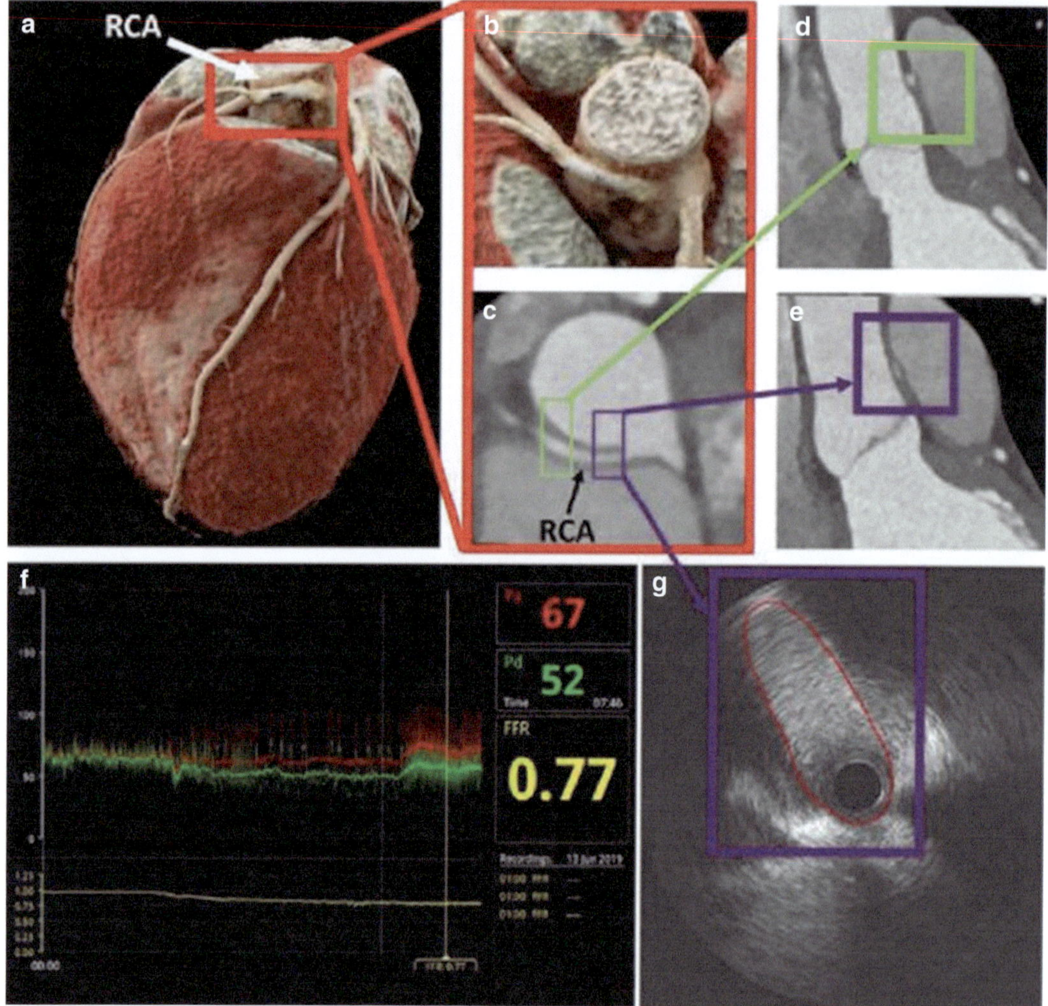

Fig. 11.18 Depiction of anatomical high-risk features in a patient with right ACAOS by coronary computed tomography angiography and invasive coronary angiography Ref [4]. Illustration of the inter-arterial course by CCTA (**a–c**). Depiction of anatomical high-risk features: acute-take off-angle, proximal narrowing, and oval vessel shape; purple box proximal segment, also called Angelini/Cheong sign, green box distal segment (**d, e**). Invasive assessment with a positive FFR and demonstration of lateral compression by intravascular ultrasound; red line depicts lumen contour (**f, g**)

ostium as a contributing ischemia-inducing mechanism [8, 9].

(c) *Intramural course* (i.e., course within the tunica media of the aortic wall). In particular, the length of the intramural segment is a significant risk factor for ischemia [5, 10–12]. Furthermore, the intramural segment may be associated with *elliptic proximal vessel shape* [defined as height/width ratio of >1.3 [13]]. Such anatomical backgrounds may be associated to the occurrence of a significant lateral compression which is dependent on the cardiac cycle being more pronounced during systole than diastole [14]. Lateral compression has been shown to increase during physical activity with augmented great vessel wall stress [14–20].

(d) The inter-arterial course has been considered as a risk factor for ischemic events. However, it itself may not be the predominant cause of ischemia, but rather represents a surrogate for other ischemia-prone anatomies which are reported above.

Double Ischemia Mechanism

Recently it has been proposed that the occurrence of ischemia in ACAOS could be related to the combination of fixed (proximal narrowing and slit-like ostium) and dynamic components (acute take-off angle, intramural course, elliptical vessel shape, dynamic changes of the ostium over the cardiac cycle). Finally, the clinical relevance could also be related to the amount of myocardial mass downstream the coronary anomaly. This could explain why right and left ACAOS may have different prognoses.

Role of Invasive Ultrasound Imaging and Fractional Flow Reserve

Catheterization laboratory evaluations are a mandatory step when dealing with anomalous origin of coronary arteries. Sometimes, even invasive coronary angiography is not conclusive in studying the clinical relevance of such anomaly. In terms of access, the radial one usually represents the preferred site. However, some degree of experience is needed to cannulate an anomalous coronary artery and perform the invasive test.

Intravascular ultrasound (IVUS) has been proposed by Angelini et al as the gold standard for the evaluation of an intramural segment. In fact, it allows to obtain clear images of the spatial relationships between structures and may show the dynamic lateral compression during simulated exercise [14, 21]. In order to perform IVUS, a guiding catheter is needed; therefore, this is the preferred option over a diagnostic catheter when dealing with ACAOS evaluation.

IVUS can provide various information about ostial morphology, proximal inter-arterial or intramural courses, degrees of hyperplasia, and coronary arteries size changes over the cardiac cycle. Ischemic symptoms are closely related to the abnormalities showed at IVUS [21]. Fractional flow reserve (FFR) is another useful tool to evaluate the clinical significance of ACAOS. The first trick is to have the catheter outside the ostium of the coronary artery since it may give obstruction by itself in small coronary arteries or on the other hand keep an intramural segment falsely open.

In. order to mimic exercise a Dobutamine test is preferred instead of Adenosine which is routinely used in case of atherosclerotic lesions. Merging together the data of IVUS and FFR it is possible to get the most comprehensive evaluation of ACAOS [15, 17–20, 22–24].

Recently, stress protocols have been proposed by different authors. In particular, Angelini and colleagues proposed a stress test called "SAD" test that aims to be equivalent to physical exercise. This pharmacological test includes rapid infusion of 500 mL saline, dobutamine stepwise infusion up to 40 µg/kg/min, and 0.5 mg atropine if the heart rate is below 140 bpm at the end of the dobutamine infusion [14, 21]. However, there are two major limitations. First of all, a heart rate of 140 bpm can be relatively low in younger patients or relatively high in older subjects. This heart rate limit is put fixed over a large age range. Secondly, dobutamine decreases the preload and then systolic arterial blood pressure, aortic wall stress, and myocardial oxygen consumption. In this setting, saline infusion is needed. However, again a fixed amount of saline infusion does not take into account the relationship between heart rate and all the physiological changes given by dobutamine during the text.

In our unit, we have created a dedicated clinic for ACAOS and a more aggressive approach has been developed. In fact, a steady infusion of saline is given during the whole invasive procedure (usually more than 1500 mL of saline to prevent a preload decrease) and attempts to reach 100% of the maximal heart rate, i.e., using atropine in addition to the ongoing dobutamine infusion to simulate vigorous physical exercise at the upper limit. The dobutamine and volume challenge is, of course, not doable for every patient but should be aimed for in order to simulate maximal physical exercise and obtain conclusive results even in the absence of ischemia (i.e., true-negative results).

References

1. Itsik Ben-Dor MD, Ron Waksman MD. Catheter selection and angiographic views for anomalous coronary arteries. A practical guide. *JACC Cardiovasc Interv*. 2021;14(9):995–1008.
2. Cheezum MK, Liberthson RR, Shah NR, Villines TC, O'Gara PT, Landzberg MJ, et al. Anomalous aortic origin of a coronary artery from the inappropriate sinus of valsalva. J Am Coll Cardiol. 2017;69:1592–608.
3. Grani C, Benz DC, Schmied C, Vontobel J, Possner M, Clerc OF, et al. Prevalence and characteristics of coronary artery anomalies detected by coronary computed tomography angiography in 5 634 consecutive patients in a single Centre in Switzerland. Swiss Med Wkly. 2016;146:w14294.
4. Angelini P. Coronary artery anomalies–current clinical issues: definitions, classification, incidence, clinical relevance, and treatment guidelines. Tex Heart Inst J. 2002;29:271–8.
5. Cheezum MK, Ghoshhajra B, Bittencourt MS, Hulten EA, Bhatt A, Mousavi N, et al. Anomalous origin of the coronary artery arising from the opposite sinus: prevalence and outcomes in patients undergoing coronary CTA. Eur Heart J Cardiovasc Imaging. 2017;18:224–35.
6. Zhang LJ, Wu SY, Huang W, Zhou CS, Lu GM. Anomalous origin of the right coronary artery originating from the left coronary sinus of Valsalva with an interarterial course: diagnosis and dynamic evaluation using dual- source computed tomography. J Comput Assist Tomogr. 2009;33:348–53.
7. Virmani R, Chun PK, Goldstein RE, Robinowitz M, McAllister HA. Acute takeoffs of the coronary arteries along the aortic wall and congenital coronary ostial valve-like ridges: association with sudden death. J Am Coll Cardiol. 1984;3:766–71.
8. Taylor AJ, Byers JP, Cheitlin MD, Virmani R. Anomalous right or left coronary artery from the contralateral coronary sinus: "high-risk" abnormalities in the initial coronary artery course and heterogeneous clinical outcomes. Am Heart J. 1997;133:428–35.
9. Nasis A, Machado C, Cameron JD, Troupis JM, Meredith IT, Seneviratne SK. Anatomic characteristics and outcome of adults with coronary arteries arising from an anomalous location detected with coronary computed tomography angiography. Int J Cardiovasc Imaging. 2015;31:181–91.
10. Jegatheeswaran A, Devlin PJ, McCrindle BW, Williams WG, Jacobs ML, Blackstone EH, et al. Features associated with myocardial ischemia in anomalous aortic origin of a coronary artery: a congenital heart surgeons' society study. J Thorac Cardiovasc Surg. 2019;158:822–34.e3.
11. Angelini P, Walmsley R, Cheong BY, Ott DA. Left main coronary artery originating from the proper sinus but with acute angulation and an intramural course, leading to critical stenosis. Tex Heart Inst J. 2010;37:221–5.
12. Kaushal S, Backer CL, Popescu AR, Walker BL, Russell HM, Koenig PR, et al. Intramural coronary length correlates with symptoms in patients with anomalous aortic origin of the coronary artery. Ann Thorac Surg. 2011;92:986–91.
13. Frommelt PC, Sheridan DC, Berger S, Frommelt MA, Tweddell JS. Ten- year experience with surgical unroofing of anomalous aortic origin of a coronary artery from the opposite sinus with an interarterial course. J Thorac Cardiovasc Surg. 2011;142:1046–51.
14. Harris MA, Whitehead KK, Shin DC, Keller MS, Weinberg PM, Fogel MA. Identifying abnormal ostial morphology in anomalous aortic origin of a coronary artery. Ann Thorac Surg. 2015;100:174–9.
15. Angelini P, Flamm SD. Newer concepts for imaging anomalous aortic origin of the coronary arteries in adults. Catheter Cardiovasc Interv. 2007;69:942–54.
16. Angelini P, Velasco JA, Ott D, Khoshnevis GR. Anomalous coronary artery arising from the opposite sinus: descriptive features and pathophysiologic mechanisms, as documented by intravascular ultrasonography. J Invasive Cardiol. 2003;15:507–14.
17. Angelini P, Uribe C. Symptomatic right coronary anomaly with dynamic systolic intramural obliteration and isolated right ventricular ischemia. Catheter Cardiovasc Interv. 2019;93:445–7.
18. Lee SE, Yu CW, Park K, Park KW, Suh JW, Cho YS, et al. Physiological and clinical relevance of anomalous right coronary artery originating from left sinus of Valsalva in adults. Heart. 2016;102:114–9.
19. Boler AN, Hilliard AA, Gordon BM. Functional assessment of anomalous right coronary artery using fractional flow reserve: an innovative modality to guide patient management. Catheter Cardiovasc Interv. 2017;89:316–20.
20. Tsujita K, Maehara A, Mintz GS, Franklin-Bond T, Mehran R, Stone GW, et al. *In vivo* intravascular ultrasonic assessment of anomalous right coronary artery arising from left coronary sinus. Am J Cardiol. 2009;103:747–51.
21. Bigler MR, Gräni C. Hemodynamic relevance of anomalous coronary arteries originating from the opposite sinus of valsalva-in search of the evidence. Front Cardiovasc Med. 2021;7:591326.
22. Sharma V, Burkhart HM, Dearani JA, Suri RM, Daly RC, Park SJ, et al. Surgical unroofing of anomalous aortic origin of a coronary artery: a single-center experience. Ann Thorac Surg. 2014;98:941–5.
23. Driesen BW, Warmerdam EG, Sieswerda GT, Schoof PH, Meijboom FJ, Haas F, et al. Anomalous coronary artery originating from the opposite sinus

of Valsalva (ACAOS), fractional flow reserve- and intravascular ultrasound- guided management in adult patients. Catheter Cardiovasc Interv. 2018;92:68–75.

24. Häner JD, Bär S, Ueki Y, Otsuka T, Gräni C, Räber L. Novel diagnostic approach to invasively confirm interarterial course of anomalous right coronary artery. JACC Cardiovasc Interv. 2020;13:132–4.

Pediatric Patients: Role of Invasive and Provocative Tests

Silvana Molossi and Tam T. Doan

Introduction

Risk stratification in anomalous aortic origin of a coronary artery (AAOCA) remains the Holy Grail that clinicians and the scientific community search continuously [1–5]. The view on management is extremely variable, ranging from standardized approach to evaluation and management to surgical intervention based solely on the presence of AAOCA from the opposite sinus [6–12]. The definition of optimal management decision is haunted by the highly variable clinical presentation, with greater than 50% of patients who presented with sudden cardiac arrest had been completely asymptomatic prior to the event, the benign nature of some AAOCA types, and the lack of long-term outcomes data in comparable large patient populations undergoing different management strategies. Therefore, identifying diagnostic tools that shed light on the potential risk of causing myocardial ischemia in the young population with AAOCA is likely the most attainable tool in hopes of optimal risk stratification.

Myocardial bridges (MBs) are common occurrences in the population and highly variable depending on the mode of imaging, and thought to be a benign finding in most patients [13, 14]. However, a small minority do present with symptoms including sudden cardiac arrest [13, 15, 16] and, unlike approaches in the adult population, committing young children and adolescents, many athletes, to long-standing medical therapy is not feasible. Moreover, identifying inducible myocardial ischemia in the presence of symptoms is key to determine management decisions that would include surgical intervention.

Testing under provocative stress includes utilizing exercise and/or pharmacologic agents to induce physiologic changes mimicking exercise, namely adenosine/regadenoson and dobutamine. Non-invasive studies include exercise stress test (EST)/cardiopulmonary exercise stress test (CPET) and imaging studies such as stress echocardiogram, nuclear perfusion imaging (NPI), and stress cardiac magnetic resonance imaging (sCMR), all of these potentially suitable to either exercise or pharmacologic inducible stress [8, 17–22]. Invasive testing in the pediatric population is performed in the cardiac catheterization laboratory under moderate sedation or general anesthesia. Angiography, measurements of coronary flow at rest and under provocative

S. Molossi (✉)
Coronary Artery Anomalies Program,
Texas Children's Hospital, Houston, TX, USA
e-mail: sxmoloss@texaschildrens.org;
smolossi@bmc.edu

T. T. Doan
The Lillie Frank Abercrombie Division of Cardiology,
Texas Children's Hospital, Baylor College of
Medicine, Houston, TX, USA
e-mail: Tam.Doan@bcm.edu

© Springer Nature Switzerland AG 2023
G. Butera, A. Frigiola (eds.), *Congenital Anomalies of Coronary Arteries*,
https://doi.org/10.1007/978-3-031-36966-7_12

pharmacologic stress, and intravascular ultrasound provide data to the understanding of hemodynamic effects of anatomic features in AAOCA and MB, and may contribute to risk stratification [6, 23, 24]. Major limitations of provocative stress testing in pediatric patients with AAOCA and MB relate to the lack of hard endpoints in this population to validate these testing modalities.

Thus, as we continue to search for tools to best risk stratify these patients and guide management decision-making, novel approaches have populated the literature in advanced imaging and invasive data under provocative stress in AAOCA and MB. This chapter will focus mainly on these two modalities in the young population (children and adolescents), with a brief mention of other diagnostic methods.

Exercise Stress Test (EST)

EST has been widely used in the evaluation of patients with coronary anomalies. It intends to elicit physiologic changes that occur with exercise and potentially unfold compromise to myocardial coronary flow leading to ischemic changes. Although frequently used, it remains a poor predictor of inducible ischemia in multiple studies reporting outcomes of cohort of patients that underwent surgical intervention. Moreover, the interpretation of inducible ischemia may vary according to different interpretations when EST is reported "abnormal", which may reflect a blunted blood pressure response, the occurrence of premature ventricular contractions, or altered ventricular repolarization such as ST segment depression/elevation [8, 10, 11, 25].

Multiple studies have described EST in AAOCA with largely inconsistent results. In 2000, Basso and colleagues described sudden cardiac death in AAOCA in patients who had undergone a normal EST. [26] Brothers and colleagues demonstrated, in the same patient with AAOCA, normal EST and abnormal ischemic changes on subsequent EST 1 week apart [4]. Current guidelines state that asymptomatic patients with right AAOCA (AAORCA) are low-risk in the presence of a normal EST. [27, 28] Intriguing data was recently presented by Qasim and colleagues demonstrating extremely poor sensitivity of EST in AAOCA which is improved with CPET data, and poor correlation with results of dobutamine stress CMR (DSCMR) [29]. Additional data by Doan et al. showed evidence of inducible myocardial ischemia in only 1% of EST in a group of 164 patients with AAORCA [30].

Yet, EST remains a valuable tool and appears to be very specific in the presence of ST segment changes suggestive of myocardial ischemia, though it seems to be undermined by its poor sensitivity. Continued data gathering and correlation with other provocative tests investigating inducible myocardial ischemia are needed to define its role in this young population.

Stress Echocardiography

The role of stress echocardiography has long been established to identify wall motion abnormalities as a surrogate of compromised coronary blood flow and suggestive of inducible ischemia upon pharmacologic stress, with dobutamine/atropine or adenosine/dipyridimole, or following EST (treadmill/cycloergometer) [31–35]. The latter poses difficulties in maintaining the desired heart rate upon echocardiographic scanning as there is need to lay supine moving quickly from the exercise equipment. This is particularly challenging in children due to rapid heart rate decrease upon cessation of exercise. On the other hand, pharmacologic stimuli allow for its use in smaller children and infants, also allowing for sustained peak heart rate [36]. The use of stress echocardiography has also been employed to detect valvular lesions/worsening of function upon provocative exercise [37, 38]. Its benefits include being readily available in most centers without needing additional equipment, it is portable, and less expensive than other advanced imaging modalities. However, expertise is paramount to detect wall motion abnormalities as an indicator of myocardial ischemia. This limits its use, particularly in centers of low patient volume and where multiple readers are employed.

Furthermore, as very high heart rates are achieved in children, a trained eye is essential for accurate interpretation and reporting of regional wall motion abnormalities.

Similar to other testing modalities, stress echocardiography has been utilized in the pediatric population with a wide variety of indications to assess impaired coronary flow, such as in acquired coronary disease (Kawasaki disease, severe/hereditary dyslipidemia, post-transplant coronary arteriopathy) and repaired and unrepaired congenital heart disease (such as AAOCA, transposition of the great arteries following arterial switch operation) [33, 34, 39, 40]. Stress echocardiography is also employed in the evaluation of children with MBs [17].

In some centers, it is utilized as the preferred method to evaluate perfusion abnormalities in children with AAOCA [10, 11, 19, 36, 41, 42]. To date, there is no data comparing multiple modalities of non-invasive testing to assess myocardial perfusion in children with AAOCA, and different centers report their specific experience with a preferred testing modality.

Advanced Imaging Upon Provocative Stress

Nuclear Perfusion Imaging (NPI)

NPI with provocative stress is established in the evaluation of ischemic heart disease in adults. Multiple reports have been published and reported its utility in the evaluation of AAOCA in the young population [8, 10, 19, 25, 43–45]. There have been concerns that in addition to patient exposure to ionizing radiation, NPI may result in a relatively high incidence of false-positive and false-negative findings, have low spatial resolution, and attenuation artifacts related to the body wall and diaphragm movement. Therefore, results should be considered in association with other clinical findings and, importantly, in those patients where intervention was indicated, repeat studies to compare with results preceding the intervention. Due to these concerns, we have transitioned to using sCMR at our center and reported its safety, feasibility, and utility in a large cohort of children with AAOCA [8, 9, 20, 46, 47].

Stress Cardiac Magnetic Resonance Imaging (sCMR)

Studies in adults with ischemic heart disease have established the clinical utility, safety profile, and prognostic value of sCMR, which improved patient outcome when used to guide revascularization [48–57]. In the pediatric population, several studies demonstrated its safety and feasibility in children with acquired coronary artery abnormalities associated with Kawasaki disease or following repair of complex congenital heart disease, such as transposition of the great arteries where translocation of coronary artery buttons is essential in the arterial switch operation [21, 58–61]. In these studies, adenosine (or regadenoson, a selective alpha-2A adenosine receptor agonist) with/without atropine, is typically employed to elicit hyperemia and unfold fixed obstructive lesions.

In the setting of AAOCA, the mechanism by which inducible ischemia may occur is postulated to relate to dynamic mechanisms influencing morphologic factors of the anomalous coronary, though arguably ostial abnormalities may represent a fixed component to this lesion. These include compression of the lumen in the intramural segment, course behind a thick inter-coronary pillar, acute angle takeoff, ostium abnormalities (slit-like, stenotic), and interarterial course between the aorta and pulmonary artery. Therefore, agents that lead solely to hyperemia may be suboptimal in the identification of perfusion abnormalities as the pathophysiology in unrepaired AAOCA is thought to incur in dynamic changes in the lumen of the anomalous coronary along the intramural and interarterial segment [49, 51, 62].

As with adenosine sCMR, DSCMR has been utilized in the adult population. Dobutamine, as a stressor agent, has the advantage of inducing positive inotropy at the same time it decreases systemic vascular resistance. It may then induce wall motion abnormalities at a time of maximal myocardial oxygen demand. It has demonstrated excellent performance with good prediction of ischemic events [55, 62, 63]. Specifically, detection of impaired perfusion has been shown to precede wall motion abnormalities in a demand ischemia cascade, thus indicating that addition of first-pass perfusion to assessment of wall motion abnormalities increases the sensitivity of this study [48, 49, 51, 57]. sCMR has advantages over NPI as it provides high-quality cardiac imaging with excellent spatial resolution and avoids ionizing radiation, a clear benefit especially in children, and its feasibility and safety have been demonstrated [64–67].

The largest series of pediatric AAOCA patients undergoing DSCMR was reported by Doan and colleagues [20]. They reported 224 studies in 182 patients <20 years and median age of 14 years in which 99% of studies were successfully completed with no major events, and 12.5% minor events observed. Most studies were completed without sedation. The interobserver variability was very good and inducible perfusion defects were seen in 14% and, of these, 42% with associated wall motion abnormalities. They concluded DSCMR is feasible and safe in the young AAOCA population and contributed to management decision-making. Similar findings were also reported in pediatric patients with MB [68, 69].

Results on DSCMR were also correlated with invasive fractional flow reserve (FFR) during cardiac catheterization in young patients with AAOCA and/or MB. Agrawal et al. reported 24 sets of DS-CMR and FFR studies in 19 patients (13 AAOCA patients) with good agreement between the two modalities (Fig. 12.1). They concluded that assessment of myocardial perfusion by DSCMR concurred with FFR and aided in the management decisions of these patients [71]. Similar data is present in isolated case reports and a series of 19 patients with intraseptal AAOCA published by Doan et al. [23, 70, 72] In this cohort, 14 patients underwent stress perfusion imaging studies and 50% had evidence of inducible perfusion abnormalities that contributed to management decisions.

DSCMR has evolved as a promising tool for detection of perfusion abnormalities in AAOCA. However, there remains a technical limitation of performing CMR at a high heart rate and in younger children. Image quality and expertise are needed for the visual assessment of first-pass perfusion of gadolinium, particularly to differentiate an inducible perfusion defect from dark rim artifacts. DSCMR has been performed successfully in patients as young as 8 years of age without general anesthesia; however, most children younger than 10 years old are not able to lie still in a CMR scanner during dobutamine infusion. In our program, unless there are exertional symptoms or other concerns for myocardial ischemia, we would defer DSCMR until patients are around 10 years of age to attempt the study without needing general anesthesia. As risk stratification remains a challenge in this population, likely a careful assessment including all clinical data is essential, and DSCMR appears to have an important role.

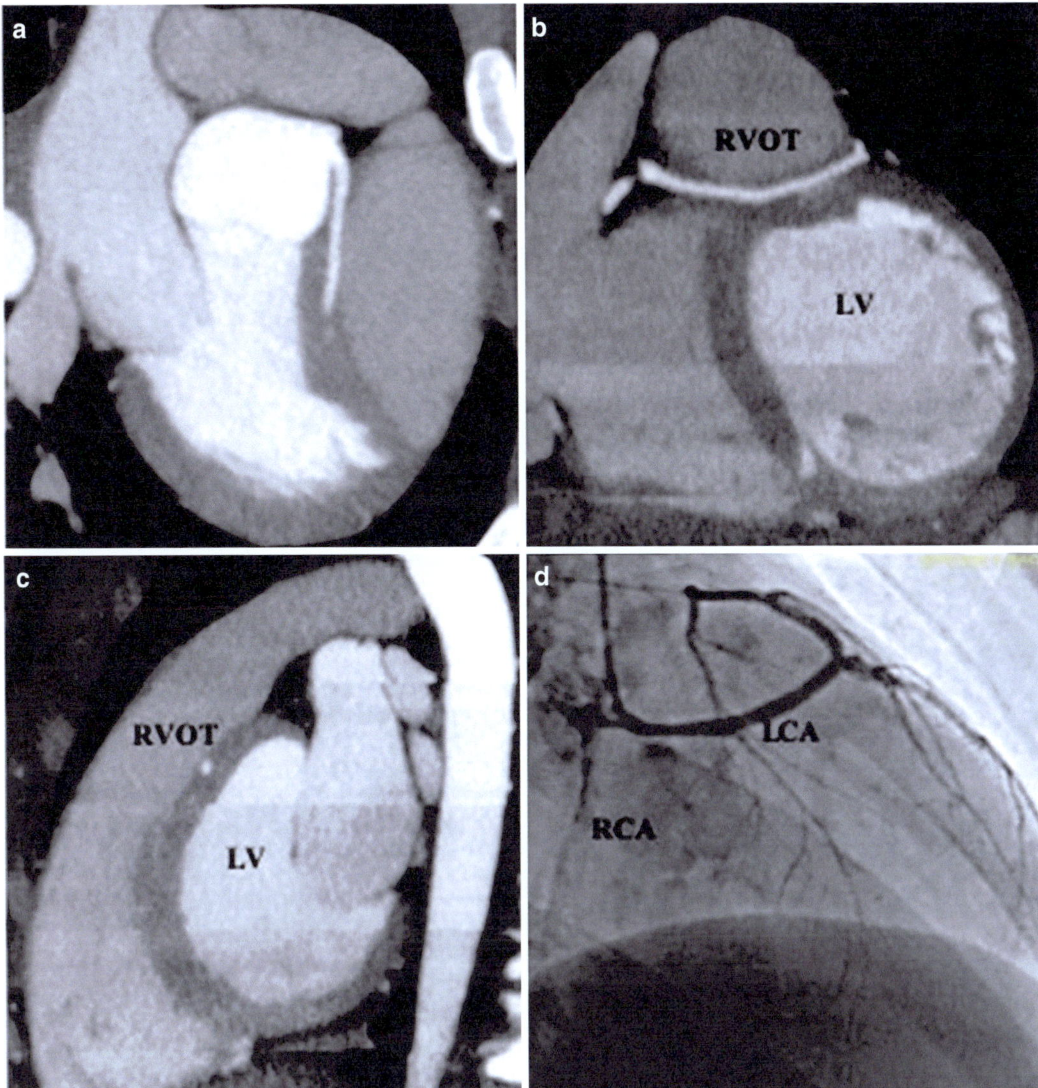

Fig. 12.1 Pre-operative assessment. CTA showing the LCA courses parallel to the aortic wall (**a**) before entering the ventricular septum (**b, c**); common origin of the RCA and LCA on angiography (**d**); DSCMR: subendocardial hypoperfusion in the anteroseptal wall (**e**) and late-gadolinium enhancement (**f**); decreased baseline iFR to 0.85 (normal >0.89) (**g**). At peak dobutamine stress, iFR further decreased to 0.65 (**h**), FFR to 0.70, and diastolic FFR 0.69 (normal >0.80) (**i**) [70]. *CTA* computed tomography angiography, *DSCMR* dobutamine stress cardiac magnetic resonance imaging, *FFR* fractional flow reserve, *iFR* instantaneous free-wave ratio, *LCA* left coronary artery, *LV* left ventricle, *RCA* right coronary artery, *RVOT* right ventricular outflow tract

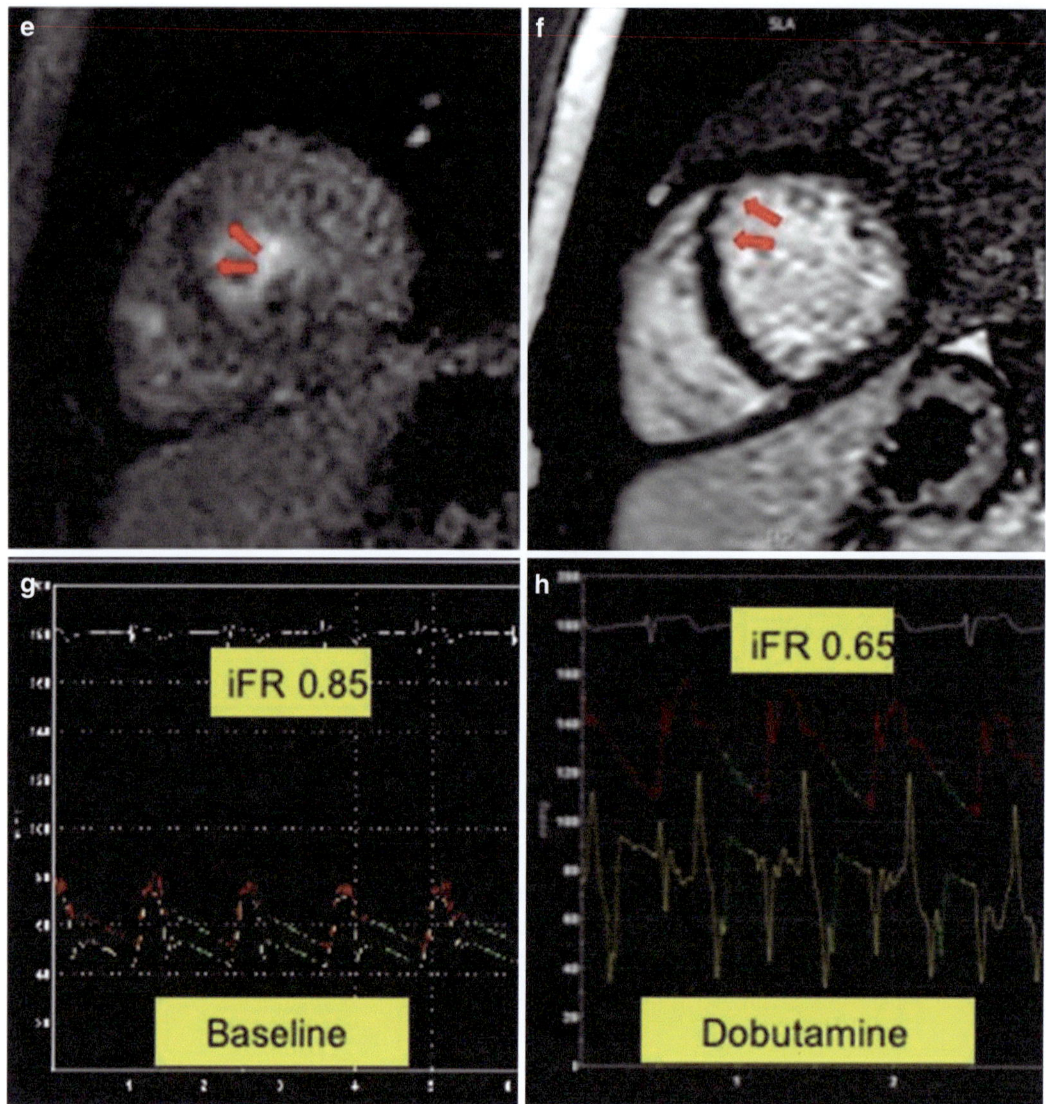

Fig. 12.1 (continued)

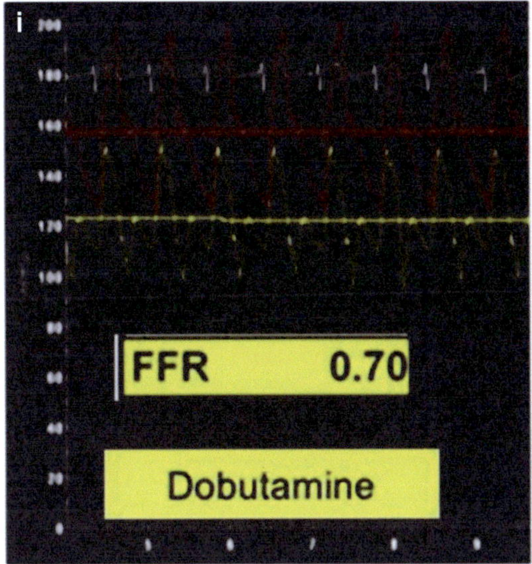

Fig. 12.1 (continued)

Cardiac Catheterization

Angiography as a means of imaging the anomalous coronary artery largely is not utilized in children, unlike adults, where angina symptoms typically trigger coronary angiography to surveil the occurrence of coronary artery disease. Thus, in the pediatric population, it is part of invasive assessment of coronary artery flow and has been performed in recent years. Clearly, this is a novel approach to determine significance of morphologic factors in coronary lesions (such as AAOCA and MB) (Fig. 12.2) that may pose a risk for myocardial ischemia when other clinical data and non-invasive studies are incongruent. It has been shown to aid in the management decision-making and need for intervention in patients with AAOCA and MB.

Invasive Angiography

Invasive angiography is an integral part of the evaluation of MB in the pediatric population; however, its value is coupled with assessment of coronary blood flow in addition to visual compression upon provocative stress.

However, in AAOCA, it may have indication only in a small subset of patients with controversial clinical findings [73, 74]. During infusion of pharmacologic stressors and increase in heart rate and blood pressure, angiography can unfold significant dynamic compression of the affected coronary vessel, contributing to the determination of a hemodynamically significant lesion that may benefit from intervention.

Fractional Flow Reserve (FFR)

FFR is a pressure-derived index of coronary artery stenosis severity. It is calculated as a ratio between mean intracoronary pressure distal to the lesion (Pd) and mean aortic pressure (Pa) obtained during the entire cardiac cycle. A vasodilator is needed to establish minimal and constant myocardial resistance and leads to sustained hyperemia resulting in unmasking a fixed coronary stenosis. It has been studied and well validated in the adult population. FFR <0.8 is indicative of a significant lesion and coronary revascularization is generally recommended. Dobutamine has been considered a pharmacologic stress agent of choice in the assessment of coronary artery anomalies in which dynamic compression during exertion is proposed as the primary mechanism of coronary flow obstruction, such as AAOCA with intramural course, intraseptal course, and MB [20, 21, 24]. Investigation in healthy, conscious dogs demonstrated that dobutamine increases heart rate and myocardial contractility as well as reduces systemic and coronary vascular resistance [75]. Non-invasive studies in healthy adults using CMR demonstrated dobutamine and exercise led to a similar rise in cardiac output with dobutamine having more significant impact on myocardial deformation and ejection fraction [76]. It was proven to fully exhaust coronary vascular resistance at a similar degree to adenosine in patients with coronary artery stenosis [77]. Diastolic FFR (dFFR) has been suggested as a better marker of intracoronary hemodynamic

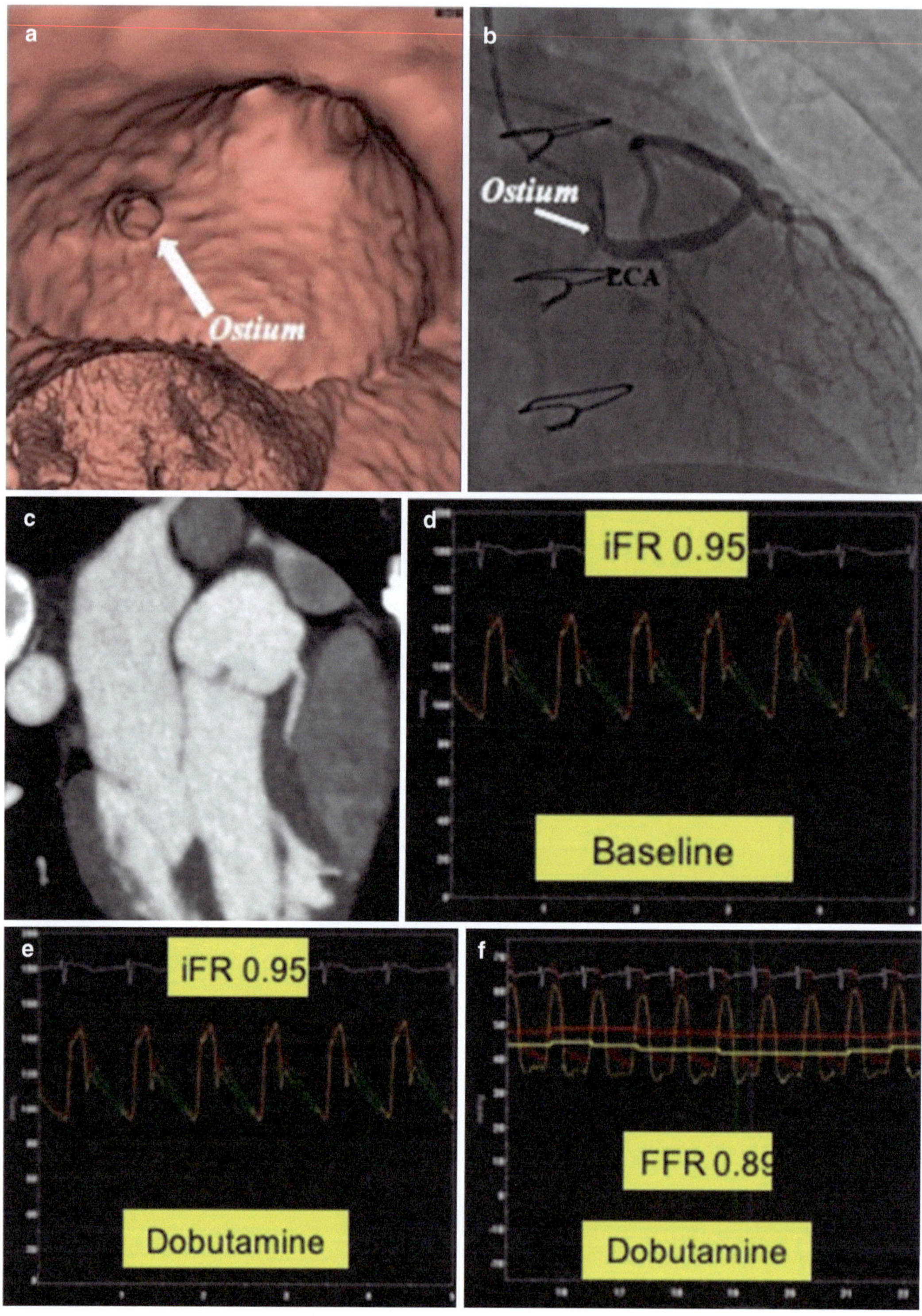

Fig. 12.2 Post-operative assessment. Widely patent LCA ostium on virtual angioscopy (**a**) and angiography (**b**); improved acute angle between the LCA and aortic wall on CTA (**c**); normalization of baseline iFR to 0.95 (**d**); at peak dobutamine stress, normal values of iFR at 0.95 (**e**), FFR at 0.96, and diastolic FFR at 0.89 (**f**) [70]. *CTA* computed tomography angiography *FFR* fractional flow reserve, *iFR* instantaneous free-wave ratio, *LCA* left coronary artery

assessment during dobutamine challenge of MB due to a potential overshooting of distal systolic pressure, which may negate a significant diastolic pressure gradient [78].

The use of FFR in children with AAOCA and MB was published initially by Agrawal et al. in 2017, when the authors described a small group of patients that included four AAOCA and four MB patients [73]. These data demonstrated safety profile of performing invasive coronary flow assessment in children, with the youngest described at the age of 2.6 years, and their contribution to management. Additional data was published by the same group correlating DSCMR findings with invasive FFR in children with AAOCA and MB with good agreement between the two testing modalities [71]. Diastolic FFR during dobutamine challenge has been used early in their adoption of the technique in the risk stratification of this challenging population [73]. A major limitation remains as dFFR is calculated manually as an average of 3 Pd/Pa ratio utilizing digital calipers at end systole. In addition, dobutamine challenge is contraindicated in patients presenting with sudden cardiac arrest, which limits the assessment of FFR. These limitations led to the addition of instantaneous wave-free ratio (iFR) which is a resting ratio derived automatically and may negate the need for a dobutamine challenge in special scenarios.

Instantaneous Wave-Free Ratio (iFR)

iFR is a drug-free pressure-derived index of coronary artery flow during a period of naturally constant and low resistance due to minimal competing pressure waves in diastole [79]. It negates the need for a vasodilator to reduce coronary vascular resistance, and has been shown to be better tolerated by the patients with shorter procedure time [80]. In the JUSTIFY-CFR study, iFR showed stronger correlation and better agreement with coronary flow velocity reserve when compared to FFR [81]. In two large multicenter randomized controlled trials, iFR was found non-inferior to FFR as it relates to health outcomes in guiding coronary revascularization in adults with ischemic heart disease [80, 82].

The adoption of resting iFR in children with AAOCA, MB, and coronary artery stenosis was first reported in 2021 by Doan et al. in 20 patients at a median age of 13 years [24]. The authors reported iFR correlated with adenosine FFR and dobutamine dFFR and they concluded it might be a useful tool without the need for vasoactive challenge in these patients, in addition to contributing to decision-making on coronary intervention. The same group of collaborators recently reported resting iFR as well as dFFR with dobutamine challenge were helpful and guided management in select patients with AAOCA and intramural course who had conflicting clinical data (either normal DSCMR and concerning symptoms or young patients with questionable high-risk left AAOCA anatomy and absence of symptoms) [83]. Additionally, abnormality in coronary flow was shown to be improved to normal levels following surgical intervention. Given dFFR was a manual process, the principles of iFR during dobutamine challenge seem ideal to overcome the systolic overshooting phenomenon in the assessment of potential dynamic compression during exertion in youths with AAOCA and MB. Tarantini et al. reported intracoronary assessment of MB using iFR was more consistent with non-invasive test results and patients' symptoms compared to FFR [84].

Ghobrial et al. recently reported their experience in 78 symptomatic adults with left and right AAOCA and MB using iFR and dobutamine challenge [85]. The authors reported significant improvement in dobutamine iFR in 18 patients who underwent surgical repair of the anomalous coronary arteries (0.70 ± 0.12 to 0.89 ± 0.06, $p = 0.0002$). In our institution, we have observed a similar pattern of provocative pharmacological stress with dobutamine affect iFR values in children with AAOCA and MB compared to those seen at rest (unpublished data). While it is promising to learn significant improvement in iFR and FFR following surgical repair of AAOCA (Fig. 12.3) and MB (Fig. 12.4) [86], it is important to recognize that these cutoffs were derived from data in adults with ischemic heart disease and there remains a strong need of longitudinal data in youth to learn if such cut off values are the most appropriate in this young population.

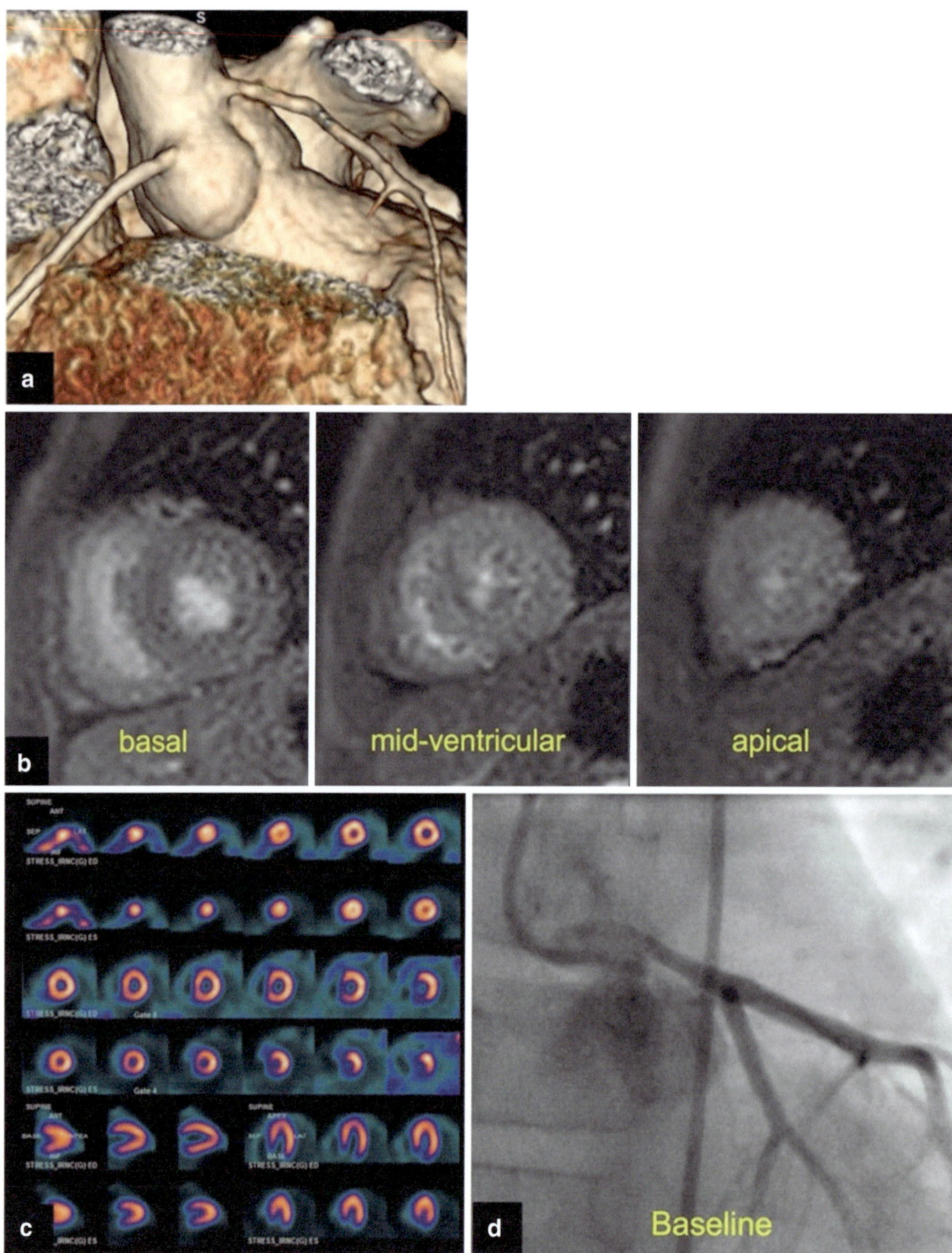

Fig. 12.3 A 9-year-old male with anomalous aortic origin of a left coronary artery (AAOLCA) at the sinotubular junction near the intercoronary commissure on CTA (**a**). Patient had a reassuring maximal exercise stress test, exercise stress echocardiogram, DSCMR (**b**), and nuclear stress perfusion study (**c**). Invasive provocative coronary assessment was recommended due to intermittent exertional chest pain and concern with high-risk anatomy. A selective angiogram confirms the diagnosis without significant coronary artery stenosis (**d**). The proximal LCA becomes severely compressed (red arrowheads) during dobutamine infusion (**e**). Baseline iFR <0.89 indicates significant coronary artery compression (**f**) and iFR is further reduced during dobutamine infusion (**g**). Diastolic FFR <0.8 is consistent with significant coronary flow impairment during provocative testing with dobutamine. *CTA* computed tomography angiography, *DSCMR* dobutamine stress cardiac magnetic resonance imaging, *FFR* fractional flow reserve, *iFR* instantaneous free-wave ration, *LCA* left coronary artery

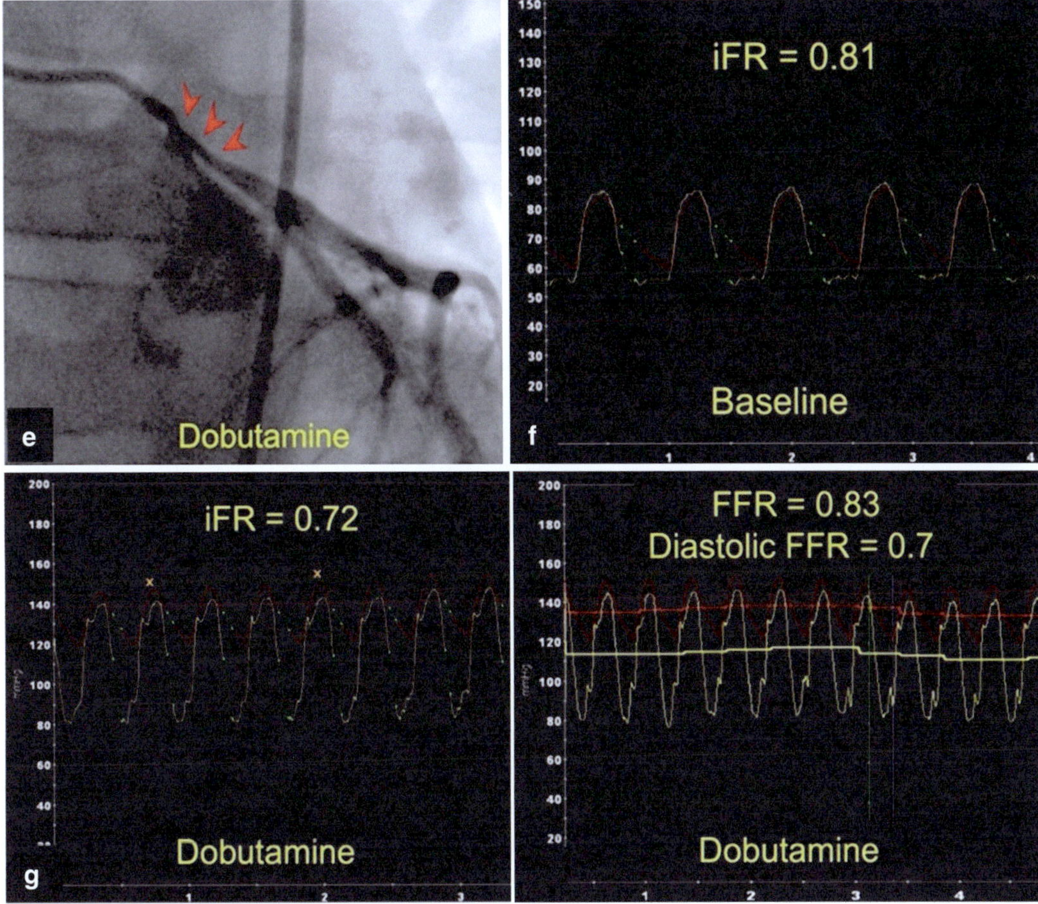

Fig. 12.3 (continued)

Intravascular Ultrasound (IVUS)

Intravascular ultrasound (IVUS) has been vastly used in adults and, in the setting of AAOCA, has been reported as the gold standard for the assessment of intramural segment, as it allows for best spatial determination and of dynamic lateral compression during provocative stress [87–90]. It has also been established in the evaluation of adult patients with typical angina in the setting of MB and absence of obstructive coronary artery disease [91]. In adults with right AAOCA, Angelini et al. used IVUS and demonstrated that the proximal RCA courses inside the aortic wall with the worst stenosis being just distal to the ostium in all patients [87]. IVUS has been performed both at baseline and during provocative testing with a SAD test, which includes 500 ml normal saline infusion over 15 min, atropine, and

dobutamine administration. The maximal and minimal diameters at the most stenotic coronary artery were measured in systole and diastole. An area ratio > 50% at baseline and/or > 60% during a SAD test have been considered significant coronary artery compression [87]. It has also been used to guide stenting in select adults with right AAOCA to attain a circular shape of the proximal intramural RCA to match the distal coronary artery size [87].

IVUS has been utilized in the pediatric population for the evaluation of congenital heart lesions [92], acquired coronary artery disease in the setting of Kawasaki disease [93–95], and in heart transplant patients [95, 96]. However, there is scant data on IVUS performed in children for evaluation of AAOCA and MB. Agrawal et al. reported feasibility and safety of performing IVUS in a small cohort of this patient population

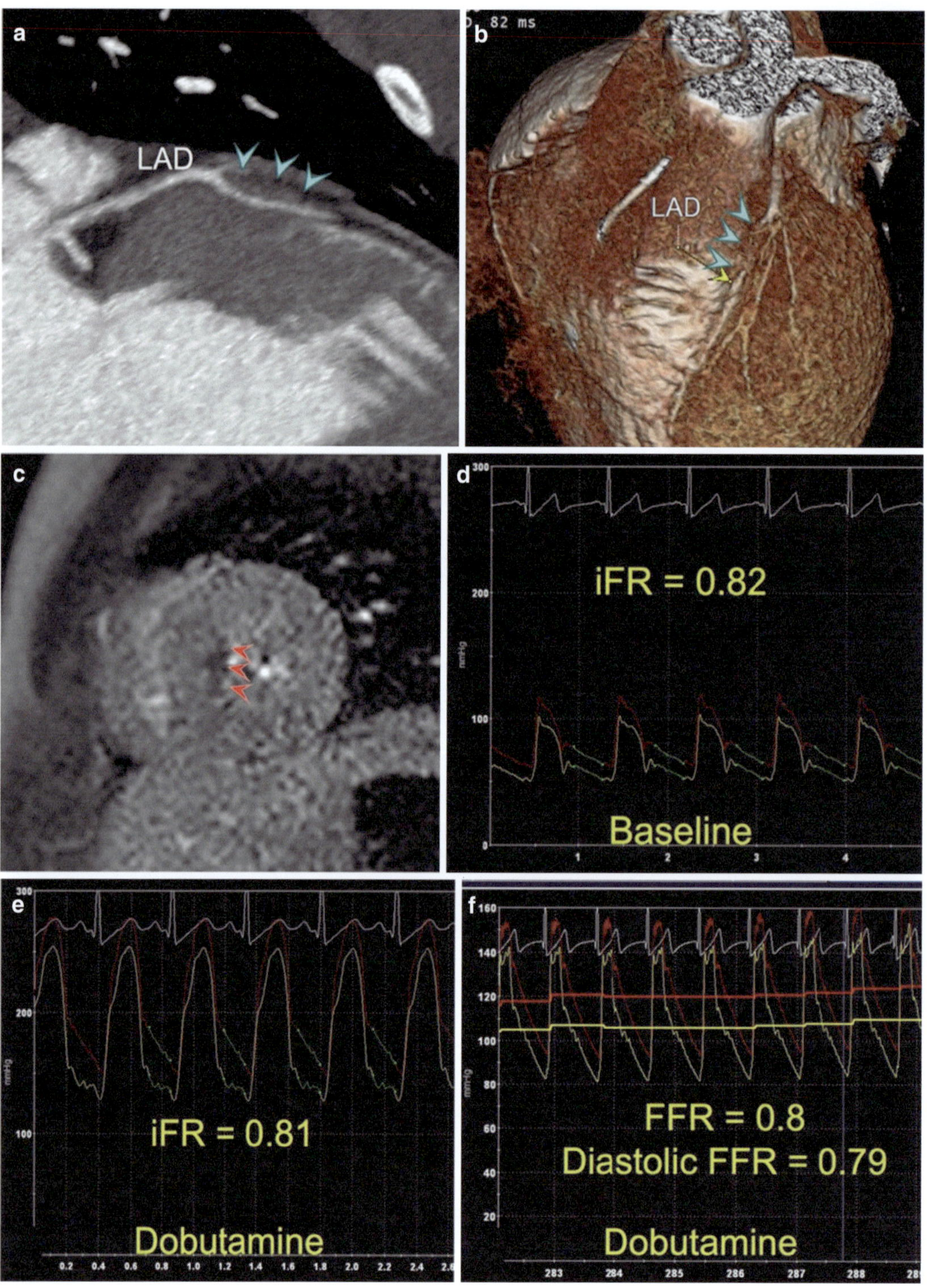

Fig. 12.4 An 11-year-old male was diagnosed with a 16-mm myocardial bridge of the left anterior descending coronary artery on CTA (**a, b**) as a result of an evaluation for exertional chest pain. A maximal exercise stress test was reassuring and a DSCMR showed inducible perfusion defect (**c**). Resting iFR (**d**) and both iFR and diastolic FFR during dobutamine infusion (**e, f**) indicated significant coronary flow impairment. The patient underwent unroof-ing of the myocardial bridge which was successful and followed by an unremarkable DSCMR and normalized iFR and FFR. He has returned to full activities and remains asymptomatic. *CTA* computed tomography angiography, *DSCMR* dobutamine stress cardiac magnetic resonance imaging, *FFR* fractional flow reserve, *iFR* instantaneous free-wave ration, *LAD* left anterior descending coronary artery

and contributing to guide management decision-making [73]. Additional data in larger cohorts of children with AAOCA and MB is needed to ascertain its role in risk stratification in this young population. At this point in time, it does not seem reasonable to justify invasive coronary artery studies in all patients with high-risk anatomy, but certainly should be considered in a small subset of patients in centers with expertise.

Conclusions

Although much remains to be unraveled on the optimal risk stratification in AAOCA and MB, most recent work utilizing non-invasive and invasive testing under provocative stress has been found helpful in the clinical approach of these children as inducible hypoperfusion tends to resolve following a successful intervention. At the same time, it adds more questions as high-risk morphologic features seem to be present in both patients with evidence of inducible myocardial ischemia and those without. The invasive assessment has been used with encouraging results, although remains a challenge in young patients. Exciting new approaches using computational and fluid-structure interaction models in AAOCA are likely to add new knowledge to the pathophysiology as it relates to morphologic features, potentially diminishing the need for invasive coronary artery studies in the young population. Only collaboration among different institutions engaged in gathering data, following outcomes, and sharing knowledge of patients with AAOCA and MB will lead to a better future for those affected by these conditions.

References

1. Molossi S, Mery CM. The search for the holy grail: risk stratification in anomalous aortic origin of a coronary artery. J Thorac Cardiovasc Surg. 2018;155(4):1758–9. https://doi.org/10.1016/j.jtcvs.2017.12.026.
2. Molossi S, Sachdeva S. Anomalous coronary arteries. Curr Opin Cardiol. 2020;35(1):42–51. https://doi.org/10.1097/HCO.0000000000000696.
3. Mery CM, Lawrence SM, Krishnamurthy R, et al. Anomalous aortic origin of a coronary artery: toward a standardized approach. Semin Thorac Cardiovasc Surg. 2014;26(2):110–22. https://doi.org/10.1053/j.semtcvs.2014.08.001.
4. Brothers J, Carter C, McBride M, Spray T, Paridon S. Anomalous left coronary artery origin from the opposite sinus of Valsalva: evidence of intermittent ischemia. J Thorac Cardiovasc Surg. 2010;140(2):e27–9. https://doi.org/10.1016/j.jtcvs.2009.06.029.
5. Schiavone M, Gobbi C, Gasperetti A, Zuffi A, Forleo GB. Congenital coronary artery anomalies and sudden cardiac death. Pediatr Cardiol. 2021;42(8):1676–87. https://doi.org/10.1007/s00246-021-02713-y.
6. Agrawal H, Mery CM, Day PE, et al. Current practices are variable in the evaluation and management of patients with anomalous aortic origin of a coronary artery: results of a survey. Congenit Heart Dis. 2017;12(5):610–4. https://doi.org/10.1111/chd.12511.
7. Rahmouni K, Bernier P-L. Current Management of Anomalous Aortic Origin of a coronary artery: a pan-Canadian survey. World J Pediatr Congenit Hear Surg. 2021;12(3):387–93. https://doi.org/10.1177/2150135121999030.
8. Molossi S, Agrawal H, Mery CM, et al. Outcomes in anomalous aortic origin of a coronary artery following a prospective standardized approach. Circ Cardiovasc Interv. 2020;13(2):e008445. https://doi.org/10.1161/CIRCINTERVENTIONS.119.008445.
9. Mery CM, De León LE, Molossi S, et al. Outcomes of surgical intervention for anomalous aortic origin of a coronary artery: a large contemporary prospective cohort study. J Thorac Cardiovasc Surg. 2018;155(1):305–319.e4. https://doi.org/10.1016/j.jtcvs.2017.08.116.
10. Brothers JA, McBride MG, Seliem MA, et al. Evaluation of myocardial ischemia after surgical repair of anomalous aortic origin of a coronary artery in a series of pediatric patients. J Am Coll Cardiol. 2007;50(21):2078–82. https://doi.org/10.1016/j.jacc.2007.06.055.
11. Sachdeva S, Frommelt MA, Mitchell ME, Tweddell JS, Frommelt PC. Surgical unroofing of intramural anomalous aortic origin of a coronary artery in pediatric patients: single-center perspective. J Thorac Cardiovasc Surg. 2018;155(4):1760–8. https://doi.org/10.1016/j.jtcvs.2017.11.003.
12. Mainwaring RD, Reddy VM, Reinhartz O, Petrossian E, Punn R, Hanley FL. Surgical repair of anomalous aortic origin of a coronary artery. Eur J Cardiothorac Surg. 2014;46(1):20–6. https://doi.org/10.1093/ejcts/ezt614.
13. Tarantini G, Migliore F, Cademartiri F, Fraccaro C, Iliceto S. Left anterior descending artery myocardial bridging: a clinical approach. J Am Coll Cardiol. 2016;68(25):2887–99. https://doi.org/10.1016/j.jacc.2016.09.973.
14. La Grutta L, Runza G, Lo Re G, et al. Prevalenza dei decorsi miocardici e relazione con l'aterosclerosi coronarica studiate mediante angiografia coronarica con TC a 64 strati. Radiol Med. 2009;114(7):1024–36. https://doi.org/10.1007/s11547-009-0446-y.

15. Corban MT, Hung OY, Eshtehardi P, et al. Myocardial bridging: contemporary understanding of pathophysiology with implications for diagnostic and therapeutic strategies. J Am Coll Cardiol. 2014;63(22):2346–55. https://doi.org/10.1016/j.jacc.2014.01.049.

16. Alegria JR, Herrmann J, Holmes DR, Lerman A, Rihal CS. Myocardial bridging. Eur Heart J. 2005;26(12):1159–68. https://doi.org/10.1093/eurheartj/ehi203.

17. Maeda K, Schnittger I, Murphy DJ, et al. Surgical unroofing of hemodynamically significant myocardial bridges in a pediatric population. J Thorac Cardiovasc Surg. 2018;156(4):1618–26. https://doi.org/10.1016/j.jtcvs.2018.01.081.

18. Lorber R, Srivastava S, Wilder TJ, et al. Anomalous aortic origin of coronary arteries in the young echocardiographic evaluation with surgical correlation. JACC Cardiovasc Imaging. 2015;8(11):1239–49. https://doi.org/10.1016/j.jcmg.2015.04.027.

19. Fabozzo A, DiOrio M, Newburger JW, et al. Anomalous aortic origin of coronary arteries: a single-center experience. Semin Thorac Cardiovasc Surg. 2016;28(4):791–800. https://doi.org/10.1053/j.semtcvs.2016.08.012.

20. Doan TT, Molossi S, Sachdeva S, et al. Dobutamine stress cardiac MRI is safe and feasible in pediatric patients with anomalous aortic origin of a coronary artery (AAOCA). Int J Cardiol. 2021;334:42–8. https://doi.org/10.1016/j.ijcard.2021.04.031.

21. Noel C. Cardiac stress MRI evaluation of anomalous aortic origin of a coronary artery. Congenit Heart Dis. 2017;12(5):627–9. https://doi.org/10.1111/chd.12501.

22. Molossi S, Agrawal H. Clinical evaluation of anomalous aortic origin of a coronary artery (AAOCA). Congenit Heart Dis. 2017;12(5):607–9. https://doi.org/10.1111/chd.12505.

23. Doan TT, Zea-Vera R, Agrawal H, et al. Myocardial ischemia in children with anomalous aortic origin of a coronary artery with Intraseptal course. Circ Cardiovasc Interv. 2020;13(3):e008375. https://doi.org/10.1161/CIRCINTERVENTIONS.119.008375.

24. Doan TT, Wilkinson JC, Agrawal H, et al. Instantaneous wave-free ratio (iFR) correlates with fractional flow reserve (FFR) assessment of coronary artery Stenoses and myocardial bridges in children. J Invasive Cardiol. 2020;32(5):176–9; http://www.ncbi.nlm.nih.gov/pubmed/32357130.

25. Cho S-H, Joo H-C, Yoo K-J, Youn Y-N. Anomalous origin of right coronary artery from left coronary sinus: surgical management and clinical result. Thorac Cardiovasc Surg. 2015;63(5):360–6. https://doi.org/10.1055/s-0034-1376256.

26. Basso C, Maron BJ, Corrado D, Thiene G. Clinical profile of congenital coronary artery anomalies with origin from the wrong aortic sinus leading to sudden death in young competitive athletes. J Am Coll Cardiol. 2000;35(6):1493–501. https://doi.org/10.1016/S0735-1097(00)00566-0.

27. Van Hare GF, Ackerman MJ, Evangelista J-AK, et al. Eligibility and disqualification recommendations for competitive athletes with cardiovascular abnormalities: task force 4: congenital heart disease: a scientific statement from the American Heart Association and American College of Cardiology. Circulation. 2015;132(22):e281–91. https://doi.org/10.1161/CIR.0000000000000240.

28. Brothers JA, Frommelt MA, Jaquiss RDB, Myerburg RJ, Fraser CD, Tweddell JS. Expert consensus guidelines: anomalous aortic origin of a coronary artery. J Thorac Cardiovasc Surg. 2017;153(6):1440–57. https://doi.org/10.1016/j.jtcvs.2016.06.066.

29. Qasim A, Doan TT, Pham TD, Reaves-O'Neal DL, Molossi S. Abstract 15075 : exercise stress testing and stress cardiac magnetic resonance imaging for detection of inducible ischemia in a large cohort of children with anomalous aortic origin of a coronary artery. Circulation. 2020;142(suppl_3):A15075. https://doi.org/10.1161/circ.142.suppl_3.15075.

30. Doan TT, Bonilla-ramirez C, Sachdeva S, et al. Abstract 13007 : myocardial ischemia in anomalous aortic origin of a right coronary artery : medium-term follow-up in a large prospective cohort. Circulation. 2020;142(suppl_3):A13007. https://doi.org/10.1161/circ.142.suppl_3.13007.

31. Paridon SM, Alpert BS, Boas SR, et al. Clinical stress testing in the pediatric age group: a statement from the American Heart Association council on cardiovascular disease in the young, committee on atherosclerosis, hypertension, and obesity in youth. Circulation. 2006;113(15):1905–20. https://doi.org/10.1161/CIRCULATIONAHA.106.174375.

32. Pellikka PA, Arruda-Olson A, Chaudhry FA, et al. Guidelines for performance, interpretation, and application of stress echocardiography in ischemic heart disease: from the American Society of Echocardiography. J Am Soc Echocardiogr. 2020;33(1):1–41.e8. https://doi.org/10.1016/j.echo.2019.07.001.

33. Chen MH, Abernathey E, Lunze F, et al. Utility of exercise stress echocardiography in pediatric cardiac transplant recipients: a single-center experience. J Heart Lung Transplant. 2012;31(5):517–23. https://doi.org/10.1016/j.healun.2011.12.014.

34. El Assaad I, Gauvreau K, Rizwan R, Margossian R, Colan S, Chen MH. Value of exercise stress echocardiography in children with hypertrophic cardiomyopathy. J Am Soc Echocardiogr. 2020;33(7):888–894.e2. https://doi.org/10.1016/j.echo.2020.01.020.

35. Badruddin SM, Ahmad A, Mickelson J, et al. Supine bicycle versus post-treadmill exercise echocardiography in the detection of myocardial ischemia: a randomized single-blind crossover trial. J Am Coll Cardiol. 1999;33(6):1485–90. https://doi.org/10.1016/S0735-1097(99)00043-1.

36. Thompson WR. Stress echocardiography in paediatrics: implications for the evaluation of anomalous aortic origin of the coronary arteries. Cardiol Young. 2015;25(8):1524–30. https://doi.org/10.1017/S1047951115002012.

37. Kimball TR. Pediatric stress echocardiography. Pediatr Cardiol. 2002;23(3):347–57. https://doi.org/10.1007/s00246-001-0198-5.

38. Armstrong WF, Zoghbi WA. Stress echocardiography: current methodology and clinical applications. J Am Coll Cardiol. 2005;45(11):1739–47. https://doi.org/10.1016/j.jacc.2004.12.078.

39. Pahl E, Duffy CE, Chaudhry FA. The role of stress echocardiography in children. Echocardiography. 2000;17(5):507–12. https://doi.org/10.1111/j.1540-8175.2000.tb01171.x.

40. Ou P, Kutty S, Khraiche D, Sidi D, Bonnet D. Acquired coronary disease in children: the role of multimodality imaging. Pediatr Radiol. 2013;43(4):444–53. https://doi.org/10.1007/s00247-012-2478-z.

41. Deng ES, O'Brien SE, Fynn-Thompson F, Chen MH. Déjà vu: recurrent sudden cardiac arrests in a child with an anomalous left coronary artery. JACC Case Reports. 2021;3(13):1527–30. https://doi.org/10.1016/j.jaccas.2021.08.015.

42. Lameijer H, Kampman MAM, Oudijk MA, Pieper PG. Ischaemic heart disease during pregnancy or post-partum: systematic review and case series. Neth Hear J. 2015;23(5):249–57. https://doi.org/10.1007/s12471-015-0677-6.

43. Mumtaz MA, Lorber RE, Arruda J, Pettersson GB, Mavroudis C. Surgery for anomalous aortic origin of the coronary artery. Ann Thorac Surg. 2011;91(3):811–5. https://doi.org/10.1016/j.athoracsur.2010.11.002.

44. Agati S, Secinaro A, Caldaroni F, et al. Perfusion study helps in the management of the Intraseptal course of an anomalous coronary artery. World J Pediatr Congenit Hear Surg. 2019;10(3):360–3. https://doi.org/10.1177/2150135119829004.

45. Blomjous MSH, Budde RPJ, Bekker MWA, et al. Clinical outcome of anomalous coronary artery with interarterial course in adults: single-center experience combined with a systematic review. Int J Cardiol. 2021;335:32–9. https://doi.org/10.1016/j.ijcard.2021.04.005.

46. Bonilla-Ramirez C, Molossi S, Sachdeva S, et al. Outcomes in anomalous aortic origin of a coronary artery after surgical reimplantation. J Thorac Cardiovasc Surg. 2021;162(4):1191–9. https://doi.org/10.1016/j.jtcvs.2020.12.100.

47. Hernandez-Pampaloni M, Allada V, Fishbein MC, Schelbert HR. Myocardial perfusion and viability by positron emission tomography in infants and children with coronary abnormalities: correlation with echocardiography, coronary angiography, and histopathology. J Am Coll Cardiol. 2003;41(4):618–26. https://doi.org/10.1016/S0735-1097(02)02867-X.

48. Charoenpanichkit C, Hundley WG. The 20 year evolution of dobutamine stress cardiovascular magnetic resonance. J Cardiovasc Magn Reson. 2010;12(1):59. https://doi.org/10.1186/1532-429X-12-59.

49. Jahnke C, Nagel E, Gebker R, et al. Prognostic value of cardiac magnetic resonance stress tests: adenosine stress perfusion and dobutamine stress wall motion imaging. Circulation. 2007;115(13):1769–76. https://doi.org/10.1161/CIRCULATIONAHA.106.652016.

50. Paetsch I, Jahnke C, Wahl A, et al. Comparison of dobutamine stress magnetic resonance, adenosine stress magnetic resonance, and adenosine stress magnetic resonance perfusion. Circulation. 2004;110(7):835–42. https://doi.org/10.1161/01.CIR.0000138927.00357.FB.

51. Gebker R, Jahnke C, Manka R, et al. Additional value of myocardial perfusion imaging during dobutamine stress magnetic resonance for the assessment of coronary artery disease. Circ Cardiovasc Imaging. 2008;1(2):122–30. https://doi.org/10.1161/CIRCIMAGING.108.779108.

52. Greenwood JP, Maredia N, Younger JF, et al. Cardiovascular magnetic resonance and single-photon emission computed tomography for diagnosis of coronary heart disease (CE-MARC): a prospective trial. Lancet. 2012;379(9814):453–60. https://doi.org/10.1016/S0140-6736(11)61335-4.

53. Schwitter J, Wacker CM, Wilke N, et al. MR-IMPACT II: magnetic resonance imaging for myocardial perfusion assessment in coronary artery disease trial: perfusion-cardiac magnetic resonance vs. single-photon emission computed tomography for the detection of coronary artery disease: a comparative. Eur Heart J. 2013;34(10):775–81. https://doi.org/10.1093/eurheartj/ehs022.

54. Ge Y, Antiochos P, Steel K, et al. Prognostic value of stress CMR perfusion imaging in patients with reduced left ventricular function. JACC Cardiovasc Imaging. 2020;13:2132. https://doi.org/10.1016/j.jcmg.2020.05.034.

55. Wahl A, Paetsch I, Gollesch A, et al. Safety and feasibility of high-dose dobutamine-atropine stress cardiovascular magnetic resonance for diagnosis of myocardial ischaemia: experience in 1000 consecutive cases. Eur Heart J. 2004;25(14):1230–6. https://doi.org/10.1016/j.ehj.2003.11.018.

56. Nagel E, Lehmkuhl HB, Bocksch W, et al. Noninvasive diagnosis of ischemia-induced wall motion abnormalities with the use of high-dose dobutamine stress MRI: comparison with dobutamine stress echocardiography. Circulation. 1999;99(6):763–70. https://doi.org/10.1161/01.CIR.99.6.763.

57. Leong-Poi H, Rim S-J, Le DE, Fisher NG, Wei K, Kaul S. Perfusion versus function: the ischemic cascade in demand ischemia: implications of single-vessel versus multivessel stenosis. Circulation. 2002;105(8):987–92. https://doi.org/10.1161/hc0802.104326.

58. Prakash A, Powell AJ, Krishnamurthy R, Geva T. Magnetic resonance imaging evaluation of myocardial perfusion and viability in congenital and acquired pediatric heart disease. Am J Cardiol. 2004;93(5):657–61. https://doi.org/10.1016/j.amjcard.2003.11.045.

59. Hauser M, Bengel FM, Kühn A, et al. Myocardial blood flow and flow reserve after coronary reimplantation in patients after arterial switch and Ross operation. Circulation. 2001;103(14):1875–80. https://doi.org/10.1161/01.CIR.103.14.1875.

60. Hauser M, Kuehn A, Hess J. Myocardial perfusion in patients with transposition of the great arteries after arterial switch operation. Circulation. 2003;107(18):2001. https://doi.org/10.1161/01.cir.0000071211.20538.25.

61. Secinaro A, Ntsinjana H, Tann O, et al. Cardiovascular magnetic resonance findings in repaired anomalous left coronary artery to pulmonary artery connection (ALCAPA). J Cardiovasc Magn Reson. 2011;13(1):1–6. https://doi.org/10.1186/1532-429X-13-27.

62. Pennell DJ, Sechtem UP, Higgins CB, et al. Clinical indications for cardiovascular magnetic resonance (CMR): consensus panel report. Eur Heart J. 2004;25(21):1940–65. https://doi.org/10.1016/j.ehj.2004.06.040.

63. Paetsch I, Jahnke C, Fleck E, Nagel E. Current clinical applications of stress wall motion analysis with cardiac magnetic resonance imaging. Eur J Echocardiogr. 2005;6(5):317–26. https://doi.org/10.1016/j.euje.2004.12.008.

64. Wilkinson JC, Doan TT, Loar RW, et al. Myocardial stress perfusion MRI using Regadenoson: a weight-based approach in infants and young children. Radiol Cardiothorac Imaging. 2019;1(4):e190061. https://doi.org/10.1148/ryct.2019190061.

65. Doan TT, Wilkinson JC, Loar RW, Pednekar AS, Masand PM, Noel CV. Regadenoson stress perfusion cardiac magnetic resonance imaging in children with Kawasaki disease and coronary artery disease. Am J Cardiol. 2019;124(7):1125–32. https://doi.org/10.1016/j.amjcard.2019.06.033.

66. Strigl S, Beroukhim R, Valente AM, et al. Feasibility of dobutamine stress cardiovascular magnetic resonance imaging in children. J Magn Reson Imaging. 2009;29(2):313–9. https://doi.org/10.1002/jmri.21639.

67. Scannell CM, Hasaneen H, Greil G, et al. Automated quantitative stress perfusion cardiac magnetic resonance in pediatric patients. Front Pediatr. 2021;9(September):1–8. https://doi.org/10.3389/fped.2021.699497.

68. Doan TT, Wilkinson JC, Loar RW, Pednekar AS, Masand PM, Noel CV. Dobutamine stress perfusion cardiac magnetic resonance imaging in children with intramyocardial coronary artery. In: Oral abstract at the 15th annual advanced symposium on pediatric cardiovascular imaging held at Nationwide Children's hospital. Columbus; 2019.

69. Doan TT, Wilkinson JC, Sachdeva S, et al. Dobutamine stress cardiac magnetic resonance imaging in 207 children with coronary artery anomaly. In: Oral abstract at the society for cardiovascular magnetic resonance annual scientific sessions. Orlando, FL; 2020.

70. Doan TT, Molossi S, Qureshi AM, McKenzie ED. Intraseptal anomalous coronary artery with myocardial infarction: novel surgical approach. Ann Thorac Surg. 2020;110(4):e271–4. https://doi.org/10.1016/j.athoracsur.2020.02.076.

71. Agrawal H, Wilkinson JC, Noel CV, et al. Impaired myocardial perfusion on stress CMR correlates with invasive FFR in children with coronary anomalies. J Invasive Cardiol. 2021;33(1):E45–51; http://www.ncbi.nlm.nih.gov/pubmed/33385986.

72. Doan TT, Qureshi AM, Sachdeva S, Noel CV, Reaves-O'Neal D, Molossi S. Beta-blockade in Intraseptal anomalous coronary artery with reversible myocardial ischemia. World J Pediatr Congenit Hear Surg. 2021;12(1):145–8. https://doi.org/10.1177/2150135120954818.

73. Agrawal H, Molossi S, Alam M, et al. Anomalous coronary arteries and myocardial bridges: risk stratification in children using novel cardiac catheterization techniques. Pediatr Cardiol. 2017;38(3):624–30. https://doi.org/10.1007/s00246-016-1559-4.

74. Bigler MR, Ashraf A, Seiler C, et al. Hemodynamic relevance of anomalous coronary arteries originating from the opposite sinus of Valsalva-in search of the evidence. Front Cardiovasc Med. 2021;7(January):591326. https://doi.org/10.3389/fcvm.2020.591326.

75. Vatner SF, McRitchie RJ, Braunwald E. Effects of dobutamine on left ventricular performance, coronary dynamics, and distribution of cardiac output in conscious dogs. J Clin Invest. 1974;53(5):1265–73. https://doi.org/10.1172/JCI107673.

76. Asrress KN, Schuster A, Ali NF, et al. Myocardial haemodynamic responses to dobutamine stress compared to physiological exercise during cardiac magnetic resonance imaging. J Cardiovasc Magn Reson. 2013;15(S1):15–6. https://doi.org/10.1186/1532-429x-15-s1-p16.

77. Bartunek J, Wijns W, Heyndrickx GR, de Bruyne B. Effects of dobutamine on coronary stenosis physiology and morphology: comparison with intracoronary adenosine. Circulation. 1999;100(3):243–9. https://doi.org/10.1161/01.cir.100.3.243.

78. Escaned J, Cortés J, Flores A, et al. Importance of diastolic fractional flow reserve and dobutamine challenge in physiologic assessment of myocardial bridging. J Am Coll Cardiol. 2003;42(2):226–33. https://doi.org/10.1016/S0735-1097(03)00588-6.

79. Sen S, Escaned J, Malik IS, et al. Development and validation of a new adenosine-independent index of stenosis severity from coronary wave–intensity analysis. J Am Coll Cardiol. 2012;59(15):1392–402. https://doi.org/10.1016/j.jacc.2011.11.003.

80. Davies JE, Sen S, Dehbi H-M, et al. Use of the instantaneous wave-free ratio or fractional flow reserve in PCI. N Engl J Med. 2017;376(19):1824–34. https://doi.org/10.1056/NEJMoa1700445.

81. Petraco R, van de Hoef TP, Nijjer S, et al. Baseline instantaneous wave-free ratio as a pressure-only estimation of underlying coronary flow reserve. Circ Cardiovasc Interv. 2014;7(4):492–502. https://doi.org/10.1161/CIRCINTERVENTIONS.113.000926.

82. Götberg M, Christiansen EH, Gudmundsdottir IJ, et al. Instantaneous wave-free ratio versus fractional flow reserve to guide PCI. N Engl J Med.

2017;376(19):1813–23. https://doi.org/10.1056/NEJMoa1616540.

83. Doan TT, Qureshi AM, Gowda S, Sachdeva S, Reaves-O'Neal DL, Molossi SM. Abstract 11876: instantaneous wave-free ratio and fractional flow reserve are helpful in the assessment of anomalous aortic origin of a coronary artery. Circulation. 2021;144(Suppl_1):A11876. https://doi.org/10.1161/circ.144.suppl_1.11876.

84. Tarantini G, Barioli A, Nai Fovino L, et al. Unmasking myocardial bridge-related ischemia by intracoronary functional evaluation. Circ Cardiovasc Interv. 2018;11(6):e006247. https://doi.org/10.1161/CIRCINTERVENTIONS.117.006247.

85. Joanna G, Ann ML, Rukmini K, et al. Physiological evaluation of anomalous aortic origin of coronary arteries and myocardial bridges. J Am Coll Cardiol. 2021;77(18_Supplement_1):514. https://doi.org/10.1016/S0735-1097(21)01873-8.

86. Aleksandric SB, Djordjevic-Đikic AD, Dobric MR, et al. Functional assessment of myocardial bridging with conventional and diastolic fractional flow reserve: vasodilator versus inotropic provocation. J Am Heart Assoc. 2021;10(13):e020597. https://doi.org/10.1161/JAHA.120.020597.

87. Angelini P, Uribe C, Monge J, Tobis JM, Elayda MA, Willerson JT. Origin of the right coronary artery from the opposite sinus of Valsalva in adults: characterization by intravascular ultrasonography at baseline and after stent angioplasty. Catheter Cardiovasc Interv. 2015;86(2):199–208. https://doi.org/10.1002/ccd.26069.

88. Angelini P. Coronary artery anomalies: an entity in search of an identity. Circulation. 2007;115(10):1296–305. https://doi.org/10.1161/CIRCULATIONAHA.106.618082.

89. Angelini P, Velasco JA, Ott D, Khoshnevis GR. Anomalous coronary artery arising from the opposite sinus: descriptive features and pathophysiologic mechanisms, as documented by intravascular ultrasonography. J Invasive Cardiol.

2003;15(9):507–14; http://www.ncbi.nlm.nih.gov/pubmed/12947211.

90. Driesen BW, Warmerdam EG, Sieswerda G-JT, et al. Anomalous coronary artery originating from the opposite sinus of Valsalva (ACAOS), fractional flow reserve- and intravascular ultrasound-guided management in adult patients. Catheter Cardiovasc Interv. 2018;92(1):68–75. https://doi.org/10.1002/ccd.27578.

91. Forsdahl SH, Rogers IS, Schnittger I, et al. Myocardial bridges on coronary computed tomography angiography - correlation with intravascular ultrasound and fractional flow reserve. Circ J. 2017;81(12):1894–900. https://doi.org/10.1253/circj.CJ-17-0284.

92. Heyden CM, Brock JE, Ratnayaka K, Moore JW, El-Said HG. Intravascular ultrasound (IVUS) provides the filling for the Angiogram's crust: benefits of IVUS in pediatric interventional cardiology. J Invasive Cardiol. 2021;33(12):E978–85; http://www.ncbi.nlm.nih.gov/pubmed/34866050.

93. Agrawal H, Qureshi AM. Cardiac catheterization in assessment and treatment of Kawasaki disease in children and adolescents. Child (Basel, Switzerland). 2019;6(2):32. https://doi.org/10.3390/children6020032.

94. Watanabe M, Fukazawa R, Ogawa S, et al. Virtual histology intravascular ultrasound evaluation of coronary artery lesions within 1 year and more than 10 years after the onset of Kawasaki disease. J Cardiol. 2020;75(2):171–6. https://doi.org/10.1016/j.jjcc.2019.06.015.

95. Sugimura T, Kato H, Inoue O, et al. Intravascular ultrasound of coronary arteries in children. Assessment of the wall morphology and the lumen after Kawasaki disease. Circulation. 1994;89(1):258–65. https://doi.org/10.1161/01.cir.89.1.258.

96. Kuhn MA, Jutzy KR, Deming DD, et al. The medium-term findings in coronary arteries by intravascular ultrasound in infants and children after heart transplantation. J Am Coll Cardiol. 2000;36(1):250–4. https://doi.org/10.1016/s0735-1097(00)00701-4.

Massimiliano Bianco, Vincenzo Palmieri,
and Paolo Zeppilli

Introduction

The anomalous aortic origin of a coronary artery (AAOCA) is a challenging topic, due to its rarity, the complexity of the pathophysiological aspects, the clinical presentation (often completely silent), the difficulty of diagnosis, and, at the same time, the potential risk of causing acute cardiovascular events up to sudden cardiac death (SCD) [1–3].

The topic becomes even more challenging if we move it to the athletic setting. Nowadays, sports practice is recommended at all ages, for healthy people and for a wide range of pathological conditions, so that an increasing portion of the population practices recreational sport. In addition, a top-level athlete is a new hero of the modern era and when he or she suffers a sport-related SCD, the individual and family drama becomes a social tragedy.

Unfortunately, clinical cardiologists are often unaware of this entity, yet. About 15 years ago,

one of the leading experts on this topic, prof. Paolo Angelini, wrote that "especially in the context of sporting or military activities, cardiologists should undergo specific training in these disorders" [2], pointing out the need to increase the knowledge on this condition, on diagnostic workup and risk assessment.

AAOCAs are a rare, heterogeneous group of malformations, isolated or associated with other congenital cardiac defects. Their prevalence in the general population (autopsy and retrospective coronary angiography studies) is around 1–2% [4, 5], even if in a prospective study conducted with precise criteria and a rigorous classification, Angelini et al. reported a fairly higher prevalence of 5.6% [6]. We can explain these apparent discrepancies by the different methods used and the fact that from the anatomical point of view defining what is "normal" or "abnormal" in the coronary tree may be difficult.

A recent prospective study on a screening program designed to identify high-risk cardiac conditions in schoolchildren using rest ECG and cardiac magnetic resonance imaging (MRI) found out that the 0.45% of the population screened had interarterial AAOCA, with 0.33% interarterial anomalous origin of right coronary artery (AAORCA) [7].

Regarding the relationship between these disorders and physical activity and sport is now widely demonstrated as some subtypes of AAOCA have a significant risk of SCD during

---

This chapter is dedicated to Salvatore Francesco Gervasi, a brilliant doctor and scientist who was taken away from his family, friends and colleagues too early

---

M. Bianco · V. Palmieri · P. Zeppilli (✉)
Sports Medicine Unit, Fondazione Policlinico Universitario A. Gemelli IRCCS - Catholic University, Rome, Italy
e-mail: massimiliano.bianco@unicatt.it;
vincenzo.palmieri@unicatt.it;
paolo.zeppilli@unicatt.it

© Springer Nature Switzerland AG 2023
G. Butera, A. Frigiola (eds.), *Congenital Anomalies of Coronary Arteries*,
https://doi.org/10.1007/978-3-031-36966-7_13

heavy exercise. Corrado et al., in a milestone of the sports medical literature, showed that the relative risk for an SCD is actually 79-fold higher in people with malignant AAOCA during strenuous exercise than at rest [8].

Before addressing the issues of this chapter, we believe it is important to define what we will focus on, that is only the AAOCAs arising from the "inappropriate," opposite, coronary sinus. Moreover, as the course of the anomalous vessel definitely impacts on the risk of SCD, we will focus only on AAOCA from the opposite sinus of Valsalva with *an interarterial course/intramural course*, being this feature considered as more malignant. Initially, some authors [1] attributed particular relevance to the hypothesis that the anomalous artery was compressed between the aorta and pulmonary trunk ("sandwich effect") during exercises with increasing cardiac output and blood pressure. Other mechanisms were proposed to explain "ischemia" as an acute angle take-off of the anomalous artery with functional closure of a slit-like orifice, sometimes with an ostial ridge and additional factors as the length, caliber, and position of the anomalous vessel in respect to the intercommissural pillar (above, under, or crossing it).

More recently, the greatest importance was attributed to *the intramural course* of the anomalous artery, especially its first tract, which, being inside the aortic wall, would be compressed (obliterated) by the expansion of the aortic itself during systole [9, 10]. All these features may explain why patients with apparently similar anatomy can have different clinical profiles and risk [1, 2, 11, 12].

Based on the now extensive literature, the anomalous aortic origin of the left coronary artery (AAOLCA) with interarterial/intramural course seems to bring the higher risk of adverse events [1, 13–17]. Other anomalies, such as a coronary artery arising from a "wrong" sinus but traveling anterior to the pulmonary artery (prepulmonic) or posterior to the aorta (posterior/retroaortic), are generally considered benign [18]. The same is deemed valid for the anomalous origin of left common trunk or the left anterior descending coronary artery alone from the inappropriate sinus running through the conal septum (intraseptal, intraconal, or intramyocardial) [12], although not all authors agree and its "absolute" benignity is still debated [19]. Finally, authors have a substantial agreement on the benign prognosis, in young people and also in athletes, of the anomalous origin of the circumflex artery from the right sinus of Valsalva or from the right coronary artery with retroaortic course [1–5, 20, 21].

Before continuing in the chapter, a last important aspect concerns the terminology to be used in the sporting context to avoid some confusion. In the following, we will define below *competitive athletes* as individuals of school age and above ($\geq$12 years of age) who regularly practice physical activity and participate in official competitions organized by a recognized Sports Federation or Association. Competitive and even more *professional* athletes place a high value on athletic excellence and typically they train at least 8–10 h per week with high exercise intensities. In contrast, we define *recreational athletes,* individuals who engage in recreational or leisure-time sports activities on a regular or intermittent basis. Usually, they train much less and do not have the pursuit of excellence as their main purpose [22].

How To Detect?

There is not a typical way of presentation for patients with AAOCA. In some cases, the first and unique presentation is, unfortunately, aborted or true SCD. In a significant number of cases, usually asymptomatic, the coronary anomaly is discovered incidentally on a transthoracic echocardiogram (TTE) or a computed tomography angiogram (CTA) that is performed for another reason, such as a heart murmur or an abnormal electrocardiogram (ECG). Finally, there are cases in which the coronary anomaly is identified by TTE, required to investigate unclear symptoms related to physical exercise (see below), and performed by cardiologists with specific experience in visualizing the coronary arteries.

Moving from our first reports in the late 1980 s [23], with some difficulties in being accepted internationally [24] and some "skepticism" by clinical cardiologists of our country, an increasing body of literature now confirms that TTE is a useful, reliable method for noninvasive in vivo detection of these anomalies, especially in young athletes, usually with training bradycardia and good acoustic windows [25–32]. However, systematic TTE-screening of all asymptomatic athletes is neither advisable nor feasible. Instead, it is time to encourage all cardiologists who perform a TTE in an athlete for whatever reason explore coronary anatomy as much as possible to verify the correct position of the ostia in and of the first tracts of the right and left coronary artery in their "appropriate" sinuses. Obviously, the echocardiographic visualization of a correct positioning of the ostia and first tracts of the coronary arteries becomes "strongly recommended" in athletes with abnormal rest and/or stress test ECG, and/or symptomatic for chest pain/discomfort or syncope on effort, or less specific symptoms as palpitations, dizziness, and breathlessness. In our experience, a not uncommon clinical presentation is the appearance of one or more episodes of cold sweating and/or presyncope during or shortly after effort. In this context, the sports physicians should make a specific request for the search of ostia and first tracts of coronary arteries and TTE should be done by personnel with specific training and expertise in visualizing coronary arteries [2, 29]. At this scope, the Color Doppler imaging may be very helpful in detecting the proximal route of coronary vessels after adequate adjustments of color flow velocity scale (Figs. 13.1, 13.2 and 13.3). In case of TTE suspicion of an AAOCA, additional imaging studies, such as cardiac MRI [7, 12, 33] and coronary CTA [34–36] are reasonable to better visualize the coronary artery anatomy and to confirm the diagnosis, with the former being the choice modality in children, to avoid radiation exposure.

This diagnostic algorithm, improved over time, allowed us to publish in 2018 a series of 23 live athletes with AAOCA (17 AAORCAs) [29] that have grown to 48 (overall, 33 AAORCAs, 13 AAOLCAs, and 2 single coronary arteries) at the time of writing this chapter. To these, we must add another 19 athletes with anomalous origin of the circumflex artery from the right sinus and 49 with myocardial bridge on the left descending artery.

When imaging studies confirm an AAOCA, a stress test should be conducted first to evaluate the presence of ischemic ECG changes, that is, mainly ST segment depression, and/or the occurrence of arrhythmias. However, rest ECG is usually normal [37], and signs of myocardial ischemia at stress testing are present only in one-third to half of cases [1, 29, 38, 39]. Other stress testing modalities include stress echocardiography (both physical or pharmacological), stress Nuclear Perfusion Imaging (NPI), MRI under pharmacological stress (adenosine or dobutamine), but all of them, over time, have frustrated clinicians by producing both low numbers of true-positive and relatively high numbers of false-positive results [40, 41].

In particular, stress NPI studies are limited by lower spatial resolution for small defects, attenuation artifacts related to the body wall and diaphragm, relatively high incidence of false-positive findings [42, 43] and potentially harmful effects of ionizing radiations. A promising minimally invasive tool seems to be the stress MRI (aside from its role in confirming the diagnosis of AAOCA as an alternative to coronary CTA [7, 12, 33]. MRI may show at rest the presence of myocardial scars as late gadolinium enhancement areas (with ischemic patterns) and, during pharmacological stress, may detect wall motion anomalies in the territory of the anomalous coronary artery. This test has proved to be more accurate than stress echocardiography and has been used both in adults (mainly in coronary artery disease patients) and children [42–47].

However, all the modalities of pharmacological stress test increase heart rate (HR) and myocardial contractility through a mechanism other than the physiological one (physical exercise) and do not allow to reach HR as high as those achieved during sports (a young soccer player can easily reach HR above 170–180 beats per minute!). This eventually may lead to a possible underestimation of real myocardial ischemia [48]. In a recent paper, Doan et al.

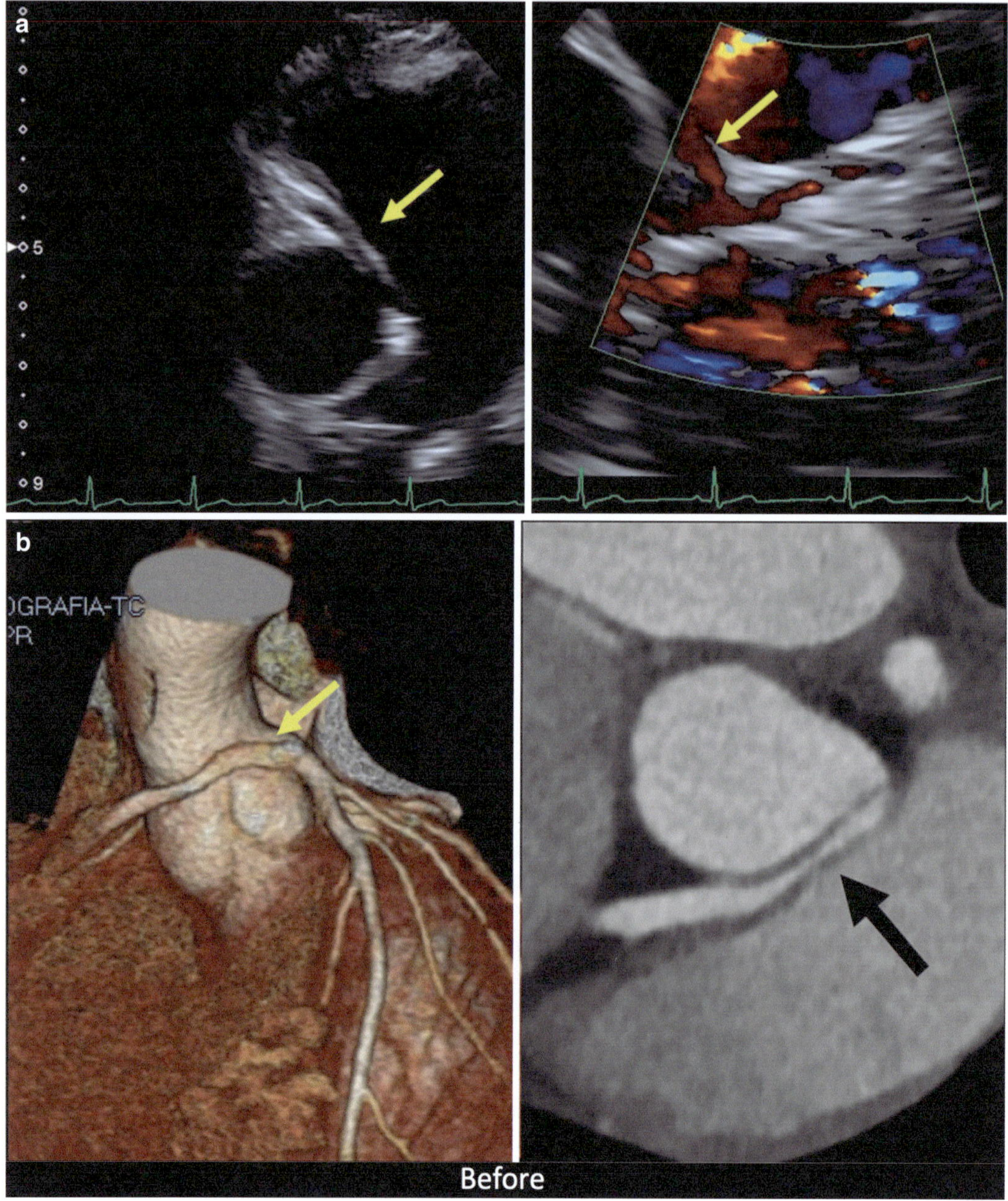

Fig. 13.1 A 13-year-old soccer player, male, with AAORCA, complaining chest discomfort and presyncope during heavy exercise. (**a**) Two-dimensional transthoracic echocardiography (off-axis view derived from the parasternal short-axis view of the aortic valve) showing the anomalous origin of the right coronary artery from the left sinus of Valsalva. The low-scale color-Doppler imaging confirmed the anomalous coronary flow. (**b**) Coronary CT-angiography (CTA) confirmed the diagnosis and helped to define the anatomical details of the anomaly. (**c**) Echocardiographic control after the surgical intervention of unroofing plus the application of a pericardial patch (Vouhé technique), showing optimal surgical results with visible and patent "new" right coronary ostium in the right sinus of Valsalva. (**d**) CTA performed after surgery confirmed these findings. (**e, f**) Cardiopulmonary exercise testing performed after surgery showed brilliant exercise tolerance and normality of all the parameters analyzed

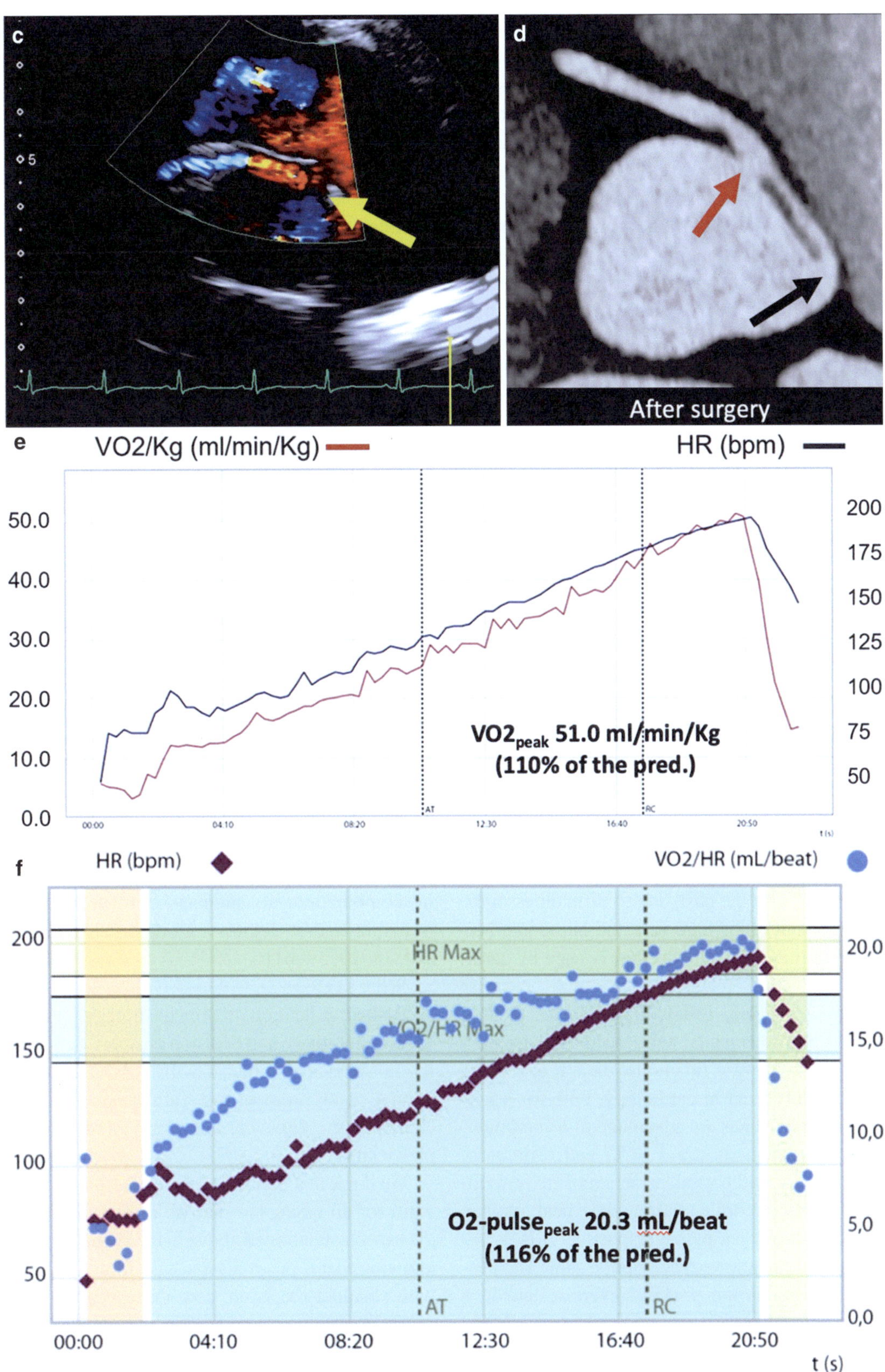

Fig. 13.1 (continued)

used dobutamine stress MRI (when needed with atropine adjunct) in a group of children with AAOCA and only in 12.1% of cases, the HR was ≥85% of their expected maximum, that, in our opinion, should be the minimum target for evaluating an athlete usually engaged in heavy physical exertion. Moreover, the higher the HR, the higher are the difficulties in interpreting the imaging results. In the same study, indeed, the authors confirmed that "at HRs >85% of age-predicted maximum there was a slight shift of the cine sequences' quality from good to adequate; however, both temporal and in-plane resolution were of diagnostic quality for interpretation" [49].

A possible alternative to stress testing is stress echocardiography [50, 51], however with all the limitations reported above for pharmacological stress. Moreover, in case of physical stress during TTE, even if the reached HR is usually higher than the one reached under pharmacological stimulus, it is lower than the HRs reached in standing positions. The adjunct of methodological difficulties in performing a TTE under physical stress (kind of ergometer, body position and movement, data interpretation, hyperventilation, sweating, pediatric patient's compliance, etc.) makes this diagnostic modality poorly used.

A long-known functional test that is returning to the attention is the cardiopulmonary exercise test (CPET). In the past, due to difficulties in the management of the hardware and in the interpretation of the results, it was poorly used by cardiologists and relegated in the exercise physiologists' lab. Today, thanks to the technological improvements and more user-friendly software to analyze functional data, it is starting to be widely used in cardiology, both for adults and children. It has the advantage of a contemporary assessment of stress ECG and respiratory gas analysis, without radiation exposure, providing indexes of cardiac output (i.e., peak oxygen uptake and oxygen pulse, respectively) [52–54]. Importantly, it allows reaching the same HR usually reached during physical exercise and in a more physiological way (Figs. 13.1, 13.2 and 13.3). In our experience, CPET has proved to be

of great utility both in the preoperative diagnosis and risk assessment, and in the rehabilitation and return to sport after any surgical correction (see below).

Finally, after an AAOCA in an athlete has been diagnosed, basically based on some anatomical features of the anomalous vessel and/or ischemic changes during stress or functional test, a cardiac catheterization should be performed with some very experienced authors proposing, during this procedure, a routine intravascular ultrasonography evaluation (IVUS) of the anomalous artery for a more precise risk assessment [55]. In the cath lab (or even during CTA), the evaluation of the fractional flow reserve (FFR) or instantaneous wave-free ratio (iFR) may be helpful in providing a functional stenosis of the anomalous artery [56–58] and in leading the treatment strategy.

Thus, all these imaging modalities, with crucial role of coronary CTA, are fundamental tools for the risk assessment of athletes with AAOCA. The presence of ostial stenosis in association with an oblique take-off from the aorta, ostial ridge, anomalous tract hypoplasia (Fig. 13.2b and 13.2d), intussusception, noncompliant pericommissural area, and compression of the anomalous coronary artery intramurally and/or between the great arteries and, in adults, coexistence of atherosclerotic coronary artery disease (Fig. 13.4) seem to be key factors, acting alone or in combination, to predispose to myocardial ischemia and/or lethal ventricular arrhythmias [10, 18, 29, 59–61].

What to Do?

Risk-stratification, treatment strategy (surgery vs. conservative), and decision on sport's eligibility in sedentary subjects with AAOCA, recreational and competitive athletes, are still challenging for cardiologists and sports physicians.

We think that there is no standardized protocol valid for all cases, but that we must evaluate all the aspects mentioned above in the single subject, knowing that it is not always easy to define them with absolute precision, considering the kind of AAOCA and the presence of symptoms or signs of myocardial ischemia at rest and mostly during functional tests. In addition, we must bear in mind that heavy exercise may trigger totally unexpected SCD [8], which is probably the end result of repeated bursts of exercise-induced acute myocardial ischemia, leading to cumulative myocardial damage, especially in AAOLCA though cases of SCD or resuscitated cardiac arrest during exercise are reported also in subjects with AAORCA [1, 2, 11, 62, 63].

Following current guidelines, individuals with AAOCA and symptoms of ischemic chest pain/discomfort, syncope suspected to be due to

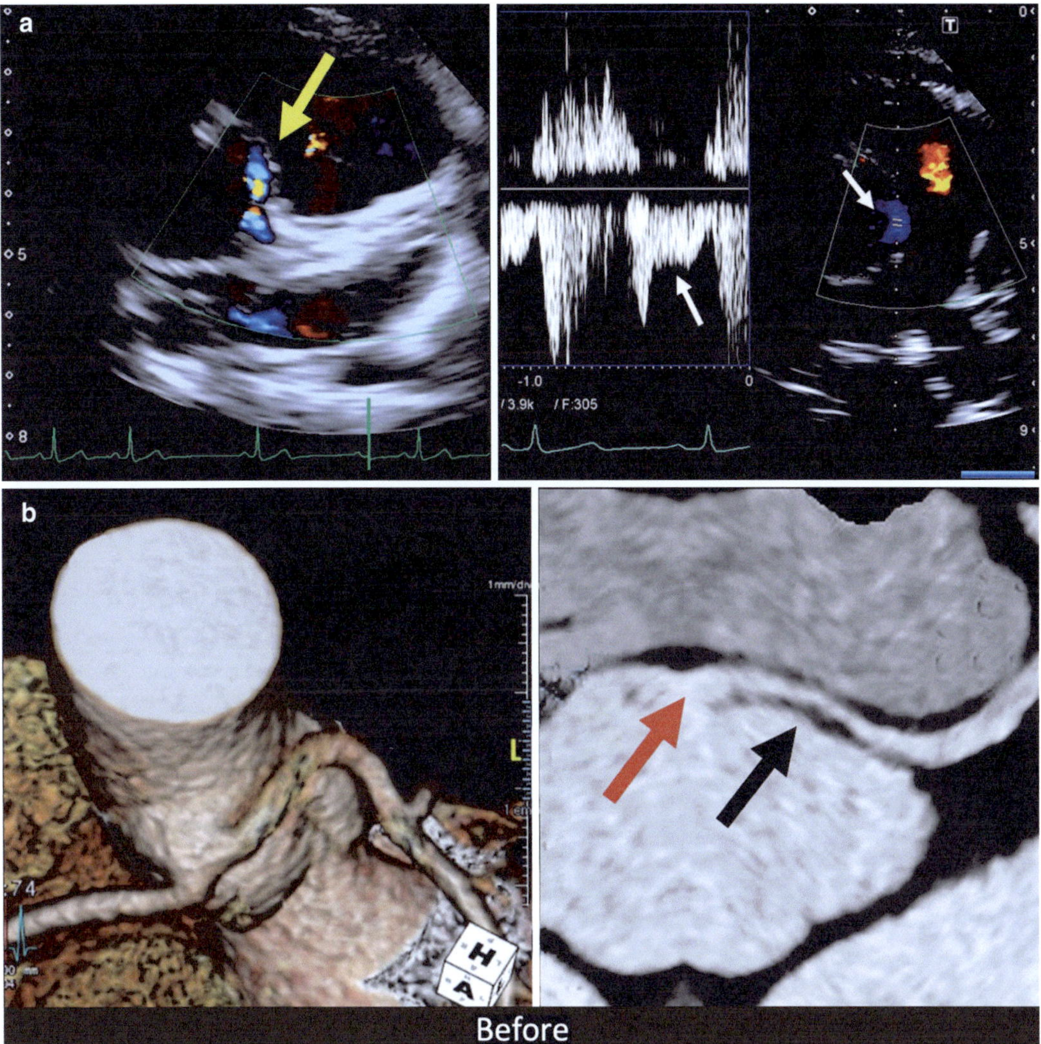

Fig. 13.2 A 13-year-old figure-skater, female, complaining dyspnea, chest discomfortm and presyncope on exertion. (**a**) Two-dimensional transthoracic echocardiography (off-axis view derived from the parasternal short-axis view of the aortic valve) showing the anomalous origin of the left coronary artery from the right sinus of Valsalva. The low-scale color-Doppler imaging confirmed the anomalous coronary flow. (**b**) Coronary CT-angiography (CTA) confirmed the diagnosis and helped to define the anatomical details of the anomaly. (**c**) Echocardiographic control after the surgical intervention of unroofing, showing apparently good surgical results with visible and patent "new" left coronary ostium in the left sinus of Valsalva. (**d**) The CTA performed after surgery revealed the persistence of a partial interarterial course and of mild proximal hypoplasia. (**e, f**) Cardiopulmonary exercise testing performed after surgery showed poor exercise tolerance, reduced $VO2/Kg_{peak}$ and $O2$-pulse$_{peak}$ values, and an early flattening of the $O2$-pulse trajectory

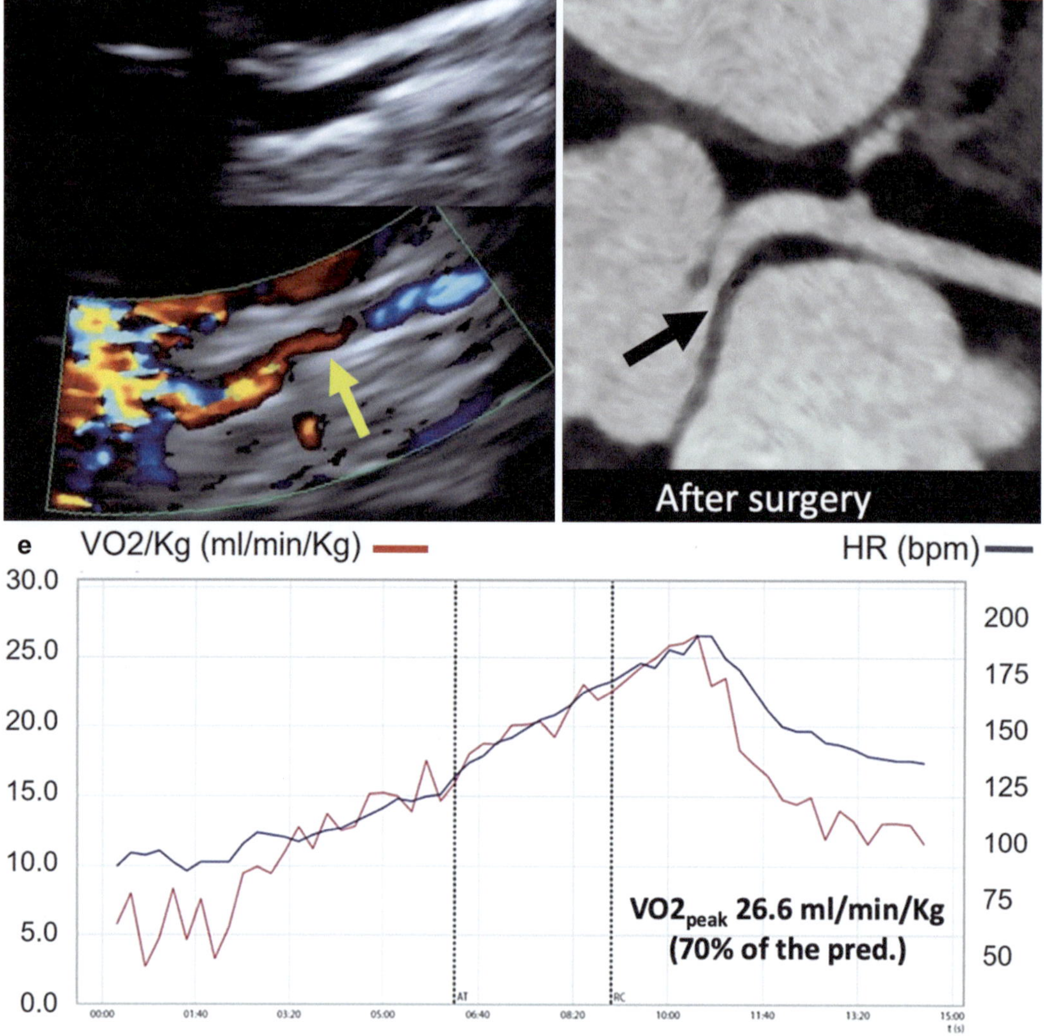

Fig. 13.2 (continued)

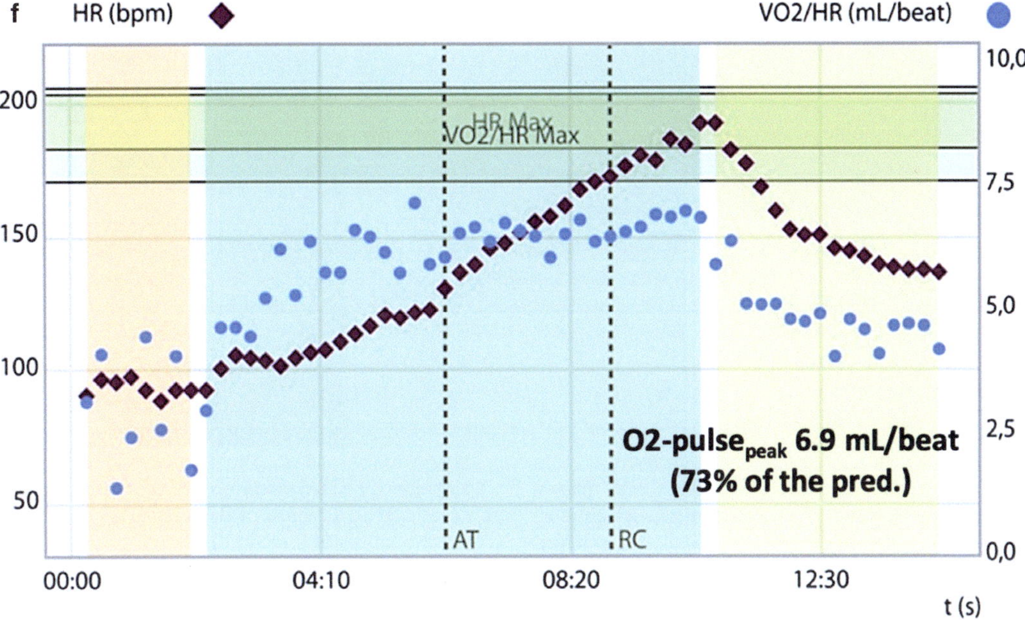

Fig. 13.2 (continued)

life-threatening ventricular arrhythmias, or a history of aborted SCD, should be restricted from participation in all sports and offered surgery [39, 60, 64–73]. Typical cases are showed in Figs. 13.1 and 13.2. The same option should be offered to athletes with an AAOLCA with an interarterial/intramural course even if asymptomatic and without any sign of myocardial ischemia at stress tests [60, 64–67, 72]. Surgery for this kind of anomalies should eliminate the intramural course and any associated ostial narrowing by unroofing, ostioplasty, or reimplantation (look, for comparison, at the surgery and functional results in Figs. 13.1 and 13.2). Repositioning of the pulmonary artery confluence away from the anomalous artery (laterally or anteriorly) may be considered as an adjunctive procedure to the previous, as it is no longer used as the only procedure in the treatment of these anomalies [71, 73–77]. In the uncommon case where surgery is not feasible, a catheter-based intervention may be considered [18]. If the athlete should refuse surgery, total exercise restriction and beta-blocking therapy seem to be the only alternative.

More problematic is the approach to athletes with AAORCA, who are generally considered to have a lower risk of SCD than individuals with AAOLCA. However, the risk exists and can't be properly quantified only based on the presence/absence of symptoms or functional testing [1, 2, 11, 13, 62, 63]. As stated above, stress NPI or MRI may have a role, but, in the general and our opinion, they suffer from important limitations, especially in pediatric patients [2, 17, 29, 78–80]. New techniques in functional assessment of inducible myocardial ischemia (i.e., FFR during coronary angiography or even CTA and iFR) [56–58] can probably open new perspectives, but conclusive evidence is still lacking.

For these reasons, we believe that risk-stratification, before and after surgery, should be multiparametric and include all available elements. Anatomical features of the anomalous artery, that is, morphology of the ostium and take-off angle, length of intra-arterial/intramural segment, and significant reduction of lumen area ("hypoplasia"), are probably crucial in making one subject "at risk" or not, but we still do not know exactly what is the specific weight of each of them. For this reason, we use to adopt a restrictive approach also for competitive athletes with AAORCA with an interarterial/intramural course,

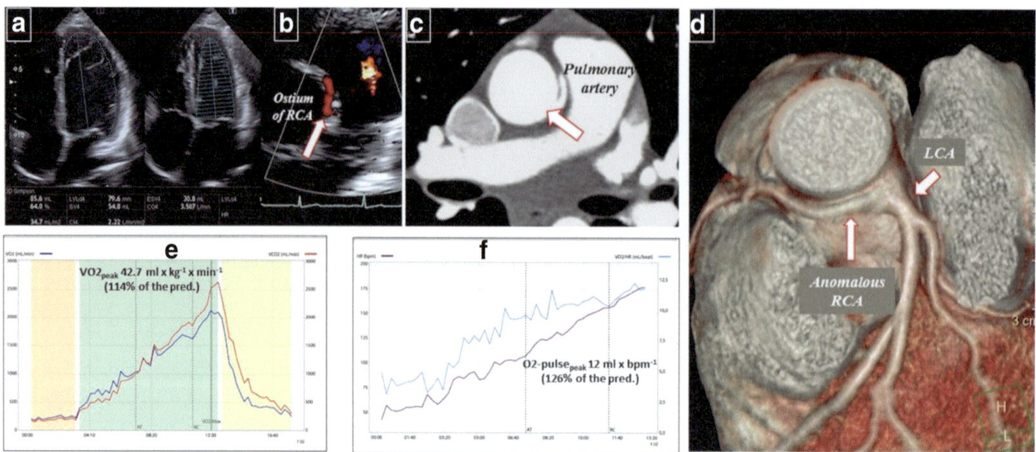

Fig. 13.3 A 22-year-old professional soccer player, female, asymptomatic. (**a**) Routine two-dimensional transthoracic echocardiography, as mandated by Italian rules for professional soccer players, shows a normal heart but (**b**) the presence of the right coronary ostium in the left sinus of Valsalva, with the anomalous tract coursing between aorta and pulmonary artery. (**c**) Coronary CT-angiography (CTA) confirmed the diagnosis, showing an intra-adventitial course of the anomalous vessel. (**d**) CTA three-dimensional reconstruction of coronary arteries. (**e**, **f**) Despite this incidental finding, the cardiopulmonary exercise testing and stress electrocardiogram (not shown) were completely normal. *RCA* right coronary artery, *LCA* left coronary artery

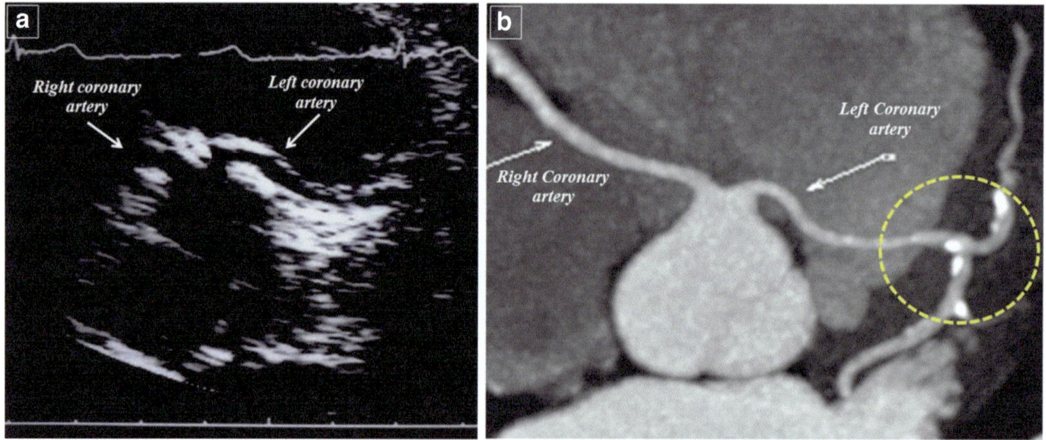

Fig. 13.4 A Long-distance master runner, male, referred to our centre for exercise-induced left bundle branch block. (**a**) At the age of 47, two-dimensional transthoracic echocardiography (TTE) showed a unique ostium in the right sinus of Valsalva originating from both the right and the left coronary arteries. The left coronary artery (LCA) had an interarterial/intramural course (TTE was executed in 1996 and this case was one of the first three published in 1998, see ref. [24]). (**b**) Eight years later, at the age of 55, Coronary CT, which in the meantime became available in our hospital, confirmed the diagnosis, also showing atherosclerotic plaques in the LCA (dashed circle)

disqualifying them from sport, although we admit that Italian law, which attributes legal responsibility to sports physicians, partially influences our behavior.

Anyhow, on the basis of our experience and literature data, we think that surgical treatment of AAORCA with interarterial/intramural course should ever be considered in case of (a) symptoms during or immediately after exertion (Figs. 13.1 and 13.2); (b) positive stress-tests for ischemia; (c) presence of an intramural proximal segment and/or critical reduction of lumen area (Figs. 13.1, 13.2 and 13.3). In other cases, exercise restriction, allowing however moderate recreational physical activity and a medical therapy (beta-blocking), seems safe enough even if beta-blocking therapy is not supported by evidence yet [18]. Nevertheless, in our series with conservative management and beta-blocking therapy (updated since our publication) [29], no athlete had recurrence of symptoms or major cardiac events during an average follow-up of 64 months. However, for these subjects and for those who refuse surgery, more specific counseling concerning the risk of SCD is always mandatory and it should be undertaken with both the athlete and family.

When to Allow Coming Back to Sport After SUGERY

Decision about returning to recreational high-intensity or competitive sports after surgery requires careful evaluation. Different surgical techniques do not have the same results in removing potential mechanisms that might cause ischemia. Currently, the "unroofing procedure" seems the most used and the more effective in most cases [63, 69, 73, 81–83], but it can have sequelae and it is not always feasible. Furthermore, in some cases, surgery can only partially resolve the problem [15]. To our knowledge, just a few cases of exercise SCD after surgery have been reported [15, 79], even if some authors have news of other pediatric deaths postoperatively, that have not been published [18]. It is interesting to note that, at least in the young, if a patient presents with resuscitated SCD and survives the surgery, he or she may still be at increased risk for an SCD when returning to sport [79].

Those who have undergone surgery will need close follow-up in the initial postoperative period: first resting ECG and TTE at 7–10 days from surgery, then at 4–6 weeks with the first functional test at 3 months. If the first controls give favorable results, after the first year from intervention the interval between medical checks can be prolonged [18]. According to the recent North American guidelines, these patients may return even to competitive sports at least 3 months postoperatively if an exercise stress test reveals no evidence of myocardial ischemia or ventricular arrhythmias [18, 72, 84]. Regarding patients who experienced an aborted SCD, it is recommended that they do not return to competitive sport for at least 1 year postoperatively if they are fully asymptomatic and have a negative exercise stress test [18].

However, all these recommendations come from experts' consensus papers, with a relatively low level of evidence [18, 72, 84]. Honestly speaking, we lack long-term follow-up of patients and athletes after surgical repair. Short- and medium-term results are encouraging; however, there are reports of issues, such as new aortic valve regurgitation that will need to be followed over time [18].

In our opinion, we can consider *return to recreational high-intensity or competitive sport* after surgery only if (a) surgery removed all mechanisms potentially responsible for exercise-induced ischemia (Figs. 13.1 and 13.3); (b) no symptoms/signs of inducible myocardial ischemia and/or significant arrhythmias or sequelae are present at least 6 months after the procedure. For this purpose, we recommend an accurate "postsurgery protocol" including at least TTE, stress test ECG (we suggest a CPET), and CT/MRI (preferably both) to evaluate the new anatomy and function of the operated coronary artery [15].

After return to competitive sport, we recommend ECG, TTE, and stress test follow-up every 6 months for the first 3 years from surgery, with Holter monitoring when needed. After this period, the time interval may be prolonged to 1 year if no alterations have been encountered over time.

In all operated cases, however, we recommend that an automated external defibrillator with trained personnel should be immediately available during competition and training, even if this should be the rule in modern sporting setting [85, 86].

Finally, those managed conservatively with exercise restriction will need follow-up annually [18, 87–89].

References

1. Basso C, Maron BJ, Corrado D, Thiene G. Clinical profile of congenital coronary artery anomalies with origin from the wrong aortic sinus leading to sudden death in young competitive athletes. J Am Coll Cardiol. 2000;35(6):1493–501.
2. Angelini P. Coronary artery anomalies: an entity in search of an identity. Circulation. 2007;115(10):1296–305.
3. Pérez-Pomares LM, de la Pompa JL, Franco D, Henderson D, Ho SY, Houyel L, Kelly RG, Sedmera D, Sheppard M, Sperling S, Thiene G, van den Hoff M, Basso C. Congenital coronary artery anomalies: a bridge from embryology to anatomy and pathophysiology—a position statement of the development, anatomy, and pathology ESC working group. Cardiovasc Res. 2016;109(2):204–16.
4. Yamanaka O, Hobbs RE. Coronary artery anomalies in 126.595 patients undergoing coronary arteriography. Catheter Cardiovasc Diagn. 1990;21:28.
5. Yuksel S, Meric M, Soylu K, Gulel O, Zengin H, Demircan S, et al. The primary anomalies of coronary artery origin and course: a coronary angiographic analysis of 16,573 patients. Exp Clin Cardiol. 2013;18(2):121–3.
6. Angelini P, Velasco JA, Flamm S. Coronary anomalies: incidence, pathophysiology, and clinical relevance. Circulation. 2002;105:2449.
7. Angelini P, Cheong BY, Lenge De Rosen VV, Lopez A, Uribe C, Masso AH, Ali SW, Davis BR, Muthupillai R, Willerson JT. High-risk cardiovascular conditions in sports-related sudden death: prevalence in 5,169 schoolchildren screened via cardiac magnetic resonance. Tex Heart Inst J. 2018;45(4):205–13.
8. Corrado D, Basso C, Rizzoli G, Schiavon M, Thiene G. Does sports activity enhance the risk of sudden death in adolescents and young adults? J Am Coll Cardiol. 2003;42(11):1959–63.
9. Angelini P. Novel imaging of coronary artery anomalies to assess their prevalence, the causes of clinical symptoms, and the risk of sudden cardiac death. Circ Cardiovasc Imaging. 2014;7:747–54.
10. Lo Rito M, Romarowski RM, Rosato A, Pica S, Secchi F, Giamberti A, Auricchio F, Frigiola A, Conti M. Anomalous aortic origin of coronary artery biomechanical modeling: toward clinical application. J Thorac Cardiovasc Surg. 2020;S0022-5223(20):32430–2.
11. Frescura C, Basso C, Thiene G, et al. Anomalous origin of coronary arteries and risk of sudden death: a study based on an autopsy population of congenital heart disease. Hum Pathol. 1998;29(7):689–95.
12. Brothers JA, Whitehead KK, Keller MS, Fogel MA, Paridon SM, Weinberg PM, Harris MA. Cardiac MRI and CT: differentiation of normal ostium and intraseptal course from slitlike ostium and interarterial course in anomalous left coronary artery in children. AJR Am J Roentgenol. 2015;204(1):W104–9.
13. Maron BJ, Doerer JJ, Haas TS, Tierney DM, Mueller FO. Sudden deaths in young competitive athletes: analysis of 1866 deaths in the United States, 1980–2006. Circulation. 2009;119(8):1085–92.
14. Brothers J, Gaynor JW, Paridon S, Lorber R, Jacobs M. Anomalous aortic origin of a coronary artery with an interarterial course: understanding current management strategies in children and young adults. Pediatr Cardiol. 2009;30(7):911–21.
15. Mery CM, Lawrence SM, Krishnamurthy R, et al. Anomalous aortic origin of a coronary artery: toward a standardized approach. Semin Thorac Cardiovasc Surg. 2014;26(2):110–22.
16. Jacobs ML. Anomalous aortic origin of a coronary artery: the gaps and the guidelines. J Thorac Cardiovasc Surg. 2017;153(6):1462–5.
17. Davis JA, Cecchin F, Jones TK, Portman MA. Major coronary artery anomalies in a pediatric population: incidence and clinical importance. J Am Coll Cardiol. 2001;37(2):593–7.
18. Brothers JA, Frommelt MA, Jaquiss RDB, Myerburg RJ, Fraser CD Jr, Tweddell JS. Expert consensus guidelines: anomalous aortic origin of a coronary artery. J Thorac Cardiovasc Surg. 2017;153(6):1440–57.
19. Duke C, Rosenthal E, Simpson JM. Myocardial infarction in infancy caused by compression of an anomalous left coronary artery arising from the right coronary artery. Cardiol Young. 2004;14:654–7.
20. Page HI, Engel HJ, Campbell WB, Thomas CS. Anomalous origin of the left circumflex coronary artery. Recognition, angiographic demonstration and clinical significance. Circulation. 1974;50:768–73.
21. West NE, McKenna CJ, Ormerod O, Forfar JC, Banning AP, Channon KM. Percutaneous coronary intervention with stent deployment in anomalously-arising left circumflex coronary arteries. Catheter Cardiovasc Interv. 2006;68(6):882–90.
22. Solberg EE, Borjesson M, Sharma S, Papadakis M, Wilhelm M, Drezner JA, et al. Sudden cardiac arrest in sports—need for uniform registration: a position paper from the sport cardiology section of the European Association for Cardiovascular Prevention and Rehabilitation. Eur J Prev Cardiol. 2016;23:657–67.
23. Zeppilli P, Rubino P, Manno V, Cameli S, Palmieri V, Gorra A. Visualizzazione ecocardiografica delle arterie coronarie in atleti di resistenza. G Ital Cardiol. 1987;17:957–65.
24. Zeppilli P, dello Russo A, Santini C, Palmieri V, Natale L, Giordano A, Frustaci A. In vivo detection of coronary artery anomalies in asymptomatic athletes by echocardiographic screening. Chest. 1998 Jul;114(1):89–93.
25. Frommelt PC, Frommelt MA, Tweddell JS, Jaquiss RD. Prospective echocardiographic diagnosis and surgical repair of anomalous origin of a coronary artery from the opposite sinus with an interarterial course. J Am Coll Cardiol. 2003;42:148–54.

26. Thankavel PP, Lemler MS, Ramaciotti C. Utility and importance of new echocardiographic screening methods in diagnosis of anomalous coronary origins in the pediatric population: assessment of quality improvement. Pediatr Cardiol. 2015;36:120–5.

27. Lee S, Uppu SC, Lytrivi ID, Sanz J, Weigand J, Geiger MK, et al. Utility of multimodality imaging in the morphologic characterization of anomalous aortic origin of a coronary artery. World J Pediatr Congenit Heart Surg. 2016;7:308–17.

28. Lorber R, Srivastava S, Wilder TJ, McIntyre S, De Campli WM, Williams WG, et al. Anomalous aortic origin of coronary arteries in the young: echocardiographic evaluation with surgical correlation. JACC Cardiovasc Imaging. 2015;8:1239–49.

29. Palmieri V, Gervasi S, Bianco M, Cogliani R, Poscolieri B, Cuccaro F, Marano R, Mazzari M, Basso C, Zeppilli P. Anomalous origin of coronary arteries from the "wrong" sinus in athletes: diagnosis and management strategies. Int J Cardiol. 2018;252:13–20.

30. Angelini P. Imaging approaches for Coronary artery anomalies: purpose and techniques. Curr Cardiol Rep. 2019;21(9):101.

31. Frommelt P, Lopez L, Dimas VV, Eidem B, Han BK, Ko HH, Lorber R, Nii M, Printz B, Srivastava S, Valente AM, Cohen MS. Recommendations for multimodality assessment of congenital Coronary anomalies: a guide from the American Society of Echocardiography: developed in collaboration with the Society for Cardiovascular Angiography and Interventions, Japanese Society of Echocardiography, and Society for Cardiovascular Magnetic Resonance. J Am Soc Echocardiogr. 2020;33(3):259–94.

32. Cantinotti M, Giordano R, Assanta N, Koestenberger M, Franchi E, Marchese P, Clemente A, Kutty S, D'Ascenzi F. Echocardiographic screening of anomalous origin of Coronary arteries in athletes with a focus on high take-off. Healthcare (Basel). 2021;9(2):231.

33. Brothers JA, Kim TS, Fogel MA, Whitehead KK, Morrison TM, Paridon SM, et al. Cardiac magnetic resonance imaging characterizes stenosis, perfusion, and fibrosis preoperatively and postoperatively in children with anomalous coronary arteries. J Thorac Cardiovasc Surg. 2016;152:205–10.

34. Marano R, Merlino B, Savino G, Natale L, Rovere G, Paciolla F, Muciaccia M, Flammia FC, Larici AR, Palmieri V, Zeppilli P, Manfredi R. Coronary computed tomography angiography in the clinical workflow of athletes with anomalous origin of Coronary arteries from the contralateral Valsalva sinus. J Thorac Imaging. 2021;36(2):122–30.

35. Savino G, Piccolo FL, Merlino B, Rovere G, Bianco M, Gervasi SF, Palmieri V, Larici AR, Manfredi R, Marano R. Cardiac-CT with the newest CT scanners: an incoming screening tool for competitive athletes? Clin Imaging. 2021;78:74–92.

36. Hirono K, Hata Y, Miyao N, Nakaoka H, Saito K, Ibuki K, et al. Anomalous origin of the right coronary artery evaluated with multidetector computed tomography and its clinical relevance. J Cardiol. 2016;68:196–201.

37. Roberts WO, Asplund CA, O'Connor FG, Stovitz SD. Cardiac preparticipation screening for the young athlete: why the routine use of ECG is not necessary. J Electrocardiol. 2015;48:311–5.

38. Eckart RE, Scoville SL, Campbell CL, Shry EA, Stajduhar KC, Potter RN, et al. Sudden death in young adults: a 25-year review of autopsies in military recruits. Ann Intern Med. 2004;141:829–34.

39. Osaki M, McCrindle BW, Van Arsdell G, Dipch and aI. Anomalous origin of a coronary artery from the opposite sinus of Valsalva with an interarterial course: clinical profile and approach to management in the pediatric population. Pediatr Cardiol. 2008;29:24–30.

40. Angelini P, Monge J. Coronary artery anomalies. In: Morsucci M Goodman's cardiac Catherization, angiography, and intervention. Riverwoods, IL: Lippincott Williams & Wilkins; 2013. p. 325–53.

41. Angelini P, Monge JU, Forstall P, Ramirez JM, Uribe C, Hernandez E. Anomalous right coronary artery from the left sinus of Valsalva: pathophysiological mechanisms studied by intravascular ultrasound, clinical presentations and response to stent angioplasty. J Am Coll Cardiol. 2013;61:E1804.

42. Noel C. Cardiac stress MRI evaluation of anomalous aortic origin of a coronary artery. Congenit Heart Dis. 2017 Sep;12(5):627–9.

43. Uebleis C, Groebner M, von Ziegler F, Becker A, Rischpler C, Tegtmeyer R, Becker C, Lehner S, Haug AR, Cumming P, Bartenstein P, Franz WM, Hacker M. Combined anatomical and functional imaging using coronary CT angiography and myocardial perfusion SPECT in symptomatic adults with abnormal origin of a coronary artery. Int J Card Imaging. 2012;28(7):1763–74.

44. Strigl S, Beroukhim R, Valente AM, et al. Feasibility of dobutamine stress cardiovascular magnetic resonance imaging in children. J Magn Reson Imaging. 2009;29:313–9.

45. Nagel E, Lehmkuhl HB, Bocksch W, et al. Noninvasive diagnosis of ischemia-induced wall motion abnormalities with the use of high-dose dobutamine stress MRI: comparison with dobutamine stress echocardiography. Circulation. 1999;99:763–70.

46. Prakash A, Powell AJ, Krishnamurthy R, Geva T. Magnetic resonance imaging evaluation of myocardial perfusion and viability in congenital and acquired pediatric heart disease. Am J Cardiol. 2004;93:657–61.

47. Buechel ER, Balmer C, Bauersfeld U, Kellenberger CJ, Schwitter J. Feasibility of perfusion cardiovascular magnetic resonance in paediatric patients. J Cardiovasc Magn Reson. 2009;11:51.

48. Scannell CM, Hasaneen H, Greil G, Hussain T, Razavi R, Lee J, Pushparajah K, Duong P, Chiribiri A. Automated quantitative stress perfusion cardiac magnetic resonance in pediatric patients. Front Pediatr. 2021;9:699497.

49. Doan TT, Molossi S, Sachdeva S, Wilkinson JC, Loar RW, Weigand JD, Schlingmann TR, Reaves-O'Neal DL, Pednekar AS, Masand P, Noel CV. Dobutamine stress cardiac MRI is safe and feasible in pediatric patients with anomalous aortic origin of a coronary artery (AAOCA). Int J Cardiol. 2021;334:42–8.

50. Kimball TR. Pediatric stress echocardiography. Pediatr Cardiol. 2002;23:347–57.

51. Lameijer H, Ter Maaten JM, Steggerda RC. Additive value of dobutamine stress echocardiography in patients with an anomalous origin of a coronary artery. Neth Hear J. 2015;23(2):139–40.

52. Glaab T, Taube C. Practical guide to cardiopulmonary exercise testing in adults. Respir Res. 2022;23(1):9.

53. Guazzi M, Adams V, Conraads V, Halle M, Mezzani A, Vanhees L, Arena R, Fletcher GF, Forman DE, Kitzman DW, Lavie CJ, Myers J, European Association, for Cardiovascular Prevention & Rehabilitation; American Heart Association. EACPR/AHA scientific statement. Clinical recommendations for cardiopulmonary exercise testing data assessment in specific patient populations. Circulation. 2012;126(18):2261–74.

54. Guazzi M, Arena R, Halle M, Piepoli MF, Myers J, Lavie CJ. 2016 focused update: clinical recommendations for cardiopulmonary exercise testing data assessment in specific patient populations. Eur Heart J. 2018;39(14):1144–61.

55. Angelini P, Uribe C, Monge J, Tobis JM, Elayda MA, Willerson JT. Origin of the right coronary artery from the opposite sinus of Valsalva in adults: characterization by intravascular ultrasonography at baseline and after stent angioplasty. Catheter Cardiovasc Interv. 2015;86(2):199–208.

56. Boler AN, Hilliard AA, Gordon BM. Functional assessment of anomalous right coronary artery using fractional flow reserve: an innovative modality to guide patient management. Catheter Cardiovasc Interv. 2017;89(2):316–20.

57. Nørgaard BL, Leipsic J, Gaur S, et al. NXT trial study group, diagnostic performance of noninvasive fractional flow reserve derived from coronary computed tomography angiography in suspected coronary artery disease: the NXT trial (analysis of coronary blood flow using CT angiography: next steps). J Am Coll Cardiol. 2014;63(12):1145–55.

58. Sheng CC, Ghobrial J, Cho L. Patients with varying courses of single coronary artery: case series. Eur Heart J Case Rep. 2021;5(10):ytab314.

59. Cheitlin MD, De Castro CM, McAllister HA. Sudden death as a complication of anomalous left coronary origin from the anterior sinus of Valsalva: a not-so-minor congenital anomaly. Circulation. 1974;50:780–7.

60. Taylor AJ, Byers JP, Cheitlin MD, Virmani R. Anomalous right or left coronary artery from the contralateral coronary sinus: "high-risk" abnormalities in the initial coronary artery course and heterogeneous clinical outcomes. Am Heart J. 1997;133:428–35.

61. Roberts WC, Siegel RJ, Zipes DP. Origin of the right coronary artery from the left sinus of Valsalva and its functional consequences: analysis of 10 necropsy patients. Am J Cardiol. 1982;49:863–8.

62. Elhmidi Y, Nöbauer C, Hörer J, Schreiber C, Lange R. Surgical unroofing of an anomalous right coronary artery arising from the posterior left sinus of Valsalva. World J Pediatr Congenit Heart Sur. 2013;4(4):433–5.

63. Muñoz-Guijosa C, Permanyer E, Leta R. Anomalous origin of right coronary artery from the left coronary sinus: sudden death and successful surgical reimplantation. Eur Heart J. 2012;33(11):1308.

64. Kragel AH, Roberts WC. Anomalous origin of either the right or left main coronary artery from the aorta with subsequent coursing between aorta and pulmonary trunk: analysis of 32 necropsy cases. Am J Cardiol. 1988;62:771–7.

65. Meyer L, Stubbs B, Fahrenbruch C, Maeda C, Harmon K, Eisenberg M, et al. Incidence, causes, and survival trends from cardiovascular-related sudden cardiac arrest in children and young adults 0 to 35 years of age: a 30-year review. Circulation. 2012;126:1363–72.

66. Pilmer CM, Kirsh JA, Hildebrandt D, Krahn AD, Gow RM. Sudden cardiac death in children and adolescents between 1 and 19 years of age. Heart Rhythm. 2014;11:239–45.

67. Marijon E, Tafflet M, Celermajer DS, Dumas F, Perier MC, Mustafic H, et al. Sports-related sudden death in the general population. Circulation. 2011;124:672–81.

68. Cho SH, Joo HC, Yoo KJ, Youn YN. Anomalous origin of right coronary artery from left coronary sinus: surgical management and clinical result. Thorac Cardiovasc Surg. 2015;63:360–6.

69. Frommelt PC, Sheridan DC, Berger S, Frommelt MA, Tweddell JS. Ten-year experience with surgical unroofing of anomalous aortic origin of a coronary artery from the opposite sinus with an interarterial course. J Thorac Cardiovasc Surg. 2011;142:1046–51.

70. Sharma V, Burkhart HM, Dearani JA, Suri RM, Daly RC, Park SJ, et al. Surgical unroofing of anomalous aortic origin of a coronary artery: a single-center experience. Ann Thorac Surg. 2014;98:941–5.

71. Davies JE, Burkhart HM, Dearani JA, Suri RM, Phillips SD, Warnes CA, et al. Surgical management of anomalous aortic origin of a coronary artery. Ann Thorac Surg. 2009;88:844–7.

72. Van Hare GF, Ackerman MJ, Evangelista JA, Kovacs RJ, Myerburg RJ, Shafer KM, et al. Eligibility and disqualification recommendations for competitive athletes with cardiovascular abnormalities: task force 4: congenital heart disease: a scientific statement from the American Heart Association and American College of Cardiology. Circulation. 2015;132:e281–91.

73. Mainwaring RD, Murphy DJ, Rogers IS, et al. Surgical repair of 115 patients with anomalous aortic origin of a coronary artery from a single institution. World J Pediatr Congenit Heart Surg. 2016;7(3):353–9.

74. Turner II, Turek JW, Jaggers J, Herlong JR, Lawson DS, Lodge AJ. Anomalous aortic origin of a coronary artery: preoperative diagnosis and surgical planning. World J Pediatr Congenit Heart Surg. 2011;2:340–5.

75. Mumtaz MA, Lorber RE, Arruda J, Pettersson GB, Mavroudis C. Surgery for anomalous aortic origin of the coronary artery. Ann Thorac Surg. 2011;91:811–4.

76. Erez E, Tam VK, Doublin NA, Stakes J. Anomalous coronary artery with aortic origin and course between the great arteries: improved diagnosis, anatomic findings, and surgical treatment. Ann Thorac Surg. 2006;82:973–7.

77. Law T, Dunne B, Stamp N, Ho KM, Andrews D. Surgical results and outcome safter reimplantation for the management of anomalous aortic origin of the right coronary artery. Ann Thorac Surg. 2016;102:192–8.

78. Labombarda F, Coutance G, Pellissier A, et al. Major congenital coronary artery anomalies in a paediatric and adult population: a prospective echocardiographic study. Eur Heart J Cardiovasc Imaging. 2014;15(7):761–8.

79. Nguyen AL, Haas F, Evens J, Breur JM. Sudden cardiac death after repair of anomalous origin of left coronary artery from right sinus of Valsalva with an inter-arterial course: case report and review of the literature. Neth Hear J. 2012;20(11):463–71.

80. Gräni C, Buechel RR, Kaufmann PA, Kwong RY. Multimodality imaging in individuals with anomalous coronary arteries. JACC Cardiovasc Imaging. 2017;10(4):471–81.

81. Bria S, Chessa M, Abella R, et al. Aborted sudden death in a young football player due to anomalous origin of the left coronary artery: successful surgical correction. J Cardiovasc Med. 2008;9(8):834–8.

82. Wittlieb-Weber CA, Paridon SM, Gaynor JW, Spray TL, Weber DR, Brothers JA. Medium-term outcome after anomalous aortic origin of a coronary artery repair in a pediatric cohort. J Thorac Cardiovasc Surg. 2014;147(5):1580–6.

83. Romp RL, Herlong JR, Landolfo CK, et al. Outcome of unroofing procedure for repair of anomalous aortic origin of left or right coronary artery. Ann Thorac Surg. 2003;76(2):589–95.

84. Warnes CA, Williams RG, Bashore TM, Child JS, Connolly HM, Dearani JA, et al. ACC/AHA 2008 guidelines for the management of adults with congenital heart disease: a report of the American College of Cardiology/American Heart Association Task Force on practice guidelines (writing committee to develop guidelines on the management of adults with congenital heart disease). Developed in collaboration with the American Society of Echocardiography, Heart Rhythm Society, International Society for Adult Congenital Heart Disease, Society for Cardiovascular Angiography and Interventions, and Society of Thoracic Surgeons. J Am Coll Cardiol. 2008;52:e143–263.

85. Link MS, Myerburg RJ, Estes NA III. Eligibility and disqualification recommendations for competitive athletes with cardiovascular abnormalities: task force 12: emergency action plans, resuscitation, cardiopulmonary resuscitation, and automated external defibrillators: a scientific statement from the American Heart Association and American College of Cardiology. Circulation. 2015;132:e334–8.

86. Fukuda T, Ohashi-Fukuda N, Kobayashi H, Gunshin M, Sera T, Kondo Y, et al. Public access defibrillation and outcomes after pediatric out-of-hospital cardiac arrest. Resuscitation. 2017;111:1–7.

87. Drezner JA, Rao AL, Heistand J, Bloomingdale MK, Harmon KG. Effectiveness of emergency response planning for sudden cardiac arrest in United States high schools with automated external defibrillators. Circulation. 2009;120:518–25.

88. Drezner JA, Toresdahl BG, Rao AL, Huszti E, Harmon KG. Outcomes from sudden cardiac arrest in US high schools: a 2-year prospective study from the National Registry for AED use in sports. Br J Sports Med. 2013;47:1179–83.

89. Kitamura T, Kiyohara K, Sakai T, Matsuyama T, Hatakeyama T, Shimamoto T, et al. Public-access defibrillation and out-of-hospital cardiac arrest in Japan. N Engl J Med. 2016;375:1649–59.

Sudden Death: Differential Diagnosis and AOCA

14

Barbara Barra and Gherardo Finocchiaro

Introduction

Sudden cardiac death (SCD) is generally defined as the unexpected death of an individual not ascribed to an extracardiac cause, usually within 1 h from the onset of symptoms in an apparently healthy subject [1] or if the deceased was known to be in good health 24 h before death occurred [2]. Sudden cardiac death can be the first manifestation of cardiac disease in apparently healthy individuals. Although considered to be relatively rare, it is a devastating event, causing a strong emotional and social impact within the community.

While atherosclerotic coronary artery disease is the predominant cause of SCD in older individuals (>35 years), in younger individuals (<35 years of age), most deaths are attributed to inherited or congenital, structural or electrical disorders of the heart, which predispose to malignant ventricular arrhythmias [3].

The true incidence of SCD is unknown and difficult to define. SCD rates range from 40 to 100 per 100,000 in the general population [2], and it is a rare event in individuals of <35 years old, with an incidence of 1 to 3 per 100,000 per year [4]. It is also well recognized that intensive exercise training and competitive sports participation are associated with a higher risk of adverse cardiovascular events, including SCD in predisposed individuals [5, 6]. One large prospective study by Corrado et al. systematically assessed the incidence of SCD in young athletes and reported it to be 2.3 in 100,000 athletes per year, compared with 0.9 in 100,000 nonathletes per year [5].

More recent studies have reported a higher incidence than previously estimated in specific populations [7]. Male athletes, African-Americans, and basketball players have been found to be at higher risk [8, 9]. Although recent studies have highlighted the high prevalence of cardiomyopathies and primary arrhythmia syndromes (which often present without structural cardiac abnormalities at postmortem examination) among cohorts of athletes who died suddenly [10–12], congenital coronary anomalies are among the most frequent causes of SCD in young and athletic individuals.

B. Barra
Sports Medicine Unit, AULSS 2 Marca Trevigiana, Treviso, Italy
e-mail: barbara.barra@aulss2.veneto.it

G. Finocchiaro (✉)
Cardiothoracic Centre, Guy's and St Thomas' Hospital, London, UK

King's College London, London, UK

Royal Brompton and Harefield Hospital, London, UK

Cardiovascular Clinical Academic Group and Cardiology Research Centre, St. George's, University of London, London, UK
e-mail: gherardo.finocchiaro@nhs.net

G. Butera, A. Frigiola (eds.), *Congenital Anomalies of Coronary Arteries*,
https://doi.org/10.1007/978-3-031-36966-7_14

Anomalous origin of a coronary artery (AOCA) has been described as the second most frequent cause of SCD in young athletes in the United States, accounting for 17% of deaths [13] with other studies reporting a prevalence between 5% [11] and 11% [14].

AOCA and SCD

Most anomalies of the coronary origin do not manifest with any significant cardiac symptom, do not have any hemodynamic implications, and are incidentally detected during diagnostic imaging or at autopsy. Although various AOCA phenotypes have been identified as normal or benign variants, a high risk of exercise-related sudden cardiac death has been reported in those with a coronary artery arising from the pulmonary artery or from the opposite sinus of Valsalva with an interarterial course [15–17] (Fig. 14.1). Anomalous left coronary artery from pulmonary artery (ALCAPA) is extremely rare and usually presents in infancy, with clinical features of myocardial ischemia and/or congestive heart failure [19]. The anomalous right coronary artery arising from the left coronary cusp (ARCA) and the anomalous left coronary artery arising from the right coronary cusp (ALCA) with interarterial course appear to be the most common anatomical variants recognized at the postmortem examination in decedents of SCD [20] (Table 14.1). When the anomalous coronary is interarterial, it may also run within the myocardial sulcus (intramyocardial) or within the anterior wall of the aorta (intramural) [21].

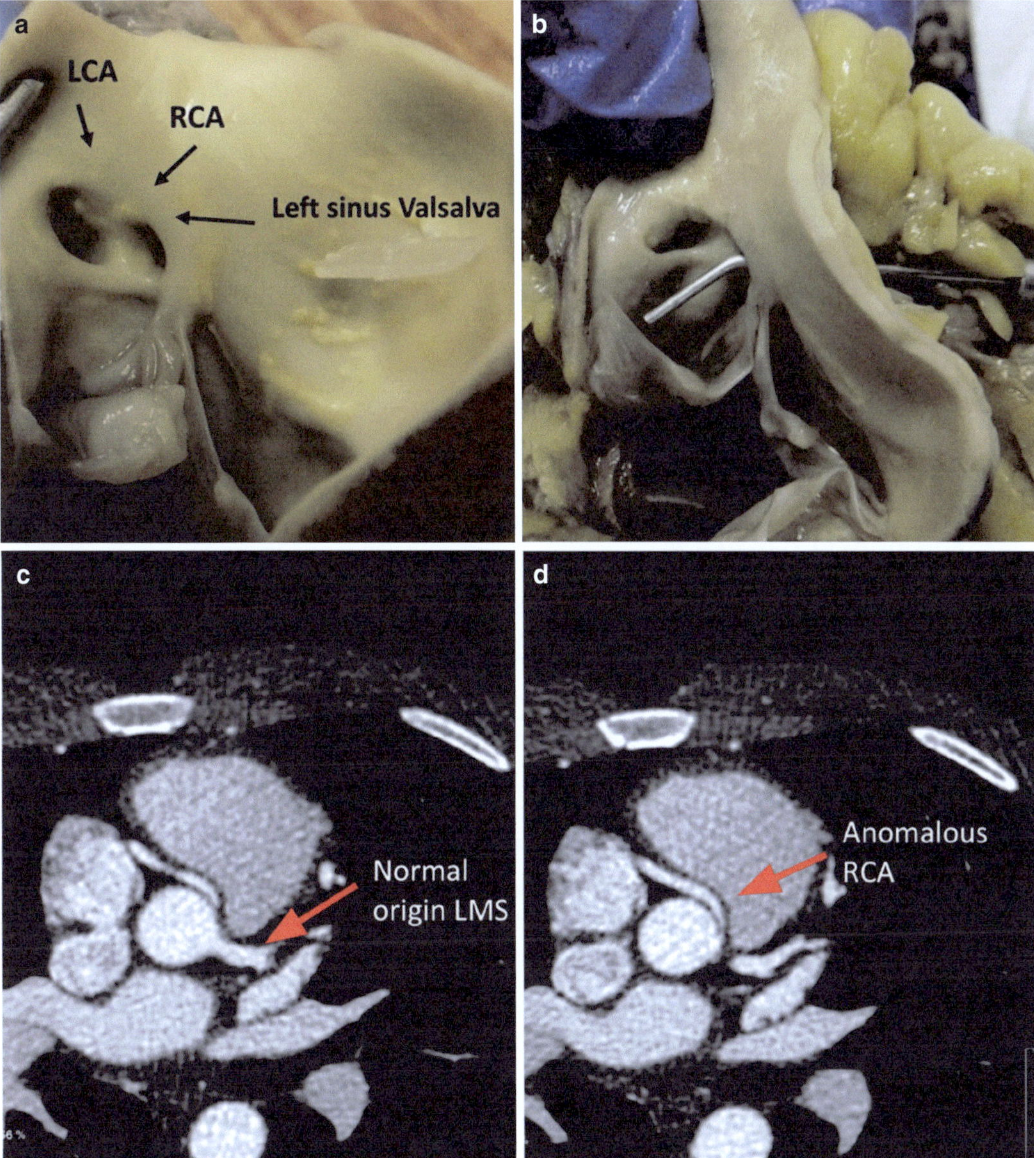

Fig. 14.1 Origin of the Right Coronary from the Left Sinus of Valsalva. (**a**) Note the right coronary artery (RCA) arising from the left sinus of Valsalva. (**b**) Intramural course of the coronary artery within the aortic wall. (**c, d**) Computerized tomography scan showing interarterial course of the right coronary artery arising from the left coronary sinus. *LCA* left coronary artery, *LMS* left main coronary artery. Modified from Finocchiaro et al. [18]

Table 14.1 Autopsy studies of SCD in ARCA/ALCA patients

Author, year	Total number		Coronary-related SCD		% of deaths during exercise	% Asymptomatic before death
	ARCA	ALCA	ARCA (%)	ALCA (%)		
Cheitlin et al. (1974)	18	33	0/18 (0)	9/33 (27)	78	Not reported
Kragel and Roberts (1988)	25	7	8/25 (32)	5/7 (71)	Not reported	38
Taylor et al. (1992)	24	28	Not reported	23/28 (82)	Not reported	66
Taylor et al., (1997)	21	9	4/21 (19)	8/9 (89)	83	66
Frescura et al. (1998)	7	4	4/7 (57)	4/4 (100)	75	50

ALCA anomalous left coronary artery, *ARCA* anomalous right coronary artery, *SCD* sudden cardiac death. Adapted from Cheezum MK, Liberthson RR, Shah NR, et al. Anomalous Aortic Origin of a Coronary Artery From the Inappropriate Sinus of Valsalva. J Am Coll Cardiol. 2017;69 (12):1592–1608. doi:10.1016/j.jacc.2017.01.031

Mechanisms of SCD in AOCA

Slit-like/fish-mouth-shaped orifice (more common in ARCA), acute angle take-off, intramural course, and interarterial course are the main anatomical patterns associated with exercise-related SCD involving AOCA [22].

In the presence of AOCA, SCD is supposed to be caused by lethal ventricular arrhythmias due to myocardial ischemia. Especially explosive bouts of exercise involve an increase in heart rate, blood pressure, cardiac output, and myocardial contractility, in order to increase the oxygen supply to the myocardium with an increased blood flow, which is compromised in the presence of AOCAs. The compression of coronary artery between the aorta and the pulmonary artery (interarterial course), the ostial obstruction of blood flow during exertion (slit-like orifice and acute angle take-off), or proximal segment occlusion (intramural course in the aortic wall) are the postulated pathophysiologic mechanisms behind reversible ischemia and malignant arrhythmias [18]. Exercise-induced expansion of the aortic root and pulmonary artery could worsen the pre-existing angulation of the coronary artery and thus reduce the diameter of the lumen in the proximal portion of the coronary artery. Finally, coronary arteries with anomalous origin can also have unstable hemodynamics, which cause blood flow turbulence and injury to vascular endothelium and may lead to arteriosclerosis; moreover, an association with coronary spasm of proximal segment of the anomalous coronary artery with an interarterial course has been reported, as the compression or kinking phenomenon could result in some degree of intimal disruption and subsequent vasospasm [23].

Implications for Cardiac Screening

The primary scope of pre-participation screening (PPS) with electrocardiography (ECG) is to identify a potentially life-threatening cardiac condition in apparently healthy individuals. Although PPS with ECG appears effective in detecting serious cardiac conditions such as cardiomyopathies and channelopathies, its value in identifying coronary artery anomalies is limited. In fact, the ECG is often normal and is not particularly useful in raising the suspicion of AOCA. Although the wide use of echocardiography in the setting of PPS is not supported by strong evidence, this test may be particularly helpful in the initial identification of AOCA, which can be confirmed by more advanced imaging techniques such as computerized tomoraphy angiography (CTA) or CMR. In a recent CMR-based population study by Angelini et al. [24], high-risk AOCAs were found in 0.44% of adolescents. Although CMR-based screening has the great advantage of accuracy, it could also capture incidental findings that do not need either intervention or disqualification from sports. Moreover, certain conditions such as cardiomyopathies may not be fully expressed especially in young individuals and therefore not detectable at CMR, a context where instead the ECG may be able to capture electrical abnormalities that predate overt structural changes [25].

Conclusions

Although rare, AOCA confers a relatively high risk of myocardial ischemia and SCD (Table 14.2), especially in young individuals and athletes. Although certain high-risk features have been identified, specific pathophysiological mechanisms related to SCD still remain poorly understood and optimal SCD risk stratification remains challenging. Because of its practical

Table 14.2 Select studies examining coronary artery anomalies and sudden cardiac death

First author, Year [Ref]	Population studied	Total population (n)	Study period	Total sudden deaths	Cardiac-related deaths	Deaths attributed to AOCA
Wren et al. (2000) [26]	Children 1–20-year old, England	806,000	1985–1994 (10 years)	270	26	0
Eckart et al. (2004) [27]	U.S. military recruits	6,300,000	1977–2001 (25 years)	126	64	21
Corrado et al. (2006) [28]	Population 12–35-year old, Italy	4,379,900	1979–2004 (26 years)	Not available[a]	320	21
Redelmeier and Greenwald, 2007 [29]	Marathoners from 26 selected U.S. marathons	3,292,268	1975–2004 (30 years)	26	21	2
Maron et al. (2009) [13]	Competitive U.S. athletes	Not available	1980–2006 (27 years)	1866	1049	119
Chugh et al. (2009) [30]	Children 0–17-year old, Oregon country	660,486[b]	2002–2005 (3 years)	8	3	0
Harris et al. (2010) [31]	U.S. triathletes	959,214	2006–2008 (3 years)	14	7[c]	1[c]
Harmon et al. (2011) [8]	NCAA athletes	393,932[d]	2004–2008 (5 years)	80	45	Not available[d]

[a] Study only looked at cardiovascular causes of sudden death

[b] Total population of Multnomah County, OR including children and adults

[c] Officially listed cause of death "drowning" (during a triathalon event) but cardiac abnormalities were identified and thought to be the causative factor

[d] Total population derived by dividing "athlete participation years" by the 5-year study period. The study did not report on specific causes of cardiac death

AOCA anomalous origin of a coronary artery, *NCAA* national collegiate athletic association. Cheezum MK, Liberthson RR, Shah NR, et al. Anomalous Aortic Origin of a Coronary Artery From the Inappropriate Sinus of Valsalva. J Am Coll Cardiol. 2017;69 (12):1592–1608. doi:10.1016/j.jacc.2017.01.031

management complexity, AOCAs require a multidisciplinary approach, which may facilitate effective risk stratification and may have implications in long-term prognosis.

References

1. Goldstein S. The necessity of a uniform definition of sudden coronary death:ss witnessed death within 1 hour of the onset of acute symptoms. Am Heart J. 1982;103(1):156–9. https://doi.org/10.1016/0002-8703(82)90552-X.
2. Fishman GI, Chugh SS, Dimarco JP, et al. Sudden cardiac death prediction and prevention: report from a National Heart, Lung, and Blood Institute and Heart Rhythm Society workshop. Circulation. 2010;122(22):2335–48. https://doi.org/10.1161/CIRCULATIONAHA.110.976092.
3. Bagnall RD, Weintraub RG, Ingles J, et al. A prospective study of sudden cardiac death among children and young adults. N Engl J Med. 2016;374(25):2441–52. https://doi.org/10.1056/NEJMoa1510687.
4. Papadakis M, Sharma S, Cox S, Sheppard MN, Panoulas VF, Behr ER. The magnitude of sudden cardiac death in the young: a death certificate-based review in England and Wales. Europace. 2009;11(10):1353–8. https://doi.org/10.1093/europace/eup229.
5. Corrado D, Basso C, Rizzoli G, Schiavon M, Thiene G. Does sports activity enhance the risk of sudden death in adolescents and young adults? J Am Coll Cardiol. 2003;42(11):1959–63. https://doi.org/10.1016/j.jacc.2003.03.002.
6. Eloi M, Muriel T, Celermajer DS, et al. Sports-related sudden death in the general population. Circulation. 2011;124(6):672–81. https://doi.org/10.1161/CIRCULATIONAHA.110.008979.
7. Asif IM, Harmon KG. Incidence and etiology of sudden cardiac death: new updates for athletic departments. Sports Health. 2017;9(3):268–79. https://doi.org/10.1177/1941738117694153.
8. Harmon KG, Asif IM, David K, Drezner JA. Incidence of sudden cardiac death in National Collegiate Athletic Association Athletes. Circulation. 2011;123(15):1594–600. https://doi.org/10.1161/CIRCULATIONAHA.110.004622.
9. Drezner JA, Harmon KG, Borjesson M. Incidence of sudden cardiac death in athletes: where did the science go? Br J Sports Med. 2011;45(12):947–8. https://doi.org/10.1136/bjsports-2011-090077.
10. Winkel BG, Holst AG, Theilade J, et al. Nationwide study of sudden cardiac death in persons aged 1-35 years. Eur Heart J. 2011;32(8):983–90. https://doi.org/10.1093/eurheartj/ehq428.
11. Finocchiaro G, Papadakis M, Robertus JL, et al. Etiology of sudden death in sports: insights from a United Kingdom regional registry. J Am Coll Cardiol. 2016;67(18):2108–15. https://doi.org/10.1016/j.jacc.2016.02.062.
12. Thiene G, Rizzo S, Schiavon M, et al. Structurally Normal hearts are uncommonly associated with sudden deaths in athletes and young people. J Am Coll Cardiol. 2019;73(23):3031–2. https://doi.org/10.1016/j.jacc.2019.03.497.
13. Maron BJ, Doerer JJ, Haas TS, Tierney DM, Mueller FO. Sudden deaths in young competitive athletes: analysis of 1866 deaths in the United States, 1980-2006. Circulation. 2009;119(8):1085–92. https://doi.org/10.1161/CIRCULATIONAHA.108.804617.
14. Harmon KG, Asif IM, Maleszewski JJ, et al. Incidence, cause, and comparative frequency of sudden cardiac death in National Collegiate Athletic Association Athletes: a decade in review. Circulation. 2015;132(1):10–9. https://doi.org/10.1161/CIRCULATIONAHA.115.015431.
15. Cheezum MK, Liberthson RR, Shah NR, et al. Anomalous aortic origin of a coronary artery from the inappropriate sinus of Valsalva. J Am Coll Cardiol. 2017;69(12):1592–608. https://doi.org/10.1016/j.jacc.2017.01.031.
16. Frescura C, Basso C, Thiene G, et al. Anomalous origin of coronary arteries and risk of sudden death: a study based on an autopsy population of congenital heart disease. Hum Pathol. 1998;29(7):689–95. https://doi.org/10.1016/s0046-8177(98)90277-5.
17. Maron BJ, Gohman TE, Aeppli D. Prevalence of sudden cardiac death during competitive sports activities in Minnesota high school athletes. J Am Coll Cardiol. 1998;32(7):1881–4. https://doi.org/10.1016/s0735-1097(98)00491-4.
18. Finocchiaro G, Behr ER, Tanzarella G, et al. Anomalous coronary artery origin and sudden cardiac death: clinical and pathological insights from a National Pathology Registry. JACC Clin Electrophysiol. 2019;5(4):516–22. https://doi.org/10.1016/j.jacep.2018.11.015.
19. Cheezum MK, Ghoshhajra B, Bittencourt MS, et al. Anomalous origin of the coronary artery arising from the opposite sinus: prevalence and outcomes in patients undergoing coronary CTA. Eur Heart J Cardiovasc Imaging. 2017;18(2):224–35; Accessed 16 Nov 2020 https://academic.oup.com/ehjcimaging/article/18/2/224/2937763.
20. Yamanaka O, Hobbs RE. Coronary artery anomalies in 126,595 patients undergoing coronary arteriography. Catheter Cardiovasc Diagn. 1990;21(1):28–40. https://doi.org/10.1002/ccd.1810210110.
21. Hill SF, Sheppard MN. A silent cause of sudden cardiac death especially in sport: congenital coronary artery anomalies. Br J Sports Med. 2014;48(15):1151–6. https://doi.org/10.1136/bjsports-2013-092195.
22. Basso C, Maron BJ, Corrado D, Thiene G. Clinical profile of congenital coronary artery anomalies with origin from the wrong aortic sinus leading to sudden death in young competitive athletes. J Am Coll Cardiol. 2000;35(6):1493–501. https://doi.org/10.1016/s0735-1097(00)00566-0.

23. Maddoux GL, Goss JE, Ramo BW, et al. Angina and vasospasm at rest in a patient with an anomalous left coronary system. Catheter Cardiovasc Diagn. 1989;16(2):95–8. https://doi.org/10.1002/ccd.1810160205.

24. Angelini P, Cheong BY, Lenge DRVV, et al. Magnetic Resonance Imaging–Based Screening Study in a General Population of Adolescents. J Am Coll Cardiol. 2018;71(5):579–80. https://doi.org/10.1016/j.jacc.2017.11.051.

25. Angelini P, Cheong BY, Lenge De Rosen VV, et al. High-risk cardiovascular conditions in sports-related sudden death: prevalence in 5,169 schoolchildren screened via cardiac magnetic resonance. Tex Heart Inst J. 2018;45(4):205–13. https://doi.org/10.14503/THIJ-18-6645.

26. Wren C, O'Sullivan JJ, Wright C. Sudden death in children and adolescents. Heart. 2000;83(4):410–3. https://doi.org/10.1136/heart.83.4.410.

27. Eckart RE, Scoville SL, Campbell CL, et al. Sudden death in young adults: a 25-year review of autopsies in military recruits. Ann Intern Med. 2004;141(11):829–34. https://doi.org/10.7326/0003-4819-141-11-200412070-00005.

28. Corrado D, Basso C, Pavei A, Michieli P, Schiavon M, Thiene G. Trends in sudden cardiovascular death in young competitive athletes after implementation of a preparticipation screening program. JAMA. 2006;296(13):1593–601. https://doi.org/10.1001/jama.296.13.1593.

29. Redelmeier DA, Greenwald JA. Competing risks of mortality with marathons: retrospective analysis. BMJ. 2007;335(7633):1275–7. https://doi.org/10.1136/bmj.39384.551539.25.

30. Chugh SS, Reinier K, Balaji S, et al. Population-based analysis of sudden death in children: the Oregon sudden unexpected death study. Heart Rhythm. 2009;6(11):1618–22. https://doi.org/10.1016/j.hrthm.2009.07.046.

31. Harris KM, Henry JT, Rohman E, Haas TS, Maron BJ. Sudden death during the triathlon. JAMA. 2010;303(13):1255–7. https://doi.org/10.1001/jama.2010.368.

Congenital Coronary Artery Anomalies: Differential Diagnosis of Ventricular Arrhythmias in Young Athletes

15

Carlo Pappone, Gabriele Negro, and Giuseppe Ciconte

Congenital coronary artery anomalies (CCAAs) are a heterogeneous group of anatomical abnormalities with a wide spectrum of clinical manifestation according to morphological aspects, severity, and localization of the defect and its functional impact on coronary flow. Dynamic change of diastolic coronary flow during increased cardiac output is the mechanism leading to myocardial ischemia and possibly inducing serious ventricular arrhythmias (VAs) and sudden cardiac death (SCD).

Because of the widespread use of noninvasive cardiovascular imaging and of the increased awareness among clinicians, prevalence of CCAAs is growing in recent years. Of note, most of the diagnoses are incidental, with limited clinical relevance as expression of benign variants. On the other hand, the anomalous aortic origin of a coronary artery has been reported as the second most common cause of SCD in young competitive athletes [1]. In particular, the origin from the opposite aortic sinus of Valsalva has shown the strongest link with sports-related SCD, as described in an Italian report [2]. The origin of a coronary artery from the pulmonary artery is often diagnosed and treated in the first year of life. A minority of patients (mainly when the defect causes hypoperfusion of a limited portion of myocardium) can survive until adulthood and present with symptoms of myocardial ischemia and fatal ventricular arrhythmias [3]. Being often triggered by strenuous exercise, life-threatening arrhythmias are one of the most feared CCAA manifestations in athletes. A high level of suspicion is pivotal when evaluating an athlete or sporty subject who manifests ominous symptoms during or shortly after exercise. This chapter will focus on ventricular arrhythmias in athletes, differential diagnosis among the most common heart diseases, and on diagnostic tests for risk stratification.

Ventricular Arrhythmias in Young Athletes

Young athletes may experience bradyarrhythmia, supraventricular and ventricular tachyarrhythmia with different clinical relevance and prognosis. Treatment is focused not only on the resolution of the arrhythmia, but also on returning to play. Ventricular arrhythmias can be an incidental finding during preparticipation screening, can cause suspicious symptoms, or manifest as sudden cardiac death. Each athlete should receive an ECG and echocardiography screening according to national guidelines and each ventricular arrhythmia should be carefully scrutinized before competitive sport participation.

C. Pappone (✉) · G. Negro · G. Ciconte
U.O. di Aritmologia Clinica ed Elettrofisiologia,
I.R.C.C.S. Policlinico San Donato, Milan, Italy
e-mail: carlo.pappone@grupposandonato.it

© Springer Nature Switzerland AG 2023
G. Butera, A. Frigiola (eds.), *Congenital Anomalies of Coronary Arteries*,
https://doi.org/10.1007/978-3-031-36966-7_15

Premature Ventricular Complexes

Isolated premature ventricular complexes (PVCs) during 24 h Holter ECG monitoring are a common finding among sedentary, sporty, and athletic people. Frequent PVCs may be a primary electrical disorder or an expression of heart disease. The main element that influences the prognosis of patients with PVCs is the presence of structural heart disease. In the absence of heart disease, PVCs rarely increase the risk of malignant ventricular arrhythmias. In the presence of heart disease, the prognosis depends on the type and severity of the structural abnormality. The number of the PVCs/24 h does not influence prognosis, while their behavior during an exercise test is useful for risk stratification: increase in number and complexity of the ectopic activity during the effort has a negative prognostic meaning.

The morphology of the PVC is another important characteristic to consider. Benign PVCs often come from the right or left ventricle outflow tract and show an inferior axis and a left bundle branch block morphology with early QRS transition in the precordial leads (Fig. 15.1). PVCs with a right bundle branch block morphology and large QRS, originating in the left ventricle, are rare in healthy people and may arise from diseased myocardial tissue (fibrosis or adipose tissue) (Fig. 15.2). When frequent PVCs are diagnosed, an echocardiogram should be performed to identify an underlying structural heart disease; an exercise test is also useful to evaluate the response to sympathetic drive. A 3-month period of detraining is suggested, because a reduction of the ectopic activity during resting period has a favorable prognostic meaning. Sports eligibility should be addressed individually, but, as a general rule, absence of organic heart disease, major symptoms, family history of sudden death, or arrhythmogenic cardiomyopathy are reliable indicators of positive prognosis. In subjects with frequent PVCs who go on train-

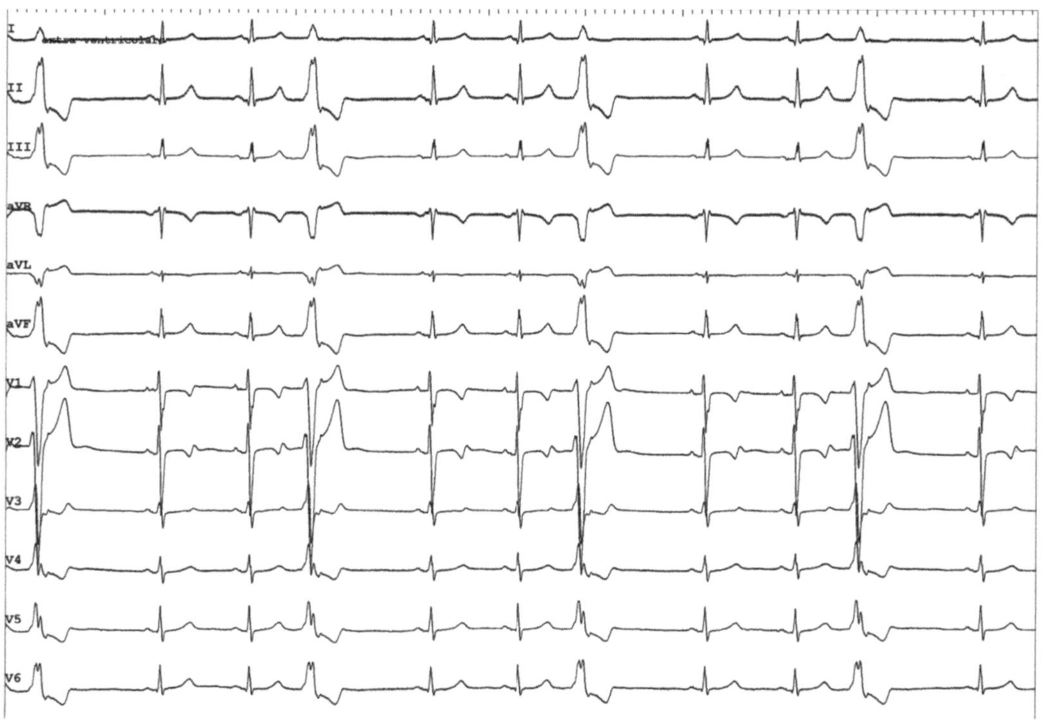

Fig. 15.1 Premature ventricular complexes originating from RVOT. Note inferior axis, left bundle branch block morphology with early (V4) QRS transition in the precordial leads

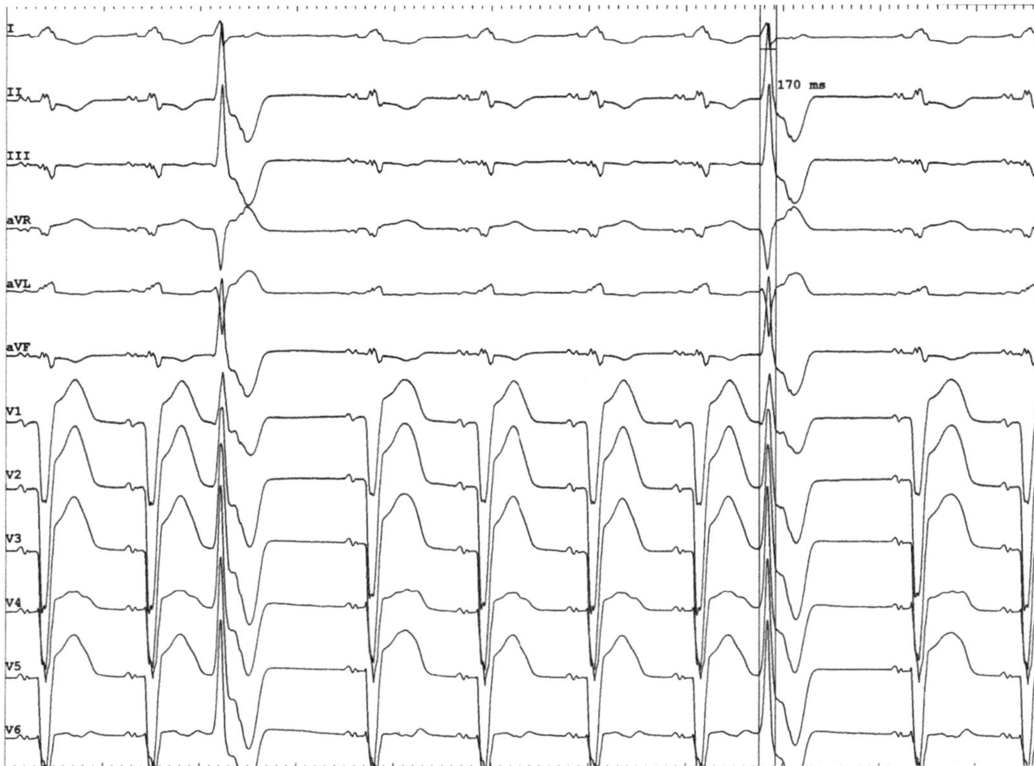

Fig. 15.2 Premature ventricular complexes in a young subject with dilated cardiomyopathy. Note the right bundle branch morphology, large QRS (170 ms) of the ectopic beat, and the intraventricular conduction delay (LBBB)

ing, an annual follow-up with exercise test, echocardiogram, and ECG Holter is recommended to monitor the arrhythmic burden over time and to identify the possible development of a tachy-myopathy.

Nonsustained Ventricular Tachycardia

Nonsustained ventricular tachycardia (NSVT) is defined as three or more beats of ectopic ventricular activity, lasting for no more than 30 s, and not leading to hemodynamic deterioration. Ventricular couplets and NSVT may be observed in healthy subjects. They can be secondary to heart disease, especially when they have an unusual morphology. For this reason, echocardiogram, exercise test, and Holter monitoring are mandatory before sport participation. Cardiac magnetic resonance imaging (MRI) provides useful anatomical details and tissue characterization and should be considered when a high level of suspicion for cardiomyopathy is present, despite a normal echocardiogram (i.e., familial history of sudden death and/or history of syncope). Cardiac MRI can identify concealed myocardial structural abnormalities involving the RV and the LV among subjects with NSVT of common morphology, including subepicardial or mid-myocardial foci of fibrosis, acute inflammation (edema), and focal fibro-fatty infiltration. Of note, the morphology of the VT is related to the presence of such abnormalities on cardiac MRI: a significant proportion (41%) of patients with RBBB morphology VTs shows myocardial structural abnormalities often involving lateral and inferior LV wall [4].

Sustained Ventricular Tachycardia

Sustained ventricular tachycardias (SVTs) are considered benign or malign, according to the presence of heart disease, their morphology, and their hemodynamic impact. The diagnosis of benign VT is one of exclusion; structural heart disease, cardiomyopathy, and coronary artery disease (including CCAA) should be excluded, with a high level of suspicion especially in young athletes.

Benign VTs include fascicular VT and right or left ventricular outflow tract VT.

Fascicular VT accounts for 10–15% of all idiopathic VTs. It is diagnosed in subjects without structural heart disease and is sustained by a macro reentry involving the left fascicular Purkinje system. The reentry circuit is most commonly (90%) located in the territory of the left posterior fascicle (RBBB + LAH morphology), infrequently (5–10%) in the region of the left anterior fascicle (RBBB + LPH morphology). Catheter ablation is highly effective (success rate of 85–90%) and is recommended in patients with frequent episodes, refractory to drug therapy with verapamil or diltiazem.

RVOT and LVOT VTs can be considered the prototype of an idiopathic focal VT. The arrhythmia arises from an automatic focus located in the outflow tract of LV or RV. The ECG shows an LBBB morphology with an inferior axis. In RVOT VTs, r wave in V1 is shorter than 30 ms, whereas in LVOT VTs, r wave in V1 is more than 30 ms. Both RVOT and LVOT can be iterative or paroxysmal, usually not fast, and often triggered by physical exercise. Assessment of subjects with SVTs of benign morphology must include exercise test, echocardiogram, Holter monitoring, and cardiac MRI to exclude the presence of structural heart disease. Particular attention is advised in order to differentiate RVOT-VTs and VTs in arrhythmogenic cardiomyopathy, because of different impact on prognostic and sport eligibility.

Differential Diagnosis

When considering a young subject with ventricular arrhythmias originating from the ventricular outflow tract, it is important to exclude structural or electrical disorders, which can also cause this type of arrhythmias. Arrhythmogenic RV cardiomyopathy (ARVC), catecholaminergic polymorphic VT (CPVT), long QT syndrome (LQTS), and idiopathic VT and VF are the main diseases to be excluded.

RVOT idiopathic ventricular arrhythmias should firstly be distinguished from ARVC, a disorder with a more negative prognosis. The distinction between these two entities is crucial, because of important prognostic and therapeutic implications. Apparently innocent, typical RVOT ectopic beats can be difficult to distinguish from the concealed phase of ARVC, in which typical ECG and imaging abnormalities are not yet manifest.

Several ECG criteria during VT can be used to discriminate between these two conditions. Longer QRS duration in lead I (>120 ms), late precordial transition (at lead V5 or V6), and the presence of a notch in QRS in multiple leads are characteristics favoring ARVC diagnosis (Fig. 15.3). QRS notching and the longer QRS duration in ARVC reflect the transmural myocardial substrate underlying the VT, a feature that is absent in idiopathic VT.

In ARVC, the resting 12-lead ECG in sinus rhythm typically shows T wave inversion in the right precordial leads. In more advanced stages, depolarization anisotropism of the right ventricle can determine a delayed ventricular activation, evident on the surface ECG as a terminal, slurred positive deflection of the QRS in the right precordial leads, namely epsilon wave. Patients with idiopathic VT, instead, always show a normal ECG and normal signal averaged ECG.

In a limited number of subjects, EP study may help to investigate the mechanism underlying the ventricular arrhythmia and discriminate between the two entities. Reentry is the mechanism of VT in most ARVC patients, whereas RVOT VT is sustained by triggered activity. The repetitive initiation of clinical VTs by programmed ventricular stimulation suggests a reentrant mechanism and is much more common in ARVC than idiopathic ventricular arrhythmias. Moreover, electro anatomical mapping during VT or SR at the site of origin of VT or other RV sites typically shows fractionated diastolic electrograms in ARVC. In addition, voltage mapping can help distinguish

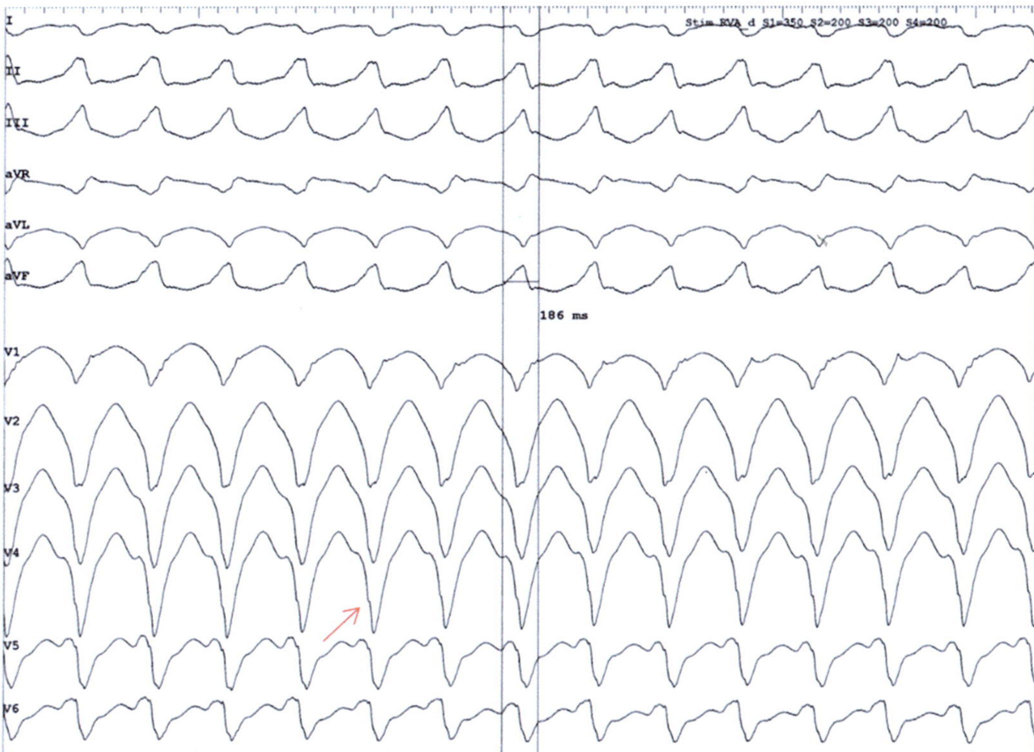

Fig. 15.3 Sustained ventricular tachycardia in a patient with ARVC (surface ECG, 50 mm/s). Note the LBBB morphology with no precordial transition, long QRS duration (186 ms), and notching in the descending branch (red arrow)

early or concealed ARVC from idiopathic VT by detecting low voltage areas, expression of the histopathological features pathognomonic of ARVC. Cardiac MRI is another important tool to be used for differential diagnosis. The presence of RV dilation or aneurysm is consistent with ARVC.

In some patients, idiopathic VT can coexist with organic heart disease and may not be related to the disease itself. On the other hand, very frequent PVCs or VTs can cause or exacerbate a dilated cardiomyopathy that can improve or disappear after elimination of the ventricular arrhythmia. A PVC related cardiomyopathy should be suspected when frequent PVCs or VTs are diagnosed at the 24 h Holter monitoring (>13% of total heart beats), monomorphic with a typical morphology, QRS duration <170 ms and without PVCs suppression at resting hours. The definite diagnosis is reached when a complete recovery of LV systolic function is observed after

PVCs elimination (usually with catheter ablation). When an athlete is diagnosed with an LV dilation and dysfunction, an Holter ECG monitoring at diagnosis and one after 3-months detraining should be recorded in order to identify arrhythmias inducing or exacerbating a cardiomyopathy.

In some cases, monomorphic focal ventricular arrhythmias can trigger sustained malignant VTs or even VF in apparently normal hearts. Despite progress in the understanding of mechanisms of arrhythmia triggering and maintenance, identification of patients presenting with focal PVCs prone to VF degeneration remains challenging. Malignant PVCs should be suspected in patients presenting with unexplained syncope. In fact, patients with idiopathic VF present with syncopal episodes before experiencing cardiac arrest [5]. Atypical sites of origin of the arrhythmias are predictive of malignant arrhythmias too. PVCs arising from the Purkinje network, RV moderator band, papillary muscles, and apical cardiac crux, for example, are more prone to induce sustained VT and VF, leading to syncope or cardiac arrest. Another prognostic factor is the PVCs coupling interval: there is no absolute coupling interval cutoff to identify ominous ventricular arrhythmias, but other secondary indexes may be used to risk stratify patients. The prematurity index (defined as the ratio of the coupling interval of the first VT beat or isolated PVC to the preceding R-R interval) and the second coupling interval may predict malignant ventricular arrhythmias [6], but these two indexes lack prospective large population validation studies.

The long QT syndrome (LQTS) is another arrhythmogenic condition to be excluded when considering a young patient experiencing syncope or cardiac arrest during exercise. The LQTS is a channelopathy causing an abnormally prolonged QT interval and characterized by an increased risk for life-threatening ventricular arrhythmias in apparently normal hearts. This syndrome is genetically determined by mutations involving cardiac ion channel genes. Most mutations are loss of function of potassium current genes (KCNQ1 gene in LQTS1 and KCNH2 gene in LQTS2), accounting for 90–95% of genetically positive patients. The remaining cases (5–10% of genetically positive patients) are mostly caused by gain of function of sodium current genes (SCN5A gene in LQTS3). The definite diagnosis of LQTS requires a positive testing for an unequivocally pathogenic mutation in one of the LQTS genes. On the other hand, the diagnosis is often a clinical one, based on clinical presentation, personal and family history and ECG measurements. Corrected QT (using the Bazett formula) above 500 ms or above 480 ms in conjunction with unexplained syncope, brings to LQTS diagnosis. The syndrome can be suspected in individuals with QTc exceeding 450 ms for men and exceeding 460 ms for women, especially in the presence of unexplained syncope and/or familial SCD (in first-degree and more distant relatives, too).

Exercise- or stress-induced polymorphic VT can be caused by a rare but highly malignant inherited arrhythmic disorder known as catecholaminergic polymorphic ventricular tachycardia (CPVT). This syndrome is caused by mutations of genes encoding for ion channels that control the release of calcium inside the myocytes; most cases are gain-of-function mutations, causing uncontrolled calcium release and accumulation inside the cell, thus facilitating delayed afterdepolarization and triggered arrhythmias. During exercise, activation of the adrenergic nervous system further influences calcium handling, often acting as initiator of calcium-mediated arrhythmogenesis. The hallmark of CPVT is "bidirectional VT," a VT characterized by an alternating beat-by-beat QRS axis with 180° rotation. The surface ECG at rest of patients with CPVT is often normal (no prolongation or shortening of the QT interval, atrioventricular and intraventricular conduction defects, or ST abnormalities), so a high level of clinical suspicion is critical for a timely diagnosis. CPVT should be considered when syncopal episodes induced by exercise or emotion occur in child or young patients with normal ECG and echocardiography. Exercise stress test is the most important step for diagnosis of CPVT. Most patients exhibit ventricular arrhythmias once heart rate exceeds an individual threshold, with worsening features as heart rate increases.

Congenital Coronary Artery Anomalies and Sudden Cardiac Death

Sudden cardiac death mainly occurs in young athletes with structural heart disease. Indeed, the more common cause of sudden death in a large series of USA athletes is hypertrophic cardiomyopathy, followed by CCAA [1]. For this reason, young patients with typical chest pain and/or syncope or aborted cardiac arrest during exercise and normal ECG and echocardiography should be suspected for CCAA.

Myocardial ischemia is considered the main cause of life-threatening events in patients with CCAA. The mechanism leading to sudden death in a patient with CCAA lies in the sudden reduction of coronary blood flow during or shortly after a strenuous exercise. Mechanical stress on the coronary artery origin is one of the recognized mechanisms by which the diastolic blood flow is severely impaired during increased cardiac output, leading to sudden, severe hypoperfusion of large areas of myocardium, ventricular sustained arrhythmias, and eventually to sudden death. The coronary artery takeoff is an important risk factor for arrhythmic events, because its oblique course inside the aortic wall is the main cause of the abrupt lumen reduction during exercise. Sympathetic activation leads to heart rate, arterial pressure, myocardial contractility increase, and, eventually, to an imbalance between oxygen demand/supply: the increased myocardial oxygen consumption is not satisfied by adequate coronary perfusion because of increased systolic expansion of the proximal aorta and mechanical stretch of the intramural course of the anomalous coronary artery. Another mechanism is the dynamic compression of the coronary lumen in those situations where the anomalous coronary passes between the aorta and the root of the main pulmonary artery or right ventricular outflow tract. However, in the absence of significant pulmonary hypertension, a relevant compression of the coronary from the pulmonary artery seems unlikely [7]. Moreover, the acute coronary takeoff could result in endothelial damage and dysfunction, leading to coronary spasm during adrenergic/sympathetic stimulation.

Repetitive, intermittent ischemic episodes during exercise may have a cumulative effect on myocardial function and structure, leading to a predisposition to ventricular arrhythmias. This hypothesis has been supported by histologic evidence. In a postmortem series, widespread areas of myocardial ischemic damage, such as myocyte necrosis and neutrophilic infiltrates, have been described in the context of chronic ischemic injury [8]. Chronic ischemia results in multiple patchy areas of myocardial fibrosis in the territory supplied by the anomalous coronary artery. These areas of slow or interrupted conduction may contribute to the development and maintenance of life-threatening ventricular arrhythmias such as ventricular fibrillation or polymorphic VT. Fatal events occur randomly after physical efforts, apparently because a critical impairment of the coronary flow takes place only under specific circumstances. For this reason, the diagnostic yield of an exercise test is limited, as the adrenergic storm experienced by the athlete during competitive performances is hard to reproduce.

Recently, an intense discussion about the precise mechanism underlying fatal events in patients with CCAA has been reignited. The main presumed mechanism is the occurrence of lethal ventricular arrhythmias caused by ischemic scars. Despite these assumptions, recent field experience suggests that episodic global left ventricular ischemia is the cause and that low cardiac output with bradycardia (up to asystole) is the mechanism leading to physical collapse. This hypothesis is supported by the evidence that hypotension, bradycardia, and transient global LV systolic impairment can be the presenting signs of an acute hypoperfusion during exercise. Recently published case reports highlight that prompt external massage resuscitation on the playing field often resolves the crisis without electric-shock cardioversion (evidence that VF was not the initial culprit) [9].

In conclusion, ventricular arrhythmias should always be carefully evaluated in athletes. First-line, noninvasive exams are usually sufficient to exclude the most dangerous cardiac abnormalities. In specific circumstances, further examinations are needed to identify concealed cardiomyopathies and to stratify the arrhythmic risk. We suggest a diagnostic workflow based on multimodal instrumental exams to investigate ventricular arrhythmias in athletes (Fig. 15.4). A high level of suspicion is pivotal in order to timely diagnose and treat potentially life-threatening heart abnormalities.

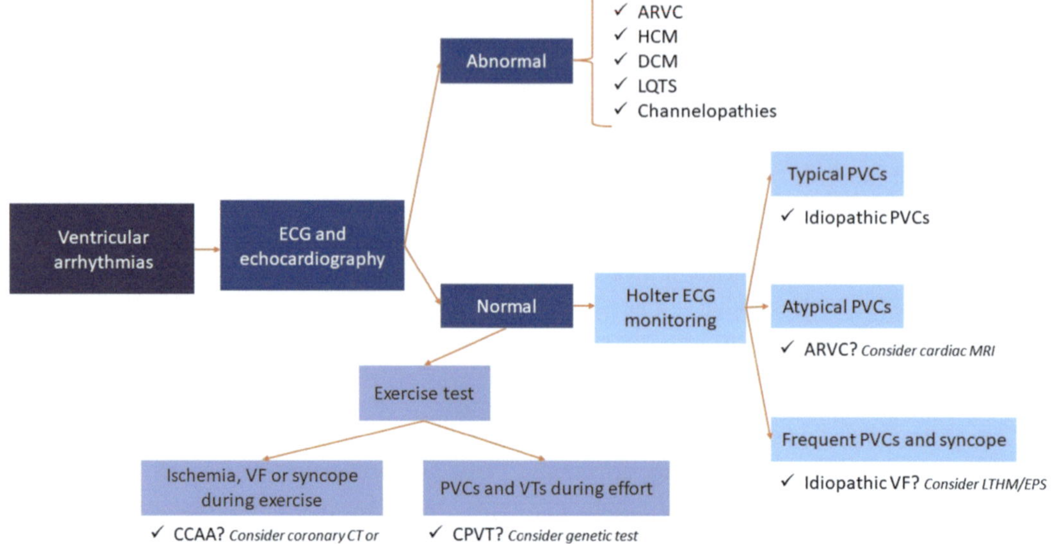

Fig. 15.4 Diagnostic workflow of a young subject with ventricular arrhythmias. *ARVC* arrhythmogenic right ventricle cardiomyopathy, *CCAA* congenital coronary artery anomaly, *CPVT* catecholaminergic polymorphic VT, *DCM* dilated cardiomyopathy, *EPS* electrophysiological study, *HCM* hypertrophic cardiomyopathy, *LQTS* long QT syndrome, *LTHM* long-term Holter monitoring

References

1. Maron BJ, Doerer JJ, Haas TS, Tierney DM, Mueller FO. Sudden deaths in young competitive athletes: analysis of 1866 deaths in the United States, 1980-2006. Circulation. 2009;119:1085–92.
2. Corrado D, Basso C, Rizzoli G, Schiavon M, Thiene G. Does sports activity enhance the risk of sudden death in adolescents and young adults? J Am Coll Cardiol. 2003;42:1959–63.
3. Romfh A, Pluchinotta FR, Porayette P, Valente AM, Sanders SP. Congenital heart defects in adults: a field guide for cardiologists. J Clin Exp Cardiolog. 2012;Suppl 8:007.
4. Nucifora G, Muser D, Masci PG, Barison A, Rebellato L, Piccoli G, Daleffe E, Toniolo M, Zanuttini D, Facchin D, Lombardi M, Proclemer A. Prevalence and prognostic value of concealed structural abnormalities in patients with apparently idiopathic ventricular arrhythmias of left versus right ventricular origin: a magnetic resonance imaging study. Circ Arrhythm Electrophysiol. 2014;7:456–62.
5. Maury P, Rollin A, Mondoly P, Duparc A. Management of outflow tract ventricular arrhythmias. Curr Opin Cardiol. 2015;30:50–7.
6. Kim YR, Nam GB, Kwon CH, Lee WS, Kim YG, Hwang KW, Kim J, Choi KJ, Kim YH. Second coupling interval of nonsustained ventricular tachycardia to distinguish malignant from benign outflow tract ventricular tachycardias. Heart Rhythm. 2014;11:2222–30.
7. Angelini P. Coronary artery anomalies: an entity in search of an identity. Circulation. Mar 13 2007;115:1296–305.
8. Basso C, Maron BJ, Corrado D, Thiene G. Clinical profile of congenital coronary artery anomalies with origin from the wrong aortic sinus leading to sudden death in young competitive athletes. J Am Coll Cardiol. 2000;35:1493–501.
9. Garcia-Arribas D, Olmos C, Higueras J, Marcos-Alberca P, de la Pedraja I, Garcia-Bouza M. Anomalous origin of left coronary artery with intramural aortic course causing symptoms in a teenaged athlete. Tex Heart Inst J. Apr 1 2020;47:165–7.

Part III

Modelling and Treatment(s)

G. M. Formato, V. Ceserani, R. M. Romarowski,
M. Lo Rito, and M. Conti

Introduction

Anomalous coronary arteries (ACAs) are congenital disorders characterized by heterogeneous anatomical arrangements of the coronary vessels.

The mechanism by which an anomalous anatomy impacts the supply of oxygenated blood to the myocardium is often not fully understood and calls for a multidisciplinary investigation. In the current clinical practice, medical imaging is essential for the diagnosis and risk stratification of ACA providing both anatomical and functional information.

The anatomical information can be obtained with noninvasive and invasive imaging techniques, which may be combined in multimodality fashion for a more accurate anatomic description [1]. The functional information can be obtained by combining different provocative tests such as cardiopulmonary stress test, exercise stress echocardiography, stress cardiac magnetic resonance (MR), or Spect. All those tests, despite having different characteristics, provide an overall assessment of the body's response to exercise and a noninvasive evaluation of the oxygen uptake [2].

However, the integration of such sources of information provides an indication of the patient's status at specific working conditions that do not fully resemble the wide range of conditions that the patient might experience during daily life or sport effort. Given such considerations, computational modeling may help to overcome such limitations and shed new light in understanding the ACA mechanism.

Modeling a particular form of ACA, which is intrinsically characterized by a complex interaction of mechanical, electrical, chemical, and biological factors, means building a simplified representation of it, and then simulating such a model under different working conditions in order to assess the impact of the selected factors on the ACA outcomes.

Solving a model translates into solving its mathematical equations. Briefly, each phenome-

G. M. Formato and M. Conti contributed equally with all other contributors.

G. M. Formato (✉)
3D and Computer Simulation Laboratory,
IRCCS Policlinico San Donato,
San Donato Milanese, Milan, Italy

V. Ceserani (✉) · R. M. Romarowski · M. Conti
Department of Civil Engineering and Architecture
(DICAr), University of Pavia, Pavia, Italy
e-mail: valentina.ceserani01@universitadipavia.it;
conmic08@unipv.it

M. Lo Rito
Department of Congenital Cardiac Surgery,
IRCCS Policlinico San Donato, San Donato
Milanese, Milan, Italy
e-mail: Mauro.LoRito@grupposandonato.it

© Springer Nature Switzerland AG 2023
G. Butera, A. Frigiola (eds.), *Congenital Anomalies of Coronary Arteries*,
https://doi.org/10.1007/978-3-031-36966-7_16

non in the model is described by one or more equations of different types depending on the complexity of the physics involved and the level of accuracy chosen by the user. As such, in a 3-D domain, the blood flow is described by the Navier-Stokes equations, and vascular wall deformation by the solid continuum mechanics equations; these are partial differential equations, whose solution in the complex vascular geometries requires the adoption of advanced numerical techniques and the help of dedicated softwares. However, the same quantities may also be computed adopting lumped parameters models (0-D models) described by simpler differential equations, obviously at the expense of accuracy. These models may be used either as stand-alone 0D representation of the coronary tree [3], or be part of more complex multiscale 3D-0D models, where the 3D part describes the domain of interest, and the 0D part describes the Windkessel effect of the peripheral vasculature [4, 5].

Computational simulations involving only mechanical phenomena are referred as biomechanical simulations, and may be subdivided into structural, computational fluid dynamic (CFD), or fluid-structure interaction (FSI) simulations, depending on if they model only the solid domain (e.g., vascular wall deformation), only the flow domain (e.g., blood flow), or the interaction of both.

Computational Modeling of Coronary Arteries

The creation of a patient-specific computational model of ACA is a process requiring several fundamental steps. The general workflow is described here, highlighting possible differences stemming from different computational methodologies (see Fig. 16.1).

Generation of Patient-Specific Coronary Geometries

The first step consists of creating a 3D geometric representation of the ACA from the patient's medical images. Such a geometry will constitute the computational domain where the model equations will be solved; therefore, the anatomy to reconstruct depends on the specific

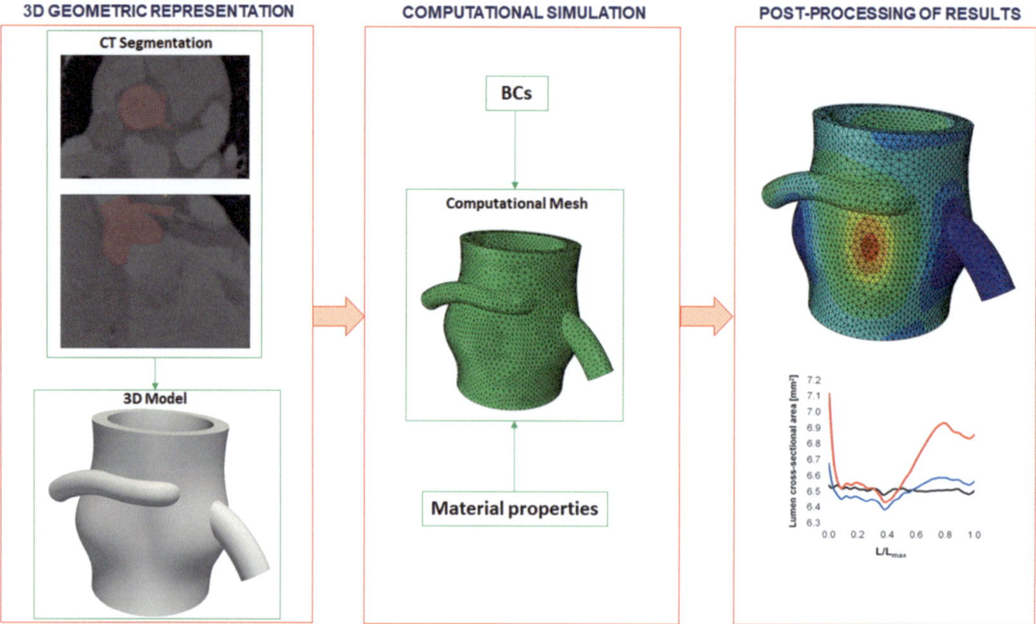

Fig. 16.1 Typical workflow of biomechanical (structural) analysis of the aortic root and anomalous coronary arteries

case: vascular wall for structural simulations, lumen for CFD simulations, and both for FSI simulations.

The choice of the specific imaging technique is fundamental during this phase: it must allow the segmentation of the anatomic structures of interest, but also ensure an adequate resolution as geometric errors will propagate and affect the reliability of the solution [6, 7].

Among noninvasive imaging techniques, computed tomography angiography (CTA) is the most used methodology to create patient-specific coronary models as it offers the best trade-off among spatial resolution ($\approx$500 µm), cost, and patient safety. Nonetheless, different phases of the cardiac cycle may be reconstructed through electrocardiographic (ECG) gating [8]. Differently, the use of noninvasive MR angiography (MRA) has been limited to ex-vivo coronary models [9, 10] due to its lower spatial resolution. Among invasive imaging techniques, X-ray angiography (XA) provides an excellent temporal resolution ($\approx$30 fps), which can be exploited to reconstruct 3-D dynamic coronary models [11, 12].

CTA, MRA, and XA allow reconstructing the 3-D configuration of the coronaries, but suffer low spatial resolution that hampers an accurate description of the cross-sectional area, affecting the simulation results [6, 13, 14].

For a more accurate assessment of the lumen morphology, Intravascular Ultrasound (IVUS) and Optical Coherence Tomography (OCT) are the two gold-standard imaging modalities. While both are catheter-based techniques, OCT has generally better spatial resolution ($\approx$10 µm), but less tissue penetrability compared to IVUS. Furthermore, IVUS has a long acquisition period that, in combination with ECG gating, allows reconstructing the investigated coronary segment at different time-points of the cardiac cycle; on the contrary, OCT acquisition is so fast that only a static model can be generated. Used alone, however, these techniques lack the 3-D spatial information of the coronary centerline, and only linearized models can be generated [15, 16].

With multimodality imaging, it is possible to fuse together two different techniques in order to obtain highly accurate models, in particular the cross-sections described by IVUS or OCT can be appropriately registered onto the 3-D centerline coming from XA or CTA modalities. Different options have been investigated: the fusion of IVUS and XA [17], IVUS and CT [18–20], OCT and XA [21–23], and OCT and CT [24, 25]. It has been shown that these models yield more accurate geometry reconstruction [26] and more reliable results from the simulations [27, 28].

Computational Mesh

The reconstructed volume is broken down into a computational mesh, a collection of elementary cells (elements) and points (nodes). This grid is adopted by the solver to discretize the model equations in order to compute its variables at the nodes. An optimal trade-off between mesh resolution and computational cost is a key aspect to consider during this phase.

Fine meshes allow to resolve the physics of the simulated phenomenon more accurately, but at the expense of increasing computational burden. A way to tackle the problem is the local mesh refinement, consisting of employing fine meshes where the solution has a clinical interest, leaving a coarser mesh elsewhere to reduce the computational cost. As the solution may change depending on the resolution of the mesh, it is good practice to carry out a "mesh sensitivity analysis": the solutions of the same problem are computed with increasingly refined meshes until no significant variation is observed between consecutive simulations, thereby achieving the spatial convergence of the results.

Material Properties

The next step consists of assigning the material properties, namely, the constitutive equations, to the coronary wall and blood tissues. So far, definitive constitutive models have not yet been determined for two main difficulties: first, human tissues are highly dishomogeneous materials made of a myriad of microscopic particles, making the mechanical characterization at microscopic level practically impossible; second, even considering the material as homogenous, a macroscopic description of its mechanical behavior has not been fully determined because of considerable variation reported among experimental studies. Again, constitutive models of increasing complexity may be used depending on the level of desired accuracy.

Coronary wall has been described using isotropic hyperelastic material models [29], or by more complex fiber-reinforced composite materials to model elastin and collagen fibers and describe tissue anisotropy [30]. Regarding the description of the blood tissue, the assumption of a Newtonian rheology is generally reliable with the high shear rates found in the large and pervious coronary arteries; however, in the microcirculatory system, and also in the presence of a coronary stenoses, the low shear rates induce the aggregation of the red blood cells to form the so-called rouleaux, and the blood becomes pseudoplastic: more complex non-Newtonian constitutive models should be used in this case [31–34].

Boundary Conditions

The model must then be completed by imposing appropriate boundary conditions (BCs). BCs are known values of the model variables prescribed at the domain boundaries, from which the solution in the whole computational domain is computed. The choice of the BCs depends on the type of simulation, model complexity, and availability of clinical data.

In structural simulations, the BCs prescribe the displacements of the nodes belonging to the boundaries of the solid part.

In CFD simulations, velocity and/or pressure waveforms have to be prescribed at the inlet and outlet of the model. Such data are not always available, as both can be acquired only through invasive catheterization procedures, and flow

measurements are often characterized by high uncertainty due to the measuring technique. Reduced-order models can be plugged at the inlet/outlet of the 3-D CFD geometry to mimic realistic flow/pressure waveforms [35]. These lumped parameters models describe the impedance of the downstream vasculature, and are independent of the morphological characteristics of the anomalous epicardial tract. Therefore, the parameters obtained from healthy models can be applied also for the study of ACA [36]. Since coronaries are constantly in motion during the cardiac cycle [37, 38], tremendous efforts have been made to perform CFD simulations where coronary arteries are treated as compliant vessels. This can be achieved by applying kinematic BCs to the nodes at the coronary walls and letting the mesh deform under such conditions [39–42].

Computational Simulation

Once the coronary geometry is discretized into a computational grid, the BCs are applied and the material properties are assigned, the model equations can be solved to simulate the physical phenomenon of interest. The computational methods used to solve the equations generally depend on the type of simulation to be performed, the most important of these are the finite element method [43] and the finite volume method [44].

For a comprehensive description of numerical methods used for cardiovascular applications, the reader can refer to the pertinent literature [45].

The choice of the type of simulation depends on the specific clinical question: if the interest is solely on wall stress/strain or flow dynamics, simple structural or CFD simulations should be performed, respectively. However, the coronaries are simultaneously exposed to pulsatile blood flow and cardiac motion, thus the link between the two physics cannot be disregarded. Therefore, FSI simulations are often performed.

With structural or CFD analyses, a key aspect to consider is whether to simulate a time-dependent model. On one hand, static (for structural simulations) or steady-state (for CFD simulations) analyses are fast but provide the description of the solution variables only in a fixed instant of the cardiac cycle; on the other hand, dynamic (for structural simulation) and transient (for CFD simulations) analyses take into account the temporal evolution of the solution variables across the whole cardiac cycle, but at the expense of increased computational cost. In FSI simulations the solid and fluid equations are always solved in time, where in particular the two solvers exchange their respective solution variables (displacement for structural simulations, forces for CFD simulations) at each time-step.

Postprocessing of Results

The final phase of the simulation workflow consists of the postprocessing of the results.

The primary outcome of structural simulations is the displacement field at each node of the computational domain, from which it is possible to compute the deformation and stress states of the coronary wall.

On the other hand, the pressure and velocity fields from the CFD simulation describe the hemodynamic status at each point of the domain. The blood pressure field can be used to compute the power loss across the coronary arteries or to derive the Fractional Flow Reserve (FFR) to evaluate the gravity of a narrowing caused by the compression of the coronary artery during the myocardial contraction [46]. The velocity field can be used to compute the total coronary blood flow, to indicate the existence of regions exposed to blood recirculation, or to calculate the wall shear stress (WSS) describing the mechanical stress on the endothelium exerted by the blood flow [47]. Regions of low WSS are prone to plaque development, while high WSS can lead to plaque rupture [48]. Other shear stress–derived indices have been proposed and correlated with specific biological effects, including time average wall shear stress (TAWSS), oscillatory shear index (OSI), and the relative residence time (RRT).

Applicative Examples

Theoretical studies on the biomechanics of ACA have been developed to understand and explain the complex mechanisms through which an anomalous anatomy impacts the coronary function. In the following, an analysis of these studies is presented, highlighting how they have contributed to understand and elucidate aspects previously unknown or unclear of the disease (See Fig. 16.2).

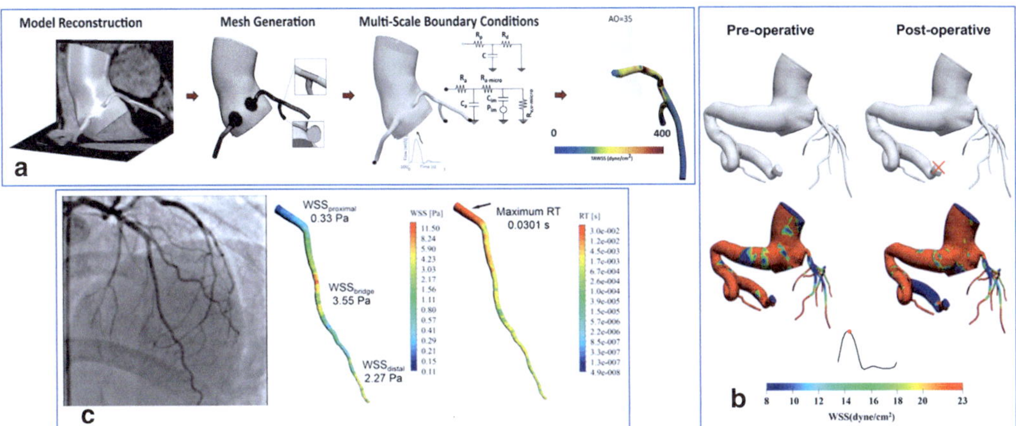

Fig. 16.2 (**a**)Workflow to set up a CFD simulation of anomalous coronary arteries with aortic origin to evaluate the hemodynamics before and after unroofing procedure [55]; (**b**) CFD simulation of coronary artery fistula before and after closure treatment with the contour plot of WSS at systolic peak [59]; (**c**) CFD simulation of a left anterior descending coronary with myocardial bridge with the contour plot of TAWSS and RT [69]

Anomalous Aortic Origin of the Coronary Artery (AAOCA)

Considering the anomalies of origin of the coronary arteries, research has predominantly focused on the anomalous origin from the aorta (AAOCA), which has a higher rate of sudden cardiac death events compared to the anomalous origin from the pulmonary artery [49].

AAOCA can cause myocardial ischemia and subsequent sudden death during physical and sports activity [50]; therefore, few studies have aimed to simulate the coronary wall deformation during effort and predict the resulting hemodynamics.

The first computational model of AAOCA was proposed by our group in 2018 [51]. We developed a structural parametric model of the aortic root and AAOCA to study the coronary narrowing at increasing efforts, investigating the impact of the intramural (IM) length and the take-off angle on the coronary expansion. The study showed that, under increasing pressures, the anomalous coronary had a reduced lumen expansion in the IM tract and a narrowing in the proximal tract compared to the healthy case, and also that the take-off angle was associated with elliptic ostial shapes. With the aim of introducing this type of analysis into the clinical practice, we subsequently simulated the computational model with the CTA-derived geometries of 5 patients with anomalous aortic origin of right coronary artery (AAORCA) and compared the results with 5 age- and sex-matched healthy controls [52]. We found that the patients with AAORCA exhibited a reduced lumen enlargement compared with controls at medium and high effort, especially in the IM course.

Although preliminary, these studies suggested that the abnormal coronary artery may fail to adapt to increasing metabolic demand from the heart muscle during effort, which might result in an inadequate blood supply and consequent ischemia. However, these studies were based only on structural simulations, which highlighted the possible mechanism of coronary narrowing, but did not provide any information on the resulting hemodynamics.

The first CFD model of AAOCA was proposed by Rigatelli et al. who investigated the diastolic coronary perfusion in 13 athletes with anomalous aortic origin of left coronary artery (AAOLCA) with IM and retroaortic (RA) courses [53]. In their simulations, the blood was treated as a non-newtonian fluid with a Carreau model for viscosity, a steady blood flow velocity was imposed at inlet, while the outlet pressure was retrieved from ergometric stress tests. The computed hemodynamic parameters seemed to confirm a compression of the IM tract during exercise, and it was speculated that such hemodynamics might propagate along the coronary tree, potentially predisposing distal coronary segments to a higher risk of spasm and thrombosis. The same group later studied the hemodynamic impact of the stent implantation in the IM segments of 21 subjects. The results underlined mechanisms of compression and torsion of the IM tract, attenuated by the stent, which, however, caused a significant decrease of WSS, vorticity magnitude, and distal pressure drop. This study suggested that the degree of twisting of the IM portion could negatively affect the compression mechanism and that the stenting procedure could bring therapeutic benefit [54]. Finally, Razavi et al. [55] compared the hemodynamics between pre- (2 patients) and post- (6 patients) unroofing procedures, highlighting the onset of hemodynamically adverse events after surgery. In particular, they observed a reduction in TAWSS in the treated coronary artery, while there were no significant differences between the contralateral coronaries.

In order to assess the impact of both structural and hemodynamic factors on the ischemic risk, Cong et al. [56] developed FSI models of 26 subjects with AAOCA and compared the cross-sectional areas and coronary blood flow against 16 control subjects. They found a threefold decrease in lumen area and a corresponding decrease in flow in abnormal subjects. In a following study, the authors also focused on assessing the impact of the take-off angle on the modification of coronary lumen and flow; however, they did not find any significant correlation [57].

Overall, the described studies suggest possible mechanisms that might occur in AAOCA albeit the number of subjects involved is often too low to draw statistically significant and clinically relevant conclusions. Nevertheless, simulations give, within a certain margin of error, absolute quantities (e.g., the compression of the intramural tract, the coronary flow) that cannot be compared with literature values, because there is still no reference range.

Coronary Arterial Fistula (CAF)

Coronary arterial fistula (CAF) consists of an atypical connection between a coronary artery and a heart cavity or another blood vessel. Such a condition can promote aneurysm formation as well as other complications including reduction of coronary blood flow, thrombosis, cardiac failure, and arrhythmias [58]. Typically, when the blood flow to the myocardium decreases by more than 30%, the fistula is occluded surgically [59]; however, thrombosis can occur also after treatment [60, 61].

The first computational study on CAF was performed by Cao et al. [59], who investigated the hemodynamics of 38 patients before and after closure procedure. The authors evidenced that CAFs were characterized by highly thrombogenic blood flow, and that the surgical operation allowed to increase the myocardial perfusion but was not able to restore physiological hemodynamics. In another study involving 4 subjects [62], the same authors aimed to assess the thrombogenic risk in CAF with terminal aneurysms depending on the treatment option. Three models were reconstructed from each patient: a first model referring to the untreated fistula, a second model referring to the postoperative CAF preserving the terminal aneurysm (distal occlusion), and a third model referring to the postoperative CAF removing the terminal aneurysm (proximal occlusion). The hemodynamic results were then compared to posttreatment follow-up. The results suggested that the procedure involving the removal of the aneurysm and the proximal

CAF closure could reduce the risk of thrombosis, and this was also confirmed by follow-up images.

Myocardial Bridging (MB)

Myocardial bridging (MB) is a congenital anomaly that occurs when a segment of a major epicardial coronary artery, that should be epicardial, runs inside the myocardium that formed a muscle bridge [63]. This condition is associated with a number of complications including myocardial ischemia, arrhythmias, acute coronary syndromes, and even sudden cardiac death. There are primarily two mechanisms that might determine the reduction of the blood flow reserve and myocardial perfusion: first, the compression of the intramyocardial segment during systolic contraction; second, the formation of an atherosclerotic plaque occluding the coronary tract proximal to the MB [64].

Nikolic et al. [65] developed a predictive model that, starting from idealized geometries reconstructed from patient-specific dynamic angiographic images, predicted the most probable location for the plaque formation based on the computation of hemodynamic features. The model was also validated against real atherosclerotic MB of 6 patients, and a good correlation was found between real and predicted positions of the plaque.

Javadzadegan et al. [66] developed a realistic patient-specific model of MB, thereby overcoming the limitation of the previous work. The study consisted of three steps: first, a moving-boundary CFD algorithm simulating the MB-associated coronary compression was developed; second, simulations were performed with and without MB to assess the hemodynamic differences; third, the model was preliminarily validated on 3 patients with different degrees of anomalous condition. The authors found atherogenic flow patterns consisting of low WSS and recirculation zone proximally to the MB, which disappeared as the MB was virtually removed, in accordance with the results from Nikolic and coworkers. The same group then exploited the developed computational methodologies on a dataset composed of 10 patients with MB in order to understand the mechanisms involved in this kind of anomaly. In particular, they showed that the presence of MB, its length, and the severity of systolic compression are all factors that likely contribute negatively to the onset of atherogenic hemodynamics and endothelial dysfunction in the proximal coronary tract [67–69].

Limitations, Conclusions, and Further Developments

This chapter has presented a series of studies about computational modeling of anomalous coronary arteries, highlighting how this approach may yield a better understanding of disease mechanisms, and potentially support diagnosis and treatment planning.

From a general point of view, computational modeling of the coronary arteries defines an extensively investigated field of biomechanics characterized by a conspicuous number of scientific studies. However, the vast majority of the developed models and methodologies have not yet found their way into clinical practice, with only a few exceptions related to CFD-derived FFR [70]. *In-silico* medicine, which consists of the application of numerical simulations in the clinical routine, demands for the development of "correct" and "trustable" models, which have to be verified and validated toward a clear clinical question and context of use. Remarkably, all the stakeholders involved in this field (from patients to clinicians, passing through biomedical industry and regulatory bodies) should direct their efforts to introduce this kind of tools at all the phases of the study of the disease, that is, in basic research, virtual clinical trials of medical devices, and diagnostic pathways [71].

Bibliography

1. Gräni C, Buechel RR, Kaufmann PA, Kwong RY. Multimodality imaging in individuals with anomalous coronary arteries. JACC Cardiovasc Imaging. 2017;10(4):471–81.

2. Pugliese NR, Fabiani I, Santini C, Rovai I, Pedrinelli R, Natali A, et al. Value of combined cardiopulmonary and echocardiography stress test to characterize the haemodynamic and metabolic responses of patients with heart failure and mid-range ejection fraction. Eur Heart J Cardiovasc Imaging. 2019;20(7):828–36.

3. Jacobs J, Algranati D, Lanir Y. Lumped flow modeling in dynamically loaded coronary vessels. J Biomech Eng. 2008;130(5):054504. https://doi.org/10.1115/1.2979877; [cited 2021 Jul 13].

4. Kim HJ, Vignon-Clementel IE, Coogan JS, Figueroa CA, Jansen KE, Taylor CA. Patient-specific modeling of blood flow and pressure in human coronary arteries. Ann Biomed Eng. 2010;38(10):3195–209.

5. Papamanolis L, Kim HJ, Jaquet C, Sinclair M, Schaap M, Danad I, et al. Myocardial perfusion simulation for coronary artery disease: a coupled patient-specific multiscale model. Ann Biomed Eng. 2021;49(5):1432–47.

6. Sankaran S, Kim HJ, Choi G, Taylor CA. Uncertainty quantification in coronary blood flow simulations: Impact of geometry, boundary conditions and blood viscosity. J Biomech. 2016;49(12):2540–7.

7. Myers JG, Moore JA, Ojha M, Johnston KW, Ethier CR. Factors influencing blood flow patterns in the human right coronary artery. Ann Biomed Eng. 2001;29(2):109–20.

8. van Zandwijk JK, Tuncay V, Vliegenthart R, Pelgrim GJ, Slump CH, Oudkerk M, et al. Assessment of dynamic change of coronary artery geometry and its relationship to coronary artery disease, based on coronary CT angiography. J Digit Imaging. 2020;33(2):480–9.

9. Huang X, Yang C, Zheng J, Bach R, Muccigrosso D, Woodard PK, et al. Higher critical plaque wall stress in patients who died of coronary artery disease compared with those who died of other causes: a 3D FSI study based on ex vivo MRI of coronary plaques. J Biomech. 2014;47(2):432–7.

10. Tang D, Yang C, Kobayashi S, Zheng J, Woodard PK, Teng Z, et al. 3D MRI-based anisotropic FSI models with cyclic bending for human coronary atherosclerotic plaque mechanical analysis. J Biomech Eng. 2009;131(6):061010.

11. Zhuk S, Smith O, Thondapu V, Halupka K, Moore S. Using contrast motion to generate patient-specific blood flow simulations during invasive coronary angiography. J Biomech Eng. 2019;142(2):021001. https://doi.org/10.1115/1.4044095; [cited 2021 Jul 13].

12. Blondel C, Malandain G, Vaillant R, Ayache N. Reconstruction of coronary arteries from a single rotational X-ray projection sequence. IEEE Trans Med Imaging. 2006;25(5):653–63.

13. Wellnhofer E, Goubergrits L, Kertzscher U, Affeld K. In-vivo coronary flow profiling based on biplane angiograms: influence of geometric simplifications on the three-dimensional reconstruction and wall shear stress calculation. Biomed Eng Online. 2006;5(1):39.

14. Berthier B, Bouzerar R, Legallais C. Blood flow patterns in an anatomically realistic coronary vessel: influence of three different reconstruction methods. J Biomech. 2002;35(10):1347–56.

15. Radu MD, Pfenniger A, Räber L, de Marchi SF, Obrist D, Kelbæk H, et al. Flow disturbances in stent-related coronary evaginations: a computational fluid-dynamic simulation study. EuroIntervention. 2014;10(1):113–23.

16. Ha J, Kim J-S, Lim J, Kim G, Lee S, Lee JS, et al. Assessing computational fractional flow reserve from optical coherence tomography in patients with intermediate coronary stenosis in the left anterior descending artery. Circ Cardiovasc Interv. 2016;9(8):e003613.

17. Shi C, Luo X, Guo J, Najdovski Z, Fukuda T, Ren H. Three-dimensional intravascular reconstruction techniques based on intravascular ultrasound: a technical review. IEEE J Biomed Health Inform. 2018;22(3):12.

18. van der Giessen AG, Schaap M, Gijsen FJH, Groen HC, van Walsum T, Mollet NR, et al. 3D fusion of intravascular ultrasound and coronary computed tomography for in-vivo wall shear stress analysis: a feasibility study. Int J Card Imaging. 2010;26(7):781–96.

19. Son J-W, Zhang Q, Choi Y. Reconstruction of blood vessel model with adventitia from CT and IVUS images for FSI analysis. Int J Precis Eng Manuf. 2013;14(4):643–8.

20. Gijsen FJH, Schuurbiers JCH, van de Giessen AG, Schaap M, van der Steen AFW, Wentzel JJ. 3D reconstruction techniques of human coronary bifurcations for shear stress computations. J Biomech. 2014;47(1):39–43.

21. Toutouzas K, Chatzizisis YS, Riga M, Giannopoulos A, Antoniadis AP, Tu S, et al. Accurate and reproducible reconstruction of coronary arteries and endothelial shear stress calculation using 3D OCT: Comparative study to 3D IVUS and 3D QCA. Atherosclerosis. 2015;240(2):510–9.

22. Migliori S, Chiastra C, Bologna M, Montin E, Dubini G, Genuardi L, et al. Application of an OCT-based 3D reconstruction framework to the hemodynamic assessment of an ulcerated coronary artery plaque. Med Eng Phys. 2020;78:74–81.

23. Wang J, Paritala PK, Mendieta JB, Komori Y, Raffel OC, Gu Y, et al. Optical coherence tomography-based patient-specific coronary artery reconstruction and fluid–structure interaction simulation. Biomech Model Mechanobiol. 2020;19(1):7–20.

24. Ellwein LM, Otake H, Gundert TJ, Koo B-K, Shinke T, Honda Y, et al. Optical coherence tomography for patient-specific 3D artery reconstruction and evaluation of wall shear stress in a left circumflex coronary artery. Cardiovasc Eng Technol. 2011;2(3):212.

25. Chiastra C, Wu W, Dickerhoff B, Aleiou A, Dubini G, Otake H, et al. Computational replication of the patient-specific stenting procedure for coronary artery bifurcations: From OCT and CT imaging to structural and hemodynamics analyses. J Biomech. 2016;49(11):2102–11.

26. Blanco PJ, Bulant CA, Bezerra CG, Talou GDM, Pinton FA, Ziemer PGP, et al. Coronary arterial geometry: A comprehensive comparison of two imaging modalities. Int J Numer Methods Biomed Eng. 2021;37(5):e3442.

27. Bulant CA, Blanco PJ, Maso Talou GD, Bezerra CG, Lemos PA, Feijóo RA. A head-to-head comparison between CT- and IVUS-derived coronary blood flow models. J Biomech. 2017;51:65–76.

28. Eslami P, Hartman EMJ, Albaghadai M, Karady J, Jin Z, Thondapu V, et al. Validation of Wall Shear Stress Assessment in Non-invasive Coronary CTA versus Invasive Imaging: A Patient-Specific Computational Study. Ann Biomed Eng. 2021;49(4):1151–68.

29. Lally C, Reid AJ, Prendergast PJ. Elastic behavior of porcine coronary artery tissue under uniaxial and equibiaxial tension. Ann Biomed Eng. 2004;32(10):1355–64.

30. Holzapfel GA, Sommer G, Gasser CT, Regitnig P. Determination of layer-specific mechanical properties of human coronary arteries with non-atherosclerotic intimal thickening and related constitutive modeling. Am J Physiol-Heart Circ Physiol. 2005;289(5):H2048–58.

31. Pinto SIS, Romano E, António CC, Sousa LC, Castro CF. The impact of non-linear viscoelastic property of blood in right coronary arteries hemodynamics — A numerical implementation. Int J Non-Linear Mech. 2020;123:103477.

32. Johnston BM, Johnston PR, Corney S, Kilpatrick D. Non-Newtonian blood flow in human right coronary arteries: steady state simulations. J Biomech. 2004;37(5):709–20.

33. Johnston BM, Johnston PR, Corney S, Kilpatrick D. Non-Newtonian blood flow in human right coronary arteries: Transient simulations. J Biomech. 2006;39(6):1116–28.

34. Razavi A, Shirani E, Sadeghi MR. Numerical simulation of blood pulsatile flow in a stenosed carotid artery using different rheological models. J Biomech. 2011;44(11):2021–30.

35. Vignon-Clementel IE, Figueroa CA, Jansen KE, Taylor CA. Outflow boundary conditions for 3D simulations of non-periodic blood flow and pressure fields in deformable arteries. Comput Methods Biomech Biomed Engin. 2010;13(5):625–40.

36. Zhang J-M, Zhong L, Su B, Wan M, Yap JS, Tham JPL, et al. Perspective on CFD studies of coronary artery disease lesions and hemodynamics: a review. Int J Numer Methods Biomed Eng. 2014;30(6):659–80.

37. Zinemanas D, Beyar R, Sideman S. Effects of myocardial contraction on coronary blood flow: An integrated model. Ann Biomed Eng. 1994;22(6):638–52.

38. Hasan M, Rubenstein DA, Yin W. Effects of Cyclic Motion on Coronary Blood Flow. J Biomech Eng. 2013;135(12):121002.

39. Yang C, Bach RG, Zheng J, Naqa IE, Woodard PK, Teng Z, et al. In Vivo IVUS-based 3-D fluid–structure interaction models with cyclic bending and anisotropic vessel properties for human atherosclerotic coro-

nary plaque mechanical analysis. IEEE Trans Biomed Eng. 2009 Oct;56(10):2420–8.

40. Ramaswamy SD, Vigmostad SC, Wahle A, Lai Y-G, Olszewski ME, Braddy KC, et al. Fluid dynamic analysis in a human left anterior descending coronary artery with arterial motion. Ann Biomed Eng. 2004;32(12):1628–41.

41. Prosi M, Perktold K, Ding Z, Friedman MH. Influence of curvature dynamics on pulsatile coronary artery flow in a realistic bifurcation model. J Biomech. 2004;37(11):1767–75.

42. Zeng D, Ding Z, Friedman MH, Ethier CR. Effects of cardiac motion on right coronary artery hemodynamics. Ann Biomed Eng. 2003;31(4):420–9.

43. Zienkiewicz OC, Taylor RL, Taylor RL. Taylor RL. the finite element method: Solid mechanics. Butterworth-Heinemann; 2000. p. 482.

44. Ferziger JH, Perić M, Street RL. Finite volume methods. In: Ferziger JH, Perić M, Street RL, editors. Computational methods for fluid dynamics. Cham: Springer International Publishing; 2020. p. 81–110. https://doi.org/10.1007/978-3-319-99693-6_4;[cited 2021 Jul 13].

45. Labrosse MR. Cardiovascular Mechanics. CRC Press; 2018. p. 401.

46. Min JK, Leipsic J, Pencina MJ, Berman DS, Koo B-K, van Mieghem C, et al. diagnostic accuracy of fractional flow reserve from anatomic CT angiography. JAMA. 2012;308(12):1237.

47. Sotelo J, Urbina J, Valverde I, Tejos C, Irarrázaval P, Andia ME, et al. 3D quantification of wall shear stress and oscillatory shear index using a finite-element method in 3D cine PC-MRI data of the thoracic aorta. IEEE Trans Med Imaging. 2016;35(6):1475–87.

48. Malek AM, Alper SL, Izumo S. Hemodynamic shear stress and its role in atherosclerosis. JAMA. 1999;282(21):2035–42.

49. Flosdorff P, Bakhtiary F, Riede FT, Suchowerskyj P, Kostelka M, Dähnert I. Anomalous origin of the left or right coronary artery from the pulmonary artery (ALCAPA/ARCAPA): A 10-year single center experience. Klin Pädiatr. 2010;222(S1):GNPI_FV_23.

50. Molossi S, Martínez-Bravo LE, Mery CM. Anomalous aortic origin of a coronary artery. Methodist DeBakey Cardiovasc J. 2019;15(2):111–21.

51. Formato GM, Lo Rito M, Auricchio F, Frigiola A, Conti M. Aortic expansion induces lumen narrowing in anomalous coronary arteries: a parametric structural finite element analysis. J Biomech Eng. 2018;140(11):111008–9.

52. Lo Rito M, Romarowski RM, Rosato A, Pica S, Secchi F, Giamberti A, et al. Anomalous aortic origin of coronary artery biomechanical modeling: Toward clinical application. J Thorac Cardiovasc Surg. 2020;S0022–5223(20):32430–2; [cited 2020 Oct 5]. http://www.sciencedirect.com/science/article/pii/S0022522320324302.

53. Rigatelli G, Zuin M, Galasso P, Carraro M, D'Elia K, Daniela L, et al. Mechanisms of myocardial ischemia inducing sudden cardiac death in athletes with anomalous coronary origin from the opposite sinus: insights from a computational fluid dynamic study. Cardiovasc Revasc Med. 2019;20(12):1112–6.

54. Rigatelli G, Zuin M. Computed tomography-based patients' specific biomechanical and fluid dynamic study of anomalous coronary arteries with origin from the opposite sinus and intramural course. Heart Int. 2020;14(2):105–11; [cited 2021 Jul 13]. https://www.touchcardio.com/imaging/journal-articles/computed-tomography-based-patients-specific--biomechanical-and-fluid-dynamic-study-of--anomalous-coronary-arteries-with-origin-from-the-opposite-sinus-and-intramural-course/.

55. Razavi A, Sachdeva S, Frommelt PC, LaDisa JF. Patient-specific numerical analysis of coronary flow in children with intramural anomalous aortic origin of coronary arteries. Semin Thorac Cardiovasc Surg. 2021;33(1):155–67.

56. Cong M, Xu X, Qiu J, Dai S, Chen C, Qian X, et al. Influence of malformation of right coronary artery originating from the left sinus in hemodynamic environment. Biomed Eng Online. 2020;19(1):59.

57. Cong M, Zhao H, Dai S, Chen C, Xu X, Qiu J, et al. Transient numerical simulation of the right coronary artery originating from the left sinus and the effect of its acute take-off angle on hemodynamics. Quant Imaging Med Surg. 2021;11(5):2062–75.

58. Qureshi SA. Coronary arterial fistulas. Orphanet J Rare Dis. 2006 Dec;1(1):1–6.

59. Cao H, Qiu Y, Yuan D, Yu J, Li D, Jiang Y, et al. A computational fluid dynamics study pre- and post-fistula closure in a coronary artery fistula. Comput Methods Biomech Biomed Engin. 2020;23(1):33–42.

60. Gowda ST, Latson LA, Kutty S, Prieto LR. Intermediate to long-term outcome following congenital coronary artery fistulae closure with focus on thrombus formation. Am J Cardiol. 2011;107(2):302–8.

61. Poretti G, Lo Rito M, Varrica A, Frigiola A. A case report of a coronary artery fistula to coronary sinus with giant aneurysm: risk does not end with repair. Eur Heart J Case Rep. 2020;4(6):1–6.

62. Cao H, Li D, Li Y, Qiu Y, Liu J, Pu H, et al. Role of occlusion position in coronary artery fistulas with terminal aneurysms: a hemodynamic perspective. Cardiovasc Eng Technol. 2020;11:394–404.

63. Alegria JR, Herrmann J, Holmes DR Jr, Lerman A, Rihal CS. Myocardial bridging. Eur Heart J. 2005;26(12):1159–68.

64. Ishikawa Y, Kawawa Y, Kohda E, Shimada K, Ishii T. Significance of the anatomical properties of a myocardial bridge in coronary heart disease. Circ J. 2011;75(7):1559–66.

65. Nikolić D, Radović M, Aleksandrić S, Tomašević M, Filipović N. Prediction of coronary plaque location on arteries having myocardial bridge, using finite element models. Comput Methods Prog Biomed. 2014;117(2):137–44.

66. Javadzadegan A, Moshfegh A, Fulker D, Barber T, Qian Y, Kritharides L, et al. Development of a compu-

tational fluid dynamics model for myocardial bridging. J Biomech Eng. 2018;140(9):091010. https://doi.org/10.1115/1.4040127;[cited 2021 Jul 13].

67. Javadzadegan A, Moshfegh A, Qian Y, Kritharides L, Yong ASC. Myocardial bridging and endothelial dysfunction—Computational fluid dynamics study. J Biomech. 2019 Mar;6(85):92–100.

68. Javadzadegan A, Moshfegh A, Mohammadi M, Askarian M, Mohammadi M. Haemodynamic impacts of myocardial bridge length: a congenital heart disease. Comput Methods Prog Biomed. 2019;1(175):25–33.

69. Javadzadegan A, Moshfegh A, Afrouzi HH. Relationship between myocardial bridge compression severity and haemodynamic perturbations. Comput Methods Biomech Biomed Engin. 2019;22(7):752–63.

70. Lee JM, Choi G, Koo B-K, Hwang D, Park J, Zhang J, et al. Identification of high-risk plaques destined to cause acute coronary syndrome using coronary computed tomographic angiography and computational fluid dynamics. JACC Cardiovasc Imaging. 2019;12(6):1032–43.

71. Viceconti M, Henney A, Morley-Fletcher E. In silico clinical trials: how computer simulation will transform the biomedical industry. Int J Clin Trials. 2016;3(2):37–46.

Computational Modeling for Decision Making

Gianluca Rigatelli and Marco Zuin

Introduction

Myocardial bridges (MBs) and anomalous origin from the opposite sinus (ACAOS) constitute the most systematically investigated pathologies among the wide spectrum of coronary artery anomalies (CAAs), since they have been related with angina, myocardial infarction, and sudden cardiac death [1]. Over the last two decades, computational fluid dynamic (CFD) analysis has been widely used in the field of cardiovascular medicine, allowing an in vivo and noninvasive evaluation of several hemodynamic features in both normal and pathological conditions [2]. CFD differs from traditional invasive and noninvasive cardiac imaging visualization (such as coronary angiography or computed tomography angiography), since it allows the simulation of different scenarios also before the genesis of an evident atherosclerotic process. Therefore, the interest of clinicians in this novel patient-specific assessment is progressively growing up, helping to understand pathophysiologic processes, surgical or percutaneous interventional treatments planning, and previewing the results of different therapeutical approaches. Three-dimensional (3D) reconstruction and printing, based on computed tomography (CT) scan, can be used in daily clinical practice to practically evaluate the technical steps of surgical interventions especially in case of very rare CAAs or when CAAs are associated with major cardiac congenital heart disease.

Computational Fluid Dynamics

Specific Definition for Coronary Vessels

In coronary hemodynamics, CFD is usually used to investigate the blood flow patterns within the vessels by considering the laws of physics that describe the fluid motion. The biological effects, such as auto-regulation, healing, growth, etc., are seldom modeled. More in detail, the governing equations of fluid motion generally used to model the blood flow in coronary arteries are represented by the continuity (Eq. 17.1), and the Navier-Stokes's equations (Eq. 17.2), derived from the mass and momentum conservation,

Permission: Obtained for all material from other works. Unless they can be used without permission under a copyright exception

G. Rigatelli (✉)
Department of Cardiology, Ospedaili Riuniti Padova Sud, Madre Teresa Hospital, Monselice, Italy

M. Zuin
Department of Translational Medicine, University of Ferrara, Ferrara, Italy

© Springer Nature Switzerland AG 2023
G. Butera, A. Frigiola (eds.), *Congenital Anomalies of Coronary Arteries*,
https://doi.org/10.1007/978-3-031-36966-7_17

respectively, which can be expressed in case of incompressible and Newtonian fluid as follows:

$$\nabla \cdot v = 0 \tag{17.1}$$

$$\rho\left[\frac{\partial v}{\partial t} + v \cdot \nabla v\right] = -\nabla p + \mu \nabla^2 v + \rho g \tag{17.2}$$

where ∇ is the gradient operator, v the velocity vector, ρ is the blood density, t is the time, p is the pressure, and g the gravity. These nonlinear, partial differential equations cannot be solved analytically in case of complex 3D geometries. Thus, numerical techniques, usually based on the finite volume or finite element method (FEM), are adopted to solve the discretized form of the equations within dedicated CFD software packages [3]. First, by means of the meshing process, the fluid domain (i.e., continuum of interest) is subdivided into smaller, nonoverlapping subdomains called elements. Secondly, the governing equations are integrated over all the elements of the domain and then converted into a system of nonlinear algebraic equations. Lastly, the resulting set of algebraic equations (often in the order of millions of equations) is solved iteratively using computer workstations or high-performance computing clusters. Nowadays, the current capability of parallel computer processing allows the solution of the governing equations of fluid motion under nonsteady condition in complex anatomies within reasonable computational time. Typically, resolving a time-accurate expression can require one or more days of computations, considering a fluid domain discretized into one million elements (or more) and few cardiac cycles, each subdivided into hundreds of time steps [4].

CFD Analysis: Workflow

The main steps of a patient-specific CFD analysis are summarized in Table 17.1 [5, 6]. Firstly, the 3D geometrical model of the vascular region of interest is reconstructed from patient-specific imaging data. Manual or semiautomatic segmentation algorithms, included in commercially available software, are used to identify the region

Table 17.1 Summary of the main steps of computational fluid dynamic analysis

Steps	Tool
1.Imaging data acquisition	Angiography, IVUS/OCT, CT
2. Segmentation	Manual-semiautomatic
3.Triangulated mesh surface	Available software
4. Meshing process	Available softwares
5.CFD setting up	Available softwares

CT computed tomography, *IVUS* intravascular ultrasound, *OCT* optical coherence tomography

of interest. As a result of the segmentation process, a first rough, triangulated mesh surface representing the vessel or cardiac chamber wall is obtained. The model is subsequently optimized by applying refinement processes such as triangle reduction and smoothing operations [4]. Secondly, the obtained geometrical model is discretized (meshing process) [4]. Typically, the computational grid is characterized by tetrahedral (or hexahedral) elements within the fluid domain and a prism layer close to the wall, which is introduced to better capture the high velocity gradients at the wall. Thirdly, the set-up of the CFD simulation is defined. In particular, the physical model (e.g., unsteady flow with or without the inclusion of a turbulent model), blood rheological properties (i.e., blood density and viscosity), boundary (i.e., inlet and outlet) conditions as well as solver settings are set. The definition of the initial and boundary conditions, which are prescribed values of the calculated quantities (i.e., velocity and pressure, generally expressed in m/s and Pa, respectively) at certain times (t_0, t_1, t_2, t_3, t_n) and locations (xyz, x_1,y_1,z_1, x_2,y_2,z_3, x_n,y_n,z_n), are mandatory for the resolution of the governing equations. These parameters can be derived both from imaging data or experimental measurements, obtained during functional magnetic resonance imaging (MRI Doppler ultrasound, catheter-based pressure and velocity measurements, or transesophageal echocardiography). Fourthly, the CFD simulation is run on a computer workstation or high-performance computing cluster by taking advantage of their parallel computing features. Lastly, the solution of the CFD analysis is obtained and the results are postprocessed to extract the hemodynamic quantities of interest, detailed in the following subsection.

CFD Analysis: Quantities of Interest

The main flow phenomena in this field that can be characterized by CFD and the corresponding hemodynamic quantities of interest are reported in Table 17.2.When CFD analysis is used for cardiac evaluation, the pressure in the vessels and chambers is generally expressed in pascal (Pa), according to the international system of units. Another important parameter is represented by the vorticity magnitude (expressed in 1/s), which is defined as the magnitude of the vorticity vector; the vorticity vector is a measure of the rotation of a fluid element as it moves through the domain and it may be representative of pathological conditions when far from the baseline [7]. The wall shear stress (WSS) (expressed in Pa) is defined as the frictional force of the flowing blood along the wall surface per unit area. WSS values deflecting from a baseline values are indexes of abnormalities leading to thrombus formation, abnormal vessel modelling and remodeling, and arterial damage [8]. Lower the WSS, higher is the chance to have atherosclerosis in the native vessels and restenosis/thrombosis after stenting procedures. Another important quantity to be evaluated is the power (energy per unit time, measured in watt) dissipated when the blood flows in arteries. Minimizing this loss of energy

Table 17.2 Parameters evaluable by computational fluid dynamic analysis

Parameters
Local pressures and flows
Flow distributions
Flow energy loss
Abnormal flow patterns
Recirculating flows, stagnation flow
Wall shear stress and normal stress
Oscillatory shear index
Impact on cardiac function and vessel wall compliance
Shear stress gradient

when designing or rerouting the blood in surgical connections is an index of a good streamlining of the blood [9].

Practical Modeling Process for Congenital Artery Anomalies

Virtual Model Segmentation

For the computational domain analysis, the coronary artery circulation of interest is usually segmented and then reconstructed based on the data of real patients investigated with coronary angiography, computed tomography (CT), intravascular ultrasound (IVUS), and optical coherence tomography (OCT).

Model Reconstruction

Vessels are virtually reconstructed based on the instrumental measurements of vessel size and length. Both the coronary circulation and the proximal segment of the aorta in case of ACAOS are reconstructed through manual segmentation using the software OsiriX (OsiriX Foundation, Geneva, Switzerland) as a plugin. Specifically, the user interface allowed setting various parameters (size of the rectangular box, resolution levels, and regularization parameters). The model is subsequently optimized using 3D modeling software, such as Rhinoceros v. 4.0 (McNeel & Associates, Indianapolis, IN) [10].

In case of ACAOS, the intramural tract deformation, defined as any geometrical (axial and radial) changes of the intramural (IM) segment in terms of movements and/or distortions, can be evaluated in terms of axial length and curvature change. Specifically, the artery length change can be quantified calculating the difference between the centreline artery's length in both the presenting and poststenting configurations. Conversely, the curvature change in the IM tract can be assessed at multiple points (25%, 50%, and 75% of the length of the IM segment, respectively) and compared to the curvature values at the same measurement position in the prestenting configuration. The elastic deformation is expressed in mm in both length and diameter in both prestenting and poststenting configurations.

As demonstrated for other coronary districts, such as bifurcations [11, 12], the IM segment is bending in correspondence of two ostia: the former is the opposite sinus ostium while the latter is the "real" ostium at the exit of the IM course. The two ostia represent two fix binding points at either end of the IM tract, which generate a resisting force. The torsion of an elastic pipe (e.g., the IM segment, because of the elastic return caused by the systolic phase) creates both a distortion and loss of energy, worsening the mechanical properties and the rheology of the flowing fluid. The parameters involved into a torsion, or twisting, are the torque (T), the diameter (r^2) of the shaft and the angle of twist (define as the angle θ generated by the displacement of M to M').

To analyze the torsion, the use of a local reference system is mandatory. For example, the x axis can be defined as the line passing through the centroids of two-cross sectional areas at 25% and 75% of the intramural tract length, respectively. Subsequently, the z axis can been set perpendicular to the x-y reference plane and point anteriorly (out of the page), following the rule of the right hand. Moreover, the two pilots' nodes have been set in correspondence of the two ostia. The drop of pressure in Pa, due to the IM course, can be converted to mmHg, because interventional cardiologists are more familiar with this measure unit.

Stent Geometry Reconstruction

While it is more difficult to simulate surgical bypass or coronary artery unroofing in case of ACAOS for the stent simulation, the strut design and linkage pattern of any kind of stent can be reconstructed. Based on stent original design and strut thickness, Computer-Aided Design (CAD) software can be used to reproduce the stented geometry as accurately as possible (SolidWorks 2009, Solid works Corp, Concord, MA). In the first step, the solid model of the ACAOS is recon-

structed and then the stent geometry is deployed. For this purpose, a hollow tube with outer diameter equal with both the nominal expanded diameter and thickness of the stent is usually created. Then, a 2-dimensional sketch with the stent's strut can be propagated and wrapped around the tube. Through a cut out, the obtained ring of the stent is propagated axially to create the full-length expanded model.

Applications of CFD Modeling for Decision Making: Data from Current Literature

Myocardial Bridge

The rheological properties of MB have been assessed by Javadzadegan et al. [13] using CFD, by dividing patient-specific MB models ($n = 10$) by length. Intriguingly, a direct relationship between MB length and hemodynamic perturbations emerged in this study. Specifically, long MB length seemed to be associated with lower WSS and higher residence time in the proximal segment to the bridge, and a higher WSS and shorter residence time within the bridge, as compared to short length. More recently Sharzehee M et al. [14]showed that increasing the MB length (by 140%) only had significant impact on the pressure drop in the severe MB (39% increase at the exercise). However, increasing the stenosis length dramatically increased the pressure drop in both moderate and severe stenoses at all flow rates (31% and 93% increase at the exercise, respectively). Both CFD and experimental results confirmed that the MB had a higher maximum and a lower mean pressure drop in comparison with the stenosis, regardless of MB/stenosis severity. As evidenced by these results, CFD findings obtained from rheological analysis of MB properties are helpful to determine patients who might benefit from a specific pharmacological treatment or need to avoid intensive efforts so as to prevent cardiac events (Fig. 17.1).

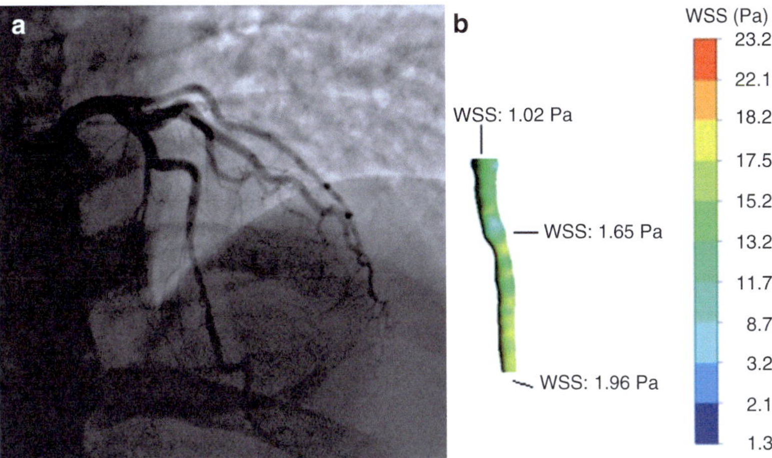

Fig. 17.1 Wall shear stress representation in a 41-year-old man with R-ACAOS-IM. (**a**) The normalization of wall shear stress (WSS) after stenting (**b**) the intramural course (from red to green -blue colour). (**c**) 3D-reconstruction of the intramural tract. Arrow: aortic wall side

Anomalous Coronary Origin Form the Opposite Sinus (ACAOS)

The description of ACAOS is currently based on the terminology introduced by Angelini et al. [15], which includes an L or R prefix to indicate the (Right or Left) coronary artery involved and a suffix to indicate the proximal course: intramural (IM), prepulmonic (PP), subpulmonic (SP), retro-aortic (RA), retrocardiac (RC), and wrapped around the apex (WA). Rigatelli et al. computationally investigated the pathophysiology of Left ACAOS with and without IM course [16]. After reviewing both the angiographic and computed tomography findings of 13 consecutive athletes, CFD models were created to simulate the conditions of extreme effort. Vorticity magnitude, static pressure, and WSS were analyzed in models of L-ACAOS with no IM course and L-ACAOS-IMat rest and during exercise. The mean vorticity magnitude and WSS significantly increased from rest to exercise in both models, in the right coronary artery, and left anterior descending and left circumflex coronary arteries. The mean static pressure (1.118e+004

vs. 1.164e+004 Pa, $p < 0.001$), as well as the mean vorticity magnitude and mean WSS (7012.78 1/s vs. 9019.56 1/s, $p < 0.001$, $\Delta = 2006.78$ 1/s and 3.02 Pa vs. 2.11 Pa, $p < 0.001$, $\Delta = 0.91$ Pa) significantly increased with exercise in the L-ACAOS-IM model. This net increment was transmitted to the entire left coronary system in L-ACAOS-IM but not in L-ACAOS with no IM. More recently, our group analyzed the pathophysiology of L- and R-ACAOS with IM course in relation to eventual stenting of the same tract [17] proving that the phasic IM squeezing phenomena change the WSS inside the IM (Fig. 17.2 and 17.3) and those alterations could be reversed after stenting (Fig. 17.4). The squeezing may be produced by a combined mechanism of compression and twisting (Fig. 17.5), which causes a net pressure drop leading to myocardial ischemia. These hypotheses seem in part confirmed by the study of Razavi et al. [18], which showed that different flow patterns exist natively between right and left anomalous coronary arteries. Unroofing may normalize Time-averaged WSS but with variance related to the AO.

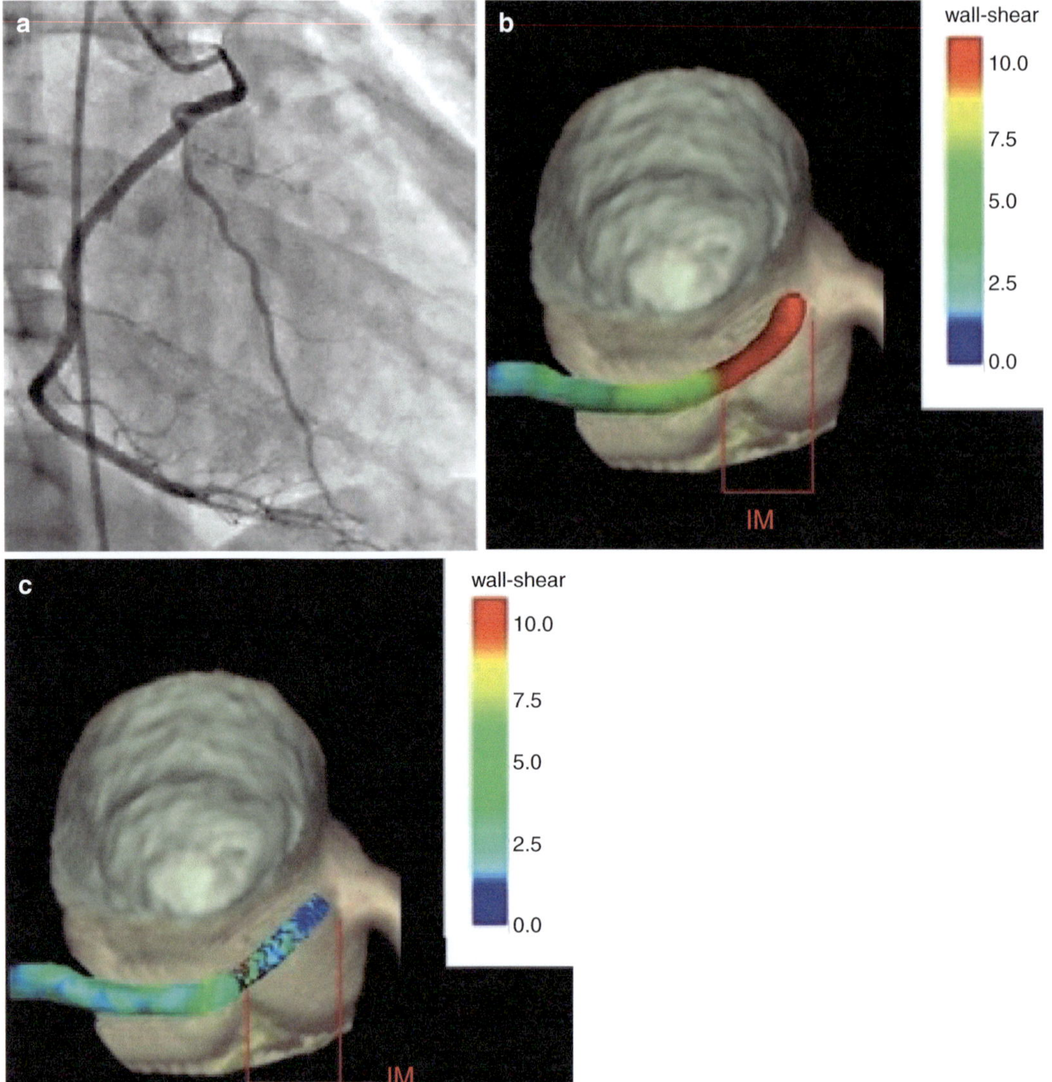

Fig. 17.2 Wall shear stress representation in a 40-year-old man with L-ACAOS-IM (**a**). Note the normalization of WSS after stenting (**b**) of the intramural course (from red to green-blue color). (**c**) 3D-reconstruction of the intramural tract. Arrow: aortic wall side

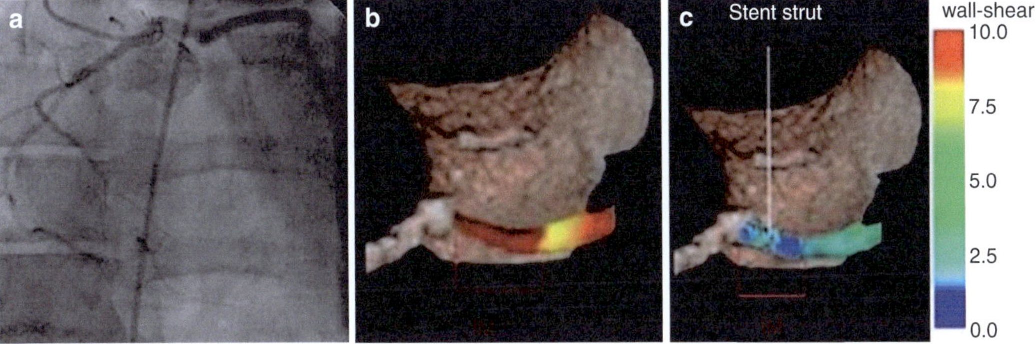

Fig. 17.3 Analysis of geometrical deformation before and after stenting within the IM segment in two patients with R-ACAOS (**a, b**) and L-ACAOS (**c**), respectively. Note the reduced deformation after stenting (from red to green-blue color)

Fig. 17.4 Mean systolic and diastolic cross-sectional deformation in patients with R-ACAOS –IM (**a, b**) and L-ACAOS-IM (**c, d**) obtained from the CFD analysis of vessels 3D reconstruction

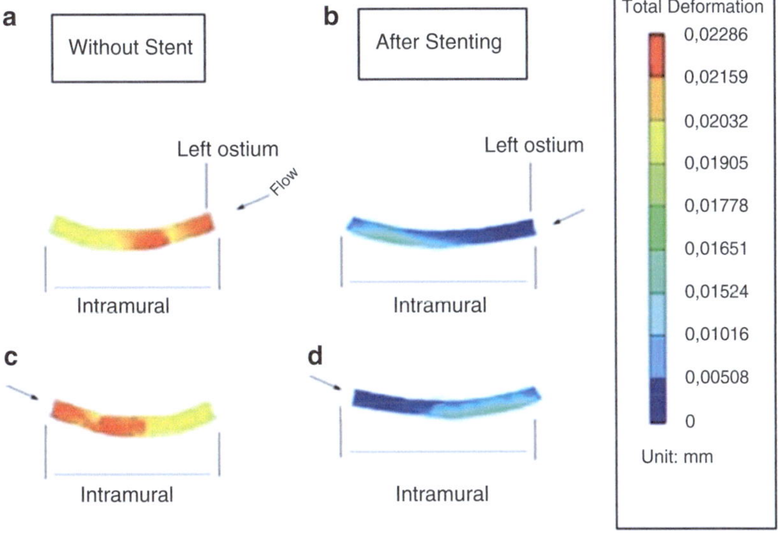

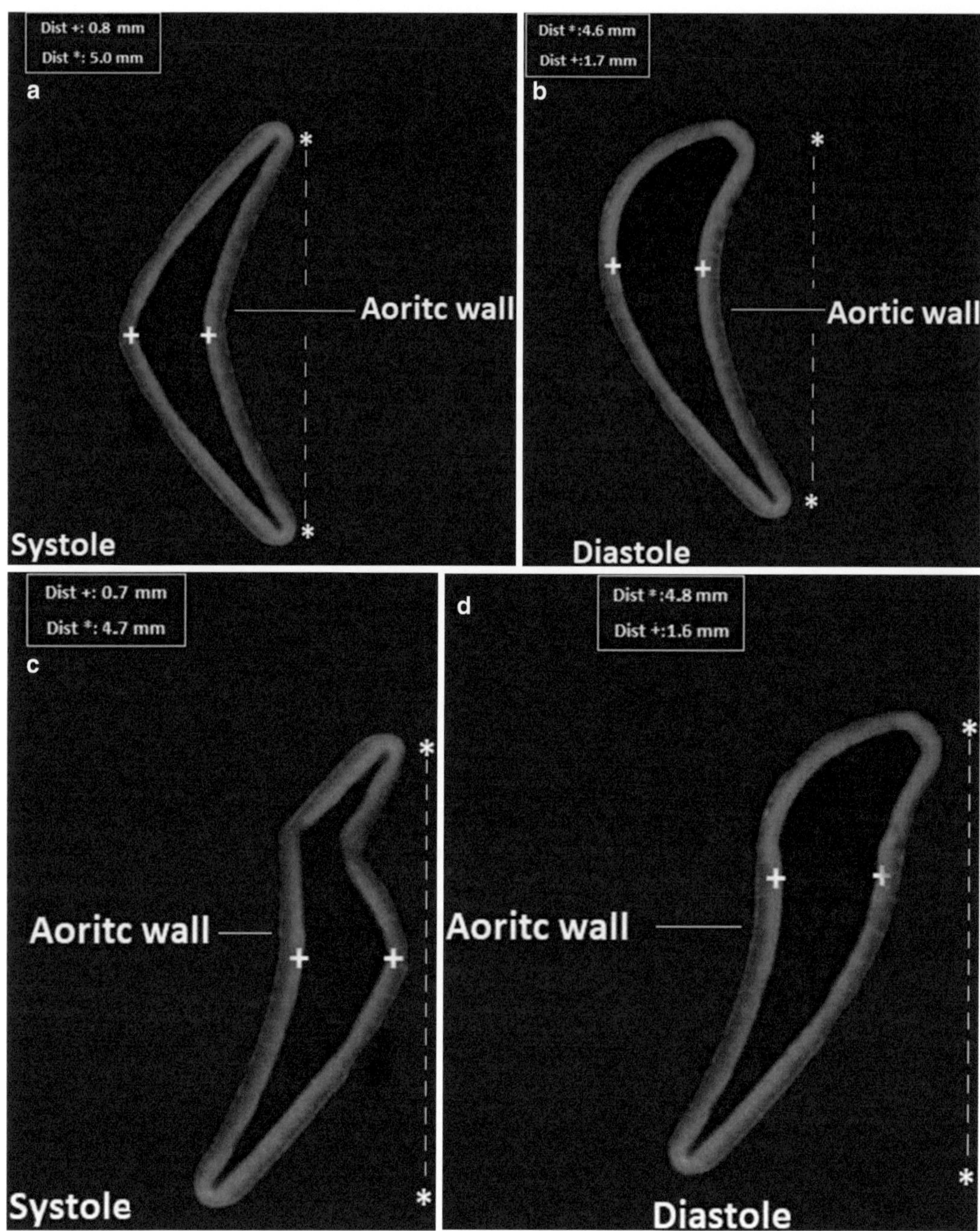

Fig. 17.5 Computational fluid dynamic of a patient without coronary atherosclerotic disease, with R-ACAOS-IM (**a**, **b**) and patients with L-ACAOS-IM (**c**, **d**). * Vertical distance in milimetres. + Horizontal distance in milimetres. *ACAOS* anomalous coronary arteries originating from the opposite sinus of Valsalva, *CFD* computational fluid dynamic, *Dist.* distance, *L* left, *R* right

Three-Dimensional Modeling and Printing

Considering the complexity of CAAs, patient-specific models can provide enhanced visuospatial appreciation of the defect in relation to other anatomical structures and increase surgeon's understanding of the anatomy. This appreciation of relational structures is particularly vital in the clinical picture of CAAs, where evaluation of the nature, and course to determine degree of abnormality of the CAA and risk of harm to the patient can significantly alter management decisions [19].

3D printing has been used to reconstruct and print the coronary arterial tree [20] and it has been demonstrated that 3D printing models were effective in visualizing the coronary arteries. Currently, CAAs are investigated primarily by CT angiography, which has an excellent detection rate and is fast becoming the imaging modality of choice [21, 22]. Although the CT scans may adequately delineate coronary anatomy, the complementary use of 3D-printed models may be useful for viewing coronary anatomy and anomalies by researchers and clinicians with imaging and cardiovascular background, and can be considered effective for increasing their understanding of the abnormality over simply viewing the CT.

3D Printing Steps

The anonymized scans are usually processed with commercial software reconstructing the 3D heart model following steps of layer masking, segmentation, and region growing. Each scan was assessed by a cardiologist [23]. The decision to remove parts of the cardiovascular anatomy is made on the basis that the direct line of sight to view and follow the coronary arteries was not obstructed. Models are usually 1:1 in size. While the accuracy of the reconstruction protocol has been previously demonstrated, the resulting 3D reconstructions should be verified visually by the cardiologist against the original CT dataset. Models are generally smoothed (3-matic

Research 11.0, Materialise) and exported as stereolithography (STL) files. The STL files are then imported into the available 3D printing software where orientation, scaffolding, and print layout were set before printing the model. Models are generally all printed in white resin. On completion of printing, the models are finally submerged in propanol for 25–30 min, and then dried in a fume cupboard for an hour. The scaffolding was removed manually.

Usefulness of the 3D Printing Models

Lee et al. [23] found in their pioneering study that CAAs associated with another major CHD, such as Transposition of great arteries, and CAAs with very unusual anatomies, such as ALCAPA (Fig. 17.6), may find benefits from 3D printing for the increase ability to understanding complex anatomical relationships with the structures of the heart. The use of different colors for different structures has been also proposed in order to help clinicians and surgeons to understand better the relationships with cardiac chambers in case of complex associated abnormalities. Other types of CAAs, such as ACAOS with intramural course, did not seem to benefit from 3D reconstruction. Coronary artery fistulas have been investigated

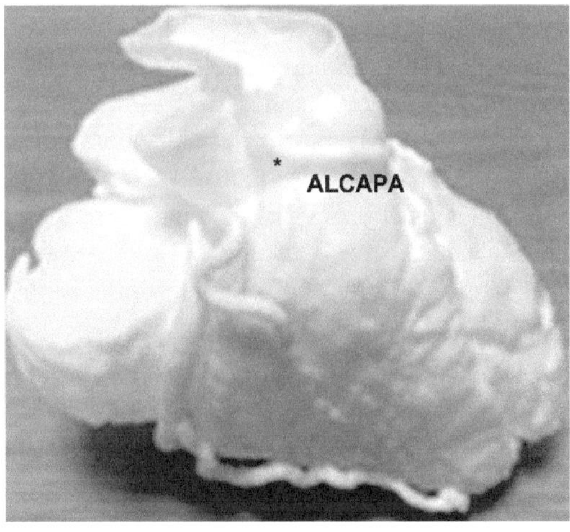

Fig. 17.6 Example of 3D printing of a coronary anomaly in a case of anomalous origin of the left coronary artery from the pulmonary trunk

with 3D printing [21, 24]. In these cases, the 3D-printed model anecdotally added value in management decisions.

Future Developments

Further improvement in the quality of available virtual simulation software and the enhanced capabilities of coupling with existing in vivo diagnostic tool such as MRI, 3DOCT reconstruction, intravascular ultrasound (IVUS) imaging, and angiographic equipment, and ultimately 3D printing are likely to push forward such a technology in the clinical practice making more effective the transition from off-line assessment and planning to on-line evaluation and treatment. Doubtless, early diagnosis, treatment, and prognosis of cardiac disease, especially those having a congenital background, could significantly reduce the related mortality and morbidity rates. CFD is considered to be a robust tool that can be used to evaluate the hemodynamic parameters. Patient-specific models obtained from subjects with CHDs can be used for various purposes, such as for (1) hemodynamic evaluation both in physiological and pathological conditions, (2) pretreatment planning, and (3) assessment of postoperative outcomes simulating the rheological effects associated with the various interventional alternatives prior to performing surgery or percutaneous procedures. However, several limiting factors that currently limit the use of such technology must be recognized. Indeed, the technical and logistic resources needed to obtain adequate data, process the images to reconstruct precise geometry, (3) and obtained patient-specific data are not yet widely available, also for related costs. Moreover, a multidisciplinary collaboration between cardiologists and engineers is required to understand the approximations, assumptions, and limitations of the numerical simulations in order to utilize CFD findings in clinical decisions [25].

References

1. Rigatelli G, Rigatelli A, Cominato S, Panin S, Nghia NT, Faggian G. A clinical-angiographic risk scoring system for coronary artery anomalies. Asian Cardiovasc Thorac Ann. 2012;20:299–303.
2. Zuin M, Rigatelli G, Faggian G, Roncon L. Mathematics and cardiovascular interventions: role of the finite element modeling in clinical decision making. JACC Cardiovasc Interv. 2016;9(5):507–8. https://doi.org/10.1016/j.jcin.2015.12.274.
3. Cho Y, Kensey KR. Effects of the non-Newtonian viscosity of blood on flows in a diseased arterial vessel. Part 1: steady flows. Biorheology. 1991;8:241–62.
4. Morris PD, Narracott A, von Tengg-Kobligk H, Silva Soto DA, Hsiao S, Lungu A, Evans P, Bressloff NW, Lawford PV, Hose DR, Gunn JP. Computational fluid dynamics modelling in cardiovascular medicine. Heart. 2016;102(1):18–28. https://doi.org/10.1136/heartjnl-2015-308044.
5. Pennati G, Corsini C, Hsia TY, Migliavacca F. Modeling of congenital hearts Alliance (MOCHA) investigators. Computational fluid dynamics models and congenital heart diseases. Front Pediatr. 2013;26(1):4. https://doi.org/10.3389/fped.2013.00004. PMID: 24432298; PMCID: PMC3882907
6. Arbia G, Esmaily Moghadam M, Marsden AL, Migliavacca F, Pennati G, Hsia TY, Vignon-Clementel IE. Modeling of congenital hearts Alliance (MOCHA) investigators. Numerical blood flow simulation in surgical corrections: what do we need for an accurate analysis? J Surg Res. 2014;186(1):44–55. https://doi.org/10.1016/j.jss.2013.07.037; Epub 2013 Aug 11.
7. Jamalidinan F, Hassanabad AF, François CJ, Garcia J. Four-dimensional-flow magnetic resonance imaging of the aortic valve and thoracic aorta. Radiol Clin N Am. 2020;58(4):753–63. https://doi.org/10.1016/j.rcl.2020.02.008.
8. Morbiducci U, Kok AM, Kwak BR, Stone PH, Steinman DA, Wentzel JJ. Atherosclerosis at arterial bifurcations: evidence for the role of haemodynamics and geometry. Thromb Haemost. 2016;115(3):484–92. https://doi.org/10.1160/TH15-07-0597.
9. de Leval MR, Dubini G, Migliavacca F, Jalali H, Camporini G, Redington A, Pietrabissa R. Use of computational fluid dynamics in the design of surgical procedures: application to the study of competitive flows in cavo-pulmonary connections. J Thorac Cardiovasc Surg. 1996;111(3):502–13. https://doi.org/10.1016/s0022-5223(96)70302-1.
10. Boutsianis E, Dave H, Frauenfelder T, Poulikakos D, Wildermuth S, Turina M, Ventikos Y, Zund G. Computational simulation of intracoronary flow

based on real coronary geometry. Eur J Cardiothorac Surg. 2004;26:248–56.

11. Pao YC, Lu JT, Ritman EL. Bending and twisting of an in vivo coronary artery at a bifurcation. J Biomech. 1992;3:287–9.

12. Basso C, Maron BJ, Corrado D, Thiene G. Clinical profile of congenital coronary artery anomalies with origin from the wrong aortic sinus leading to sudden death in young competitive athletes. J Am Coll Cardiol. 2000;35:1493–501.

13. Javadzadegan A, Moshfegh A, Fulker D, Barber T, Qian Y, Kritharides L, Yong ASC. Development of a computational fluid dynamics model for myocardial bridging. J Biomech Eng. 2018;140:in press. https://doi.org/10.1115/1.4040127.

14. Sharzehee M, Seddighi Y, Sprague EA, Finol EA, Han HC. A hemodynamic comparison of myocardial bridging and coronary atherosclerotic stenosis: a computational model with experimental evaluation. J Biomech Eng. 2020;143(3):031013. https://doi.org/10.1115/1.4049221; Epub ahead of print.

15. Angelini P, Uribe C. Anatomic spectrum of left coronary artery anomalies and associated mechanisms of coronary insufficiency. Catheter Cardiovasc Interv. 2018;92(2):313–21. https://doi.org/10.1002/ccd.27656.

16. Rigatelli G, Zuin M, Galasso P, Carraro M, D'Elia K, Daniela L, Roncon L, Truyen TTTT, Nguyen T. Mechanisms of myocardial ischemia inducing sudden cardiac death in athletes with anomalous coronary origin from the opposite sinus: insights from a computational fluid dynamic study. Cardiovasc Revasc Med. 2019;20(12):1112–6. https://doi.org/10.1016/j.carrev.2019.01.031.

17. Rigatelli G, Zuin M. Computed tomography-based patient-specific biomechanical and fluid dynamic study of anomalous coronary arteries with origin from the opposite sinus and intramural course. Heart Int. 2020;14(2):105–11.

18. Razavi A, Sachdeva S, Frommelt PC, LaDisa JF Jr. Patient-specific numerical analysis of coronary flow in children with intramural anomalous aortic origin of coronary arteries. Semin Thorac Cardiovasc Surg. 2020;S1043–0679(20):30271–9. https://doi.org/10.1053/j.semtcvs.2020.08.016; Epub ahead of print.

19. Smith ML, McGuinness J, O'Reilly MK, et al. The role of 3D printing in preoperative planning for heart transplantation in complex congenital heart disease. Ir J Med Sci. 2017;186:753–6.

20. Hinton TJ, Jallerat Q, Palchesko RN, et al. Three-dimensional printing of complex biological structures by freeform reversible embedding of suspended hydrogels. Sci Adv. 2015;1:e1500758.

21. Velasco Forte MN, Byrne N, Valverde Perez I, et al. 3D printed models in patients with coronary artery fistulae: anatomical assessment and interventional planning. Euro Intervention. 2017;13:e1080–3.

22. Aroney N, Lau K, Daniele L, et al. Three-dimensional printing: to guide management of a right coronary artery to left ventricular fistula. Eur Heart J Cardiovasc Imaging. 2018;19:268.

23. Lee M, Moharem- Elgamal S, Beckingham R, et al. Evaluating 3D-printed models of coronary anomalies: a survey among clinicians and researchers at a university hospital in the UK. BMJ Open. 2019;9:e025227. https://doi.org/10.1136/bmjopen-2018-025227.

24. Aroney N, Lau K, Daniele L, et al. Three-dimensional printing: to guide management of a right coronary artery to left ventricular fistula. Eur heart J Cardiovasc Imaging. 2018;19:268.

25. Cebral JR, Meng H. Counterpoint: realizing the clinical utility of computational fluid dynamics—closing the gap. Am J Neuroradiol. 2012;33(3):396–8. https://doi.org/10.3174/ajnr.A2994.

Anomalous Aortic Origin of Coronary Arteries Data from the Registries

Registries for Anomalous Aortic Origin of Coronary Arteries

Massimo A. Padalino and Matteo Ponzoni

Abbreviations

AAOCA	Anomalous aortic origin of coronary artery
AAOLCA	Anomalous aortic origin of left coronary artery
AAORCA	Anomalous aortic origin of right coronary artery
SCD	Sudden cardiac death

Introduction

Anomalous aortic origin of coronary arteries represents a rare clinical condition, with some anatomycal variants being the second cause of unexpected and sudden death in children and adolescents. [1]. Still, it represents the second

M. A. Padalino (✉)
Pediatric and Congenital Cardiac Surgery,
Department of Cardio-thoracic, Vascular Sciences
and Public Health, University of Padova, Medical
School, Padova, Italy

UOC Cardiochirurgia Pediatrica e Cardiopatie
Congenite, Centro "Vincenzo Gallucci", Padova, Italy
e-mail: massimo.padalino@unipd.it

M. Ponzoni
Pediatric and Congenital Cardiac Surgery,
Department of Cardio-thoracic, Vascular Sciences
and Public Health, University of Padova, Medical
School, Padova, Italy

leading cause of sudden cardiac death (SCD) in healthy children or young athletes, especially during exercise, often with no prodromes [1–7]. The most common and clinically relevant anomaly is the anomalous origin from the opposite sinus of Valsalva, including the more common anomalous aortic origin of the right coronary artery from the left sinus (Fig. 18.1), and the

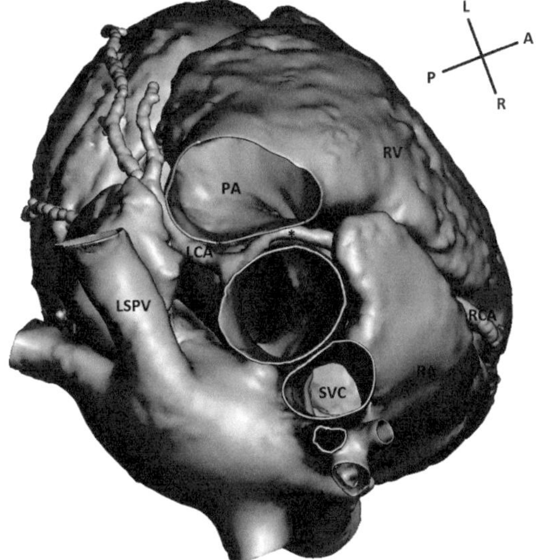

Fig. 18.1 3D reconstruction of a CT scan of an anomalous aortic origin of the right coronary artery from the opposite (left) sinus of Valsalva, with interarterial course (*). *AO* Aorta, *LSPV* left superior pulmonary vein, *PA* pulmonary artery, *RA* right atrium, *RCA* right coronary artery, *RV* right ventricle, *SVC* superior vena cava

© Springer Nature Switzerland AG 2023
G. Butera, A. Frigiola (eds.), *Congenital Anomalies of Coronary Arteries*,
https://doi.org/10.1007/978-3-031-36966-7_18

more morbid anomalous aortic origin of the left coronary artery arising from the right sinus [1].

The risk of death seems to be much higher when the left coronary artery arises from the wrong location, while it is reported to be lower when it is the right coronary to arise from the wrong sinus. However, the etiopathological mechanism, which causes SCD, is still not completely understood. It may well be a mixture of anatomy and physiological response to physical effort and increased blood pressure and aortic wall stress. As described elsewhere [1–6], in the past, the associated interarterial course has been considered as the most risky anatomical pattern because of the hypothesized compression (scissor like) exerted by the aortic and pulmonary arteries in the interarterial coronary segment during effort and rise of blood pressure. Currently, this phenomemenon is considered less important in the ethiopathogenesis of coronary ischemia. On the contrary, a greater role is played by the anaomycal features of the ostial shape (round vs. slit-like) and the intramural coronary course. (Fig. 18.2).

Diagnosis of AAOCA is nowadays easier due the advanced imaging technology. However, discerning which is the most dangerous anatomyc type is a very challenging task, because most patients do not present with obvious symptoms or complaints. Whenever symptomatic, the patients most commonly complain of chest pain, palpitations, dizziness, or fainting during or just after exercise. Also, SCD may be the first and only symptom occurring.

Furthermore, an increasing number of children and young adults are being *incidentally* found to have AAOCA on imaging studies, performed as part of screening campaigns or for other reasons.

Surgical treatment has been proposed in order to remove any risk of myocardial ischemia and SCD. Although single-center studies describe promising early and medium-term results, with excellent survival and safetyness [8–12], late effects on symptoms and risk of SCD are undefined and concerns about the surgical effectiveness and possible surgery-related complications remain [13].

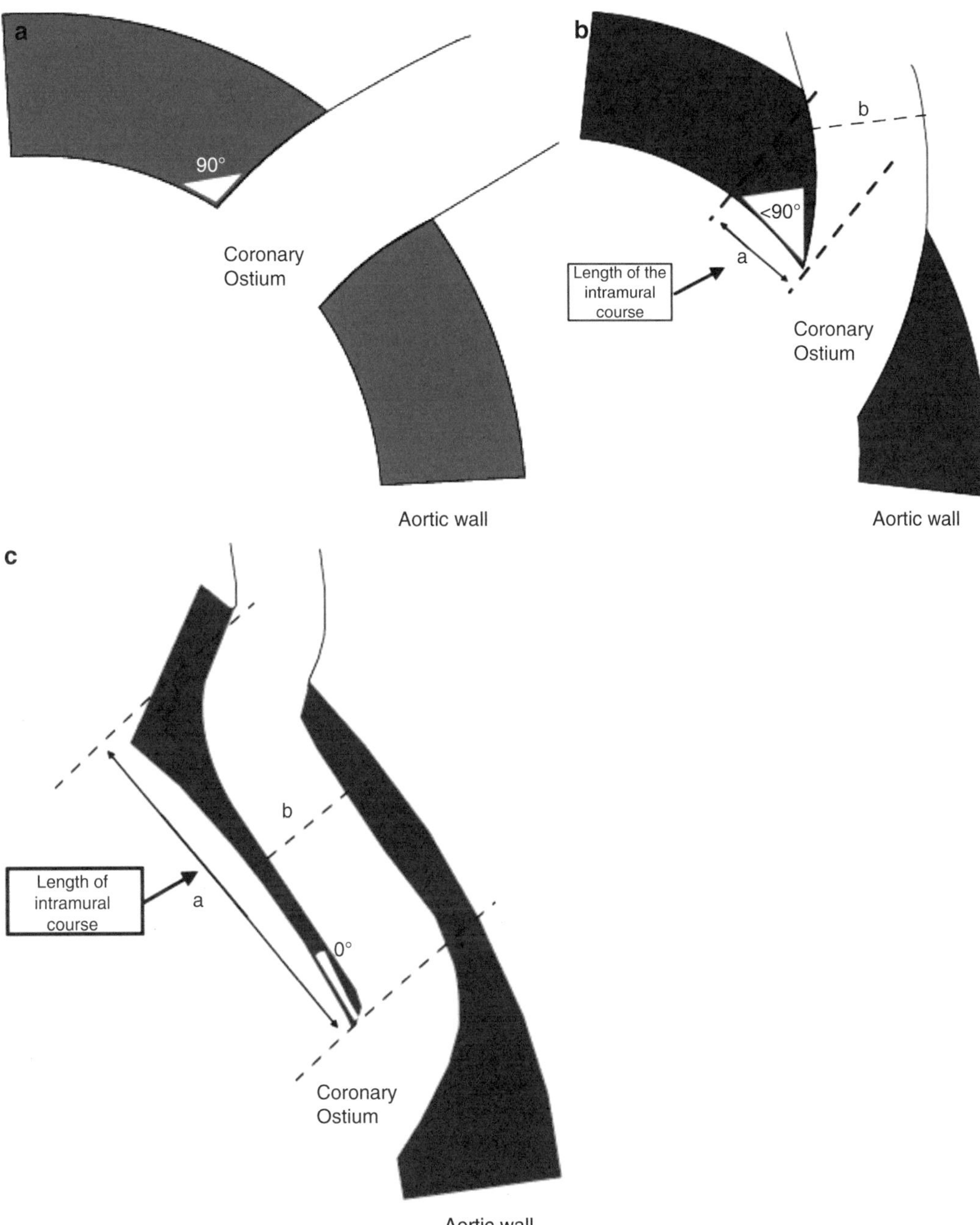

Fig. 18.2 Diagram showing: (1) the normal anatomical origin and intraparietal aortic wall course of a coronary artery, and the exit-angle is equal to 90°; (**b**) the abnormal angulated orifice: the coronary vessel passes obliquely through the aortic wall for a distance, (**a**) which is equal or inferior to the coronary artery's diameter (**b**), and the exit-angle is <90°; (**c**) the abnormal intramural course: the coronary vessel passes obliquely through the aortic wall for a distance, (**a**) which is greater than the coronary artery's diameter (**b**), and the exit-angle is about 0°

Gaps in Evidence

Currently, the majority of literature about AAOCA consists of single-center retrospective surgical reports (Table 18.1), which describe institutional experiences with relatively small number of cohorts collected over long periods of surgical activity [21, 25–30]. Most of these series account for less than 100 patients over a median period of 10 years, revealing that incidence of surgical

Table 18.1 Main surgical experiences reported in current literature

Single center surgical series	Pts n.	Age range (years)	Technique (n, %)	Early mortality (n, %)	Major early surgical complications (n, %)	FU (yrs, mean/ median)	Late cardiac mortality (n, %)	Late reinterventions (n, %)
Romp et al. (2003) [14]	9	7–65	Unroofing (9, 100)	0	0	2.4	0	1 (11%) Ross operation
Gulati et al. (2007) [15]	18	0.1–16	Unroofing (11, 61) Reimplantation (3, 16) PA translocation (4, 22)	0	0	2.2	0	1 (5.5%) OHT
Frommelt et al. (2011) [7]	27	4–20	Unroofing (27, 100)	0	0	1.8	0	0
Mumtaz et al. (2011) [8]	22	5–54	Unroofing (22, 100)	0	0	1.4	0	0
Wittlieb-Weber et al. (2014) [10]	24	5–18	Unroofing (23, 96) Reimplantation (1, 4)	0	0	5.25	0	0
Sharma et al. (2014) [16]	75	13–70	Unroofing (63, 84) Unroofing + CABG(3, 4) CABG or reimplantation (9, 12)	0	1 (1.3%) AICD	1.56	1 (CVA)	1 (1.3%) AVR
Kooij et al. (2015) [17]	31	9–66	Unroofing (17, 55) Unroofing + reimplantation (8, 26) CABG (1, 3) Ostioplasty (4, 13) Reimplantation +IV septal release (1, 3)	0	3 (9.6%) had VF postop.	6	0	0
Law et al. (2016) [45]	16	17–70	Reimplantation (16, 100)	0	1(6.2%) CABG +MVR	5	0 (cancer)	1 (1.6%) stent
Mainwaring et al. (2016) [11]	115	0.1–65	Unroofing (86, 75) Reimplantation (9, 8) PA translocation (20, 17)	0	0	6	0	2 (1.7%) coronary
Fabozzo et al. (2016) [19]	72	0.1–50.1	Unroofing (64, 89) Reimplantation (8, 11)	0	4(6%)	1.9	0	1 (1.3) AV repair
Nees et al. (2018) [12]	60	0.3–68	Unroofing (56, 93) Reimplantation (4, 7)	0	0	Median 1.6	0	3 (5%) AVR 1, coronary in 2*) *ECPR for SCD

Mery et al. (2018) [20]	44	8–18	Unroofing (35) Reimplantation (7) Ostioplasty (1) Side-to-side anastomosis (1)	0	1 (2.2%) CABG	Median 2	0	1 (2.2%) repair of myocardial bridge
Sachdeva S et al. (2018) [21]	63	0.5–18	Unroofing (63, 100)	0	0	Median 3.1	1 SCD (2%)	0
Ibraheem et al. (2019) [22]	16	Mean age 34.8 + 4.6	Off pump CABG with coronary ligation(16,100)	1 (3%)	0	5.25	1 (3%)	1 (1.6%) redo CABG on pump
Gaillard et al. (2020) [23]	61	3.7–66.1	Anatomical repair ostioplasty (37, 61) Reimplantation (19, 31) Intraseptal relief (5, 8)	0	1 (1.6%) ECMO and revision for thrombosis 2 (3.2%) stenting	3.1	0	1 (1.6%) revision for patch aneurysm
Jiang et al. (2021) [46]	36	Mean 50.5 ± 16.1	Unroofing (17, 47) CABG (12, 33) Reimplantation (3, 8) Aortocoronary window (3, 8)	0	0	Median 2.5	0	0
Bonilla-Ramirez et al. (2021) [24]	61	Median 14 (11–17)	Unroofing (45, 74) Transection and reimplantation (16, 26)	0	1 (1.6%) CABG	Median 4	0	1 (1.6%) reoperation for unknown myocardial bridge

ICD implantable cardiac defibrillator, *AVR* aortic valve replacement, *CVA* cerebro vascular attack, *CABG* coronary artery bypass graft, *ECMO* extracorporeal membrane oxygenation, *ECPR* ECMO cardiopulmonary resuscitation, *MVR* mitral valve replacement, *OHT* orthotopic heart transplant, *PA* pulmonary artery, *SCD* sudden cardiac death

AAOCA is *less than 10 patients/year* [25–27]. As an example, Mainwaring et al. described the conjunct surgical experience of three pediatric cardiac surgical centers referring to the Stanford University in three reports since 2011 [12, 28, 29]. In the first publication, the group reported the outcomes of 50 patients over 10 years of activity (1999–2010 [28]), increasing to 76 cases over 14 years (1999–2013 [29]) and to 115 patients over 16 years (1999–2015 [12]). From this experience, it is evident that surgical incidence of AAOCA also in a third-level surgical center is low, and approximately 5 to 10 patients are referred for surgical correction each year.

The limited dimensions of single-center cohorts may affect the reliability of data in terms of the actual incidence of complications and mortality, as well as decreases the statistical power of analyses and survival estimates. To date, incidence of early (i.e., postoperative) and late deaths after any surgical repair of AAOCA has been reported to be low worldwide [10, 18, 21, 30–32]. However, concerns have been raised regarding the long-term efficacy and durability of surgery. In fact, as stated by the most recent AATS Guidelines [25], one of the major gaps in actual knowledge is the *lack of long-term follow-up.* From pediatric series, the longest available follow-up is a retrospective study by Balasubramanya et al. [33], on 66 patients treated from 2006 to 2014, in which they described a median follow-up of *5.6 years*, which is still too short to speculate about the real durability of surgery in patients with supposed decades of life expectancy.

Furthermore, open debate is still going on in the following topics.

1. The *type of surgical repair:* which one to prefer and for which patient? Specific technical indications are still lacking, and often the chosen surgical technique depends on the institutional surgical experience. Current consensus guidelines [25] suggest to treat AAOCA with intramural course by means of unroofing, ostioplasty, or reimplantation techniques (Class I, level B), while pulmonary artery translocation may be considered as an adjunctive surgery (Class IIb, level C) .

2. The *association of AAOCA with myocardial bridges: is there a* need for combined correction? These two entities have been proven to present together with a certain frequency, thus some authors recommend a complete evaluation of the whole coronary tree and eventual surgical treatment of both lesions concomitantly whenever possible [12].

3. The risk of *postoperative residual myocardial ischemia* and sudden cardiac events: up to 50% of patients with transeptal AAOCA present inducible myocardial hypoperfusion during provocative testing [34], which may persist following successful surgical correction, despite demonstrated patent neo-ostia or absence of symptoms [11, 23]. Postoperative myocardial ischemic events may impose surgical or interventional revision in a minority of patients [35] and, more rarely, they could be fatal [21, 31]. Nees et al. stressed this concept in their report of 60 operated cases of AAOCA in which they experienced a not so negligible rate of major complications (reoperation for coronary stenosis in 3%, aborted SCD in 2%, significant aortic regurgitation in 12%, requiring aortic valve replacement in 2%) in a relatively short period (median follow-up of 1.6 years), emphasizing the critical need of strict clinical surveillance [13]. However, from single-center limited series, we are not able to determine if these complications are isolated and remote events or if they represent a real threat for a significant quote of patients.

4. The risk of *aortic regurgitation* following aortic valve commissure resuspension. Several authors described a consistent risk of postoperative aortic regurgitation after commissure resuspension, recommending avoiding this procedure whenever possible [11, 13, 36]. On the other hand, Yerebakan et al. who resuspended the aortic commissure routinely during the unroofing operation reported an even inferior incidence of novel aortic regurgitation with this approach [32]. Thus, scientific literature has not been conclusive yet in defining the real impact of such surgical procedure.

5. The possibility to *return to normal physical activity* for operated patients. Physical activity is a well-known determinant of the quality of life of patients with AAOCA and their parents, especially in young patients [20]. Current guidelines allow operated patients to conclude their physical activity restriction after 3 months from surgery if asymptomatic, or after 1 year if the presentation of AAOCA was an aborted SCD [25]. However, the level of evidence is low (level C) and all these recommendations and cut-off times are based on expert consensus opinions, rather than clinically proven evidence, and may vary according to different regulations in different countries (ie. Europe vs USA).

Why a Registry for AAOCA

A *registry* is a collection of information about individuals, usually focused on a specific diagnosis or condition. A *patient registry* is an organized system that uses observational study methods to collect uniform data (clinical and other) to evaluate specified outcomes for a population defined by a particular disease or exposure and that serves predetermined scientific, clinical, or policy purpose(s). A *national registry* centralizes this data for an entire country to avoid duplication of names.

The purpose of a registry is to study incidence, prevalence, outcomes, and course of a specific disease or condition, and possibly to evaluate the risk of its adverse events, that is, sudden death, in the long term. Furthermore, registries are used for comparing the effectiveness of different treatments, evaluating different approaches to a procedure, and monitoring the safety of implanted devices.

Because AAOCA is rare and postoperative adverse events are even rarer, we can only accomplish this goal through the collaboration of multiple hospitals and institutions, which is a registry. Data from a national registry can provide health outcome information to monitor patient needs and identify health problems that need prompt attention, improving health-care quality and safety.

As noted before, the small number of single-center experiences is one of the major determinants, which limits the implementation of AAOCA guidelines with a high level of evidence. Thus, the importance of *multi-institutional registries* is evident. The main objectives of this kind of registry are to augment the dimension of cohorts, to create the basis for a prospective collection of data and patients, in order to expand follow-up times. This knowledge will help us to assess most of the above-mentioned limits of current reports, allowing the formulation of more evidence-based recommendations for the diagnosis and treatment of AAOCA.

To date, 1 prospective single-center and 2 international multicenter registries are present:

- A prospective single-center data collection, named as *Coronary Anomalies Program*, ongoing at Texas's Children Hospital [37].
- A multicenter northern American registry enrolling patients from 29 institutions of the *Congenital Heart Surgeons' Society* [38], started more than 10 years ago.
- A more recent multicenter *European AAOCA registry, including a growing number of centers across Europe* [39].

Coronary Anomalies Program

This single center registry has been recruiting prospectively all consecutive patients treated at Texas Children Hospital since 2012, as a part of a standardized pre- and postoperative management protocol [24]. In 2017, Mery et al. published the first results from 44 patients enrolled from 2012 to 2017, who underwent surgical correction of AAOCA [37]. Twenty percent of them presented an anomalous aortic origin of left coronary artery (AAOLCA) and 80% an anomalous aortic origin of right coronary artery (AAORCA). The majority of patients were symptomatic (73%) and all but one had an intramural coronary course. Surgical strategy consisted in unroofing of the intramural segment in 80% of cases, coronary translocation in 16%, ostioplasty in 2%, and side-to-side anastomosis in 2%. Results were excellent, with *absent early and late mortality* at a median follow-up of 2 years. Two patients required early reoperation: one for surgical bleeding and one for saphenous vein coronary artery bypass for residual myocardial ischemia. During follow-up, another patient presented an aborted SCD and he was found to have an unrecognized myocardial bridge, which was subsequently treated. At last follow-up, 91% of patients were free of symptoms and 95% returned to full physical activity without restrictions.

From these results, the authors concluded that if individualized according to patient's anatomy, surgical treatment of AAOCA is safe and presents a low rate of complications. However, the efficacy of surgery in the prevention of SCD still needs to be assessed with a longer follow-up. Furthermore, the single-center nature of this program may expose to the risk of *selection bias* of patients, which could be empathized by the exclusion of patients above 20 years of age as a part of the institutional protocol [24]. The Coronary Anomalies Program was recently updated, reaching a total of 61 operated patients between 2012 and 2019 with no mortality, *93%* of whom have been released to *unrestricted physical activity* [40].

The Northern American Experience

The need for a multi-institutional database of AAOCA was firstly emphasized in 2009 by Brothers et al. who investigated the practitioners' opinions on treatment and management of patients with AAOCA [41]. This survey across the Congenital Heart Surgeons' Society (CHSS) members unmasked the wide heterogeneity regarding diagnostic tools and treatment strategies for AAOCA. In this report, the authors claimed the need to develop more cohesive and evidence-based guidelines, and the CHSS AAOCA registry was established to serve to this purpose.

Thus, in the participating CHSS institutions, all patients under 30 years of age with a diagnosis of AAOCA (any type), between 1998 and 2009, were *retrospectively* enrolled in the registry, and then *prospectively* since 2009. In a first publication by Poynter et al. in 2014 [42], the registry had collected *198 patients*, with a median age at diagnosis of 10 years. About half (54%) of patients were symptomatic at presentation, and in 2 cases, the diagnosis was made from autopsy following SCD. At diagnostic imaging, AAORCA was present in 73% of cases, AAOLCA in 26%, and both in 1%. Surgical repair was carried out in 52% of patients with a diagnosed AAORCA and in 67% with an AAOLCA. The decision for a surgical approach correlated with symptoms, older age, and presence of an intramural course.

A following report focused on surgical management performed in *113 patients* (median age 12.6 years) enrolled retrospectively from 1998 to 2008 and prospectively from 2009 to 2012 in 29 CHSS institutions [43]. The proportion of AAOLCA to AAORCA was 1:2, and 89% of patients presented an intramural course. *Unroofing* was the procedure of choice (88% of cases), followed by coronary reimplantation, pulmonary artery translocation, and ostioplasty, while a coronary artery bypass graft (CABG) was performed in a minority of patients. Although unroofing seemed to be a uniformly adopted strategy, this procedure was not standardized across centers, where different surgical variations were encompassed. The common wall of the anomalous coronary artery was incised with subsequent intimal tacking in most of the cases, while complete excision (endarterectomy) was performed in others. On the other hand, the major variations in surgical approach were described in the case of an anomalous coronary artery without an intramural segment, where various solutions were adopted.

The CHSS registry grew up across the years, reaching *560 patients* enrolled from 40 institutions in 2019 [44], when the authors analyzed the anatomical features of AAOCA associated with myocardial ischemia at provocative tests. Important findings were that the patients with ischemia were more likely to have AAOLCA than AAORCA (38% vs. 10%), an intramural course, a high and slit-like coronary orifice, and a longer intramural course (in those with AAORCA). Otherwise, the occurrence of SCD was not shown to have any associated anatomic features. The authors concluded that the real determinant of myocardial ischemia in AAOCA is not the interarterial course per se. Instead, various anatomic features such as the coronary artery involved, intramural course and its length, and orifice anomalies (slit-like, high take-off) were associated with evidence of myocardial ischemia and these may importantly inform risk stratification and decisions regarding surgical management.

The last registry's update encompassed 682 patients from 45 CHSS centers during the period 2000–2018 [31]. Among these, 375 patients (57%) underwent surgical correction (mainly using the unroofing procedure), with 4 reported deaths (1%), at a median follow-up of 2.8 years from surgery. New onset of moderate or greater than moderate aortic regurgitation was detected in 2% of patients, and this finding was found to be associated with surgical manipulation of aortic commissure. Interestingly, in 80% of patients with preoperative signs of myocardial ischemia, surgery allowed the resolution of ischemia. However, there were 15 coronary-related reoperations (4%), and freedom from any reoperation was 93% at 1 year, and 90% at 7 years. The authors concluded that, although surgery was found to be safe and effective in resolving myocardial ischemia in most patients, there are few patients who can experience serious postoperative complications. Thus, the question whether the risks of SCD outweigh the risks of surgery is still to be answered, and the authors stress the importance of understanding the eventuality of these risks in the surgical decision-making.

The European Experience

The European experience started later in 2016, with a retrospective data collection among the members of the European Congenital Heart Surgeons' Association (ECHSA). In 2019, the early results from the first European multicenter registry of AAOCA were published, including *217 patients*, which had been collected retrospectively from 16 institutions [39]. Patients were divided into two groups according to treatment strategy: surgical (72%) versus medical (28%). Incidence of AAOLCA to AAORCA was 1:2 to 1:3 in both groups.

Patients who underwent surgery were mostly those with an anomalous left coronary artery, symptomatic (87%), and with an intramural course (63%). The unroofing procedure was the technique of choice in most cases (56%) followed by reimplantation (19%) and CABG (15%), whose incidence was slightly higher than other reports, since the median age of the patients was higher and mostly were adult patients. Nevertheless, operative mortality was confirmed to be very low (*1.3%*), occurring mostly in patients with compromised preoperative clinical conditions. Specifically, in this series, 1 occurred after emergency surgery for aborted SCD, the other in an infant after a rescue CABG. At a median follow-up of *18 months,* there were 3 additional deaths. Patients who did not undergo surgery, and were followed up with medical treatment only, were presenting symptoms less frequently (44% vs. 87%), and had a low-risk anatomy. Noticeably, at the short follow-up available, there were no deaths in the medical group. However, the occurrence of overall and coronary-related adverse events did not differ in a statistically significant way between the two groups. On the other hand, surgery clearly turned out to be an effective option in allowing patients to return to unrestrained life and sport activity. In fact, 48% of surgical patients returned to practice sports, compared to only 18% of medical patients ($p < 0.001$).

Despite the evident limitations, the results from this registry support that surgery, especially the unroofing procedure, is safe and effective to resume physical restrictions, improving patients' quality of life. However, as in the other reports, the protective effect of surgery cannot be confirmed yet, since the incidence of coronary-related cardiac events was unrelated to treatment strategy. As a conclusion, because of the limited number of patients and the short follow-up available, an accurate and constant clinical surveillance is mandatory to assess the real long-term impact of surgical treatment on the risk of SCD in patients with AAOCA. The study is ongoing as prospective study, and some answers to the many questions are expected.

Conclusions

As a rare disease with an unknown real incidence, AAOCA represents a clinical condition where recommendations and guidelines lack of adequate levels of evidence. Single-center experiences, limited by small-number series and short follow-up times, are insufficient to answer if and in which cases AAOCA merits a surgical attention, and more importantly, the safety and efficacy of this approach is still only hypothesized.

Multi-institutional prospective registries can help in providing a solid platform for a large collection of patients and information. To date, an "older and experienced" Northern American registry and a "younger and growing" European registry have been created, and early and medium-term results have been published and are helping in refining year-by-year definitions and indications.

From both these experiences, surgical correction of AAOCA emerges to be a procedure that can be accomplished with low mortality and complications, and it is effective in resuming myocardial ischemia and physical activity restrictions. However, however, it can result in a variety of important morbidities, varying by the group evaluated. Also, follow-up times are still too limited to allow for further speculations on long-term durability and safety of this surgery, especially in younger patients. Future data from these registries might help us to solve these issues.Conflicts of interestNone declared.

References

1. Cheezum MK, Liberthson RR, Shah NR, Villines TC, O'Gara PT, Landzberg MJ, et al. Anomalous aortic origin of a coronary artery from the inappropriate sinus of Valsalva. J Am Coll Cardiol. 2017;69:1592–608.
2. Angelini P, Villason S, Chan AV Jr, et al. Normal and anomalous coronary arteries in humans. In: Angelini P, editor. Coronary artery anomalies: a comprehensive approach. Philadelphia, PA: Lippincoat Williams &Wilkins; 1999. p. 27–150.
3. Pérez-Pomares JM, de la Pompa JL, Franco D, Henderson D, Ho SY, Houyel L, et al. Congenital coronary artery anomalies: a bridge from embryology to anatomy and pathophysiology--a position statement of the development, anatomy, and pathology ESC Working Group. Cardiovasc Res. 2016;109:204–16.
4. Basso C, Maron BJ, Corrado D, et al. Clinical profile of congenital coronary artery anomalies with origin from the wrong aortic sinus leading to sudden death in young competitive athletes. J Am Coll Cardiol. 2000;35:1493–501.
5. Maron BJ, Doerer JJ, Haas TS, et al. Sudden deaths in young competitive athletes: analysis of 1866 deaths in the United States, 1980-2006. Circulation. 2009;119:1085–92.
6. Corrado D, Basso C, Rizzoli G, Schiavon M, Thiene G. Does sports activity enhance the risk of sudden death in adolescents and young adults? J Am Coll Cardiol. 2003;42(11):1959–63.
7. Palmieri V, Gervasi S, Bianco M, Cogliani R, Poscolieri B, Cuccaro F, et al. Anomalous origin of coronary arteries from the "wrong" sinus in athletes: diagnosis and management strategies. Int J Cardiol. 2018;252:13–20.
8. Frommelt PC, Sheridan DC, Berger S, Frommelt MA, Tweddell JS. Ten-year experience with surgical unroofing of anomalous aortic origin of a coronary artery from the opposite sinus with an interarterial course. J Thorac Cardiovasc Surg. 2011;142(5):1046–51.
9. Mumtaz MA, Lorber RE, Arruda J, Pettersson GB, Mavroudis C. Surgery for anomalous aortic origin of the coronary artery. Ann Thorac Surg. 2011;91:811–4.
10. Davies JE, Burkhart HM, Dearani JA, Suri RM, Phillips SD, Warnes CA, et al. Surgical management of anomalous aortic origin of a coronary artery. Ann Thorac Surg. 2009;88:844–7.
11. Wittlieb-Weber CA, Paridon SM, Gaynor JW, Spray TL, Weber DR, Brothers JA. Medium-term outcome after anomalous aortic origin of a coronary artery repair in a pediatric cohort. J Thorac Cardiovasc Surg. 2014;147:1580–6.
12. Mainwaring RD, Murphy DJ, Rogers IS, Chan FP, Petrossian E, Palmon M, et al. Surgical repair of 115 patients with anomalous aortic origin of a coronary artery from a single institution. World J Pediatr Congenit Heart Surg. 2016;7:353–9.
13. Nees SN, Flyer JN, Chelliah A, Dayton JD, Touchette L, Kalfa D, et al. Patients with anomalous aortic origin of the coronary artery remain at risk after surgical repair. J Thorac Cardiovasc Surg. 2018;155:2554–2564.e3.
14. Romp RL, Herlong JR, Landolfo CK, Sanders SP, Miller CE, Ungerleider RM, et al. Outcome of unroofing procedure for repair of anomalous aortic origin of left or right coronary artery. Ann Thorac Surg. 2003;76:589–95.

15. Gulati R, Reddy VM, Culbertson C, Helton G, Suleman S, Reinhartz O, et al. Surgical management of coronary artery arising from the wrong coronary sinus, using standard and novel approaches. J Thorac Cardiovasc Surg. 2007;134:1171–8.

16. Sharma V, Burkhart HM, Dearani JA, Suri RM, Daly RC, Park SJ, et al. Surgical unroofing of anomalous aortic origin of a coronary artery: a single-center experience. Ann Thorac Surg. 2014;98:941–5.

17. Kooij M, Vliegen HW, de Graaf MA, Hazekamp MG. Surgical treatment of aberrant aortic origin of coronary arteries. Eur J Cardiothorac Surg. 2015;48:724–30.

18. Jegatheeswaran A, Devlin PJ, Williams WG, Brothers JA, Jacobs ML, DeCampli WM, Fleishman CE, Kirklin JK, Mertens L, Mery CM, Molossi S, Caldarone CA, Aghaei N, Lorber RO, McCrindle BW. Outcomes after anomalous aortic origin of a coronary artery repair: a congenital heart Surgeons' Society study. J Thorac Cardiovasc Surg. 2020;160(3):757–771.e5.

19. Fabozzo A, DiOrio M, Newburger J, Powell A, Liu H, Fynn-Thompson F, et al. Anomalous aortic origin of coronary arteries: a single-center experience. Semin Thorac Cardiovasc Surg. 2016;28:791–800.

20. Sing AC, Tsaur S, Paridon SM, Brothers JA. Quality of life and exercise performance in unoperated children with anomalous aortic origin of a coronary artery from the opposite sinus of valsalva. Cardiol Young. 2017;27(5):895–904.

21. Nguyen AL, Haas F, Evens J, Breur JM. Sudden cardiac death after repair of anomalous origin of left coronary artery from right sinus of Valsalva with an interarterial course : case report and review of the literature. Neth Heart J. 2012;20(11):463–71.

22. Ibraheem WI, Abass OA, Toema AM, Yehia AM. Coronary artery bypass grafting experience in the setting of an anomalous origin of the right coronary artery from the left sinus of Valsalva: midterm results. J Card Surg. 2019;34:1162–71.

23. Brothers JA, McBride MG, Seliem MA, Marino BS, Tomlinson RS, Pampaloni MH, Gaynor JW, Spray TL, Paridon SM. Evaluation of myocardial ischemia after surgical repair of anomalous aortic origin of a coronary artery in a series of pediatric patients. J Am Coll Cardiol. 2007;50(21):2078–82.

24. Molossi S, Agrawal H, Mery CM, Krishnamurthy R, Masand P, Sexson Tejtel SK, Noel CV, Qureshi AM, Jadhav SP, McKenzie ED, Fraser CD Jr. Outcomes in anomalous aortic origin of a coronary artery following a prospective standardized approach. Circ Cardiovasc Interv. 2020;13(2):e008445.

25. Brothers JA, Frommelt MA, Jaquiss RDB, Myerburg RJ, Fraser CD Jr, Tweddell JS. Expert consensus guidelines: anomalous aortic origin of a coronary artery. J Thorac Cardiovasc Surg. 2017 Jun;153(6):1440–57.

26. Karangelis D, Mylonas KS, Loggos S, Adreanides E, Tzifa A, Mitropoulos F. Surgical repair of anomalous aortic origin of coronary artery in adults. Asian Cardiovasc Thorac Ann. 2021;29(1):51–8.

27. Baumgartner H, De Backer J, Babu-Narayan SV, Budts W, Chessa M, Diller GP, Lung B, Kluin J, Lang IM, Meijboom F, Moons P, Mulder BJM, Oechslin E, Roos-Hesselink JW, Schwerzmann M, Sondergaard L. Zeppenfeld K; ESC scientific document group. 2020 ESC guidelines for the management of adult congenital heart disease. Eur Heart J. 2021;42(6):563–645.

28. Mainwaring RD, Reddy VM, Reinhartz O, Petrossian E, MacDonald M, Nasirov T, Miyake CY, Hanley FL. Anomalous aortic origin of a coronary artery: medium-term results after surgical repair in 50 patients. Ann Thorac Surg. 2011;92(2):691–7.

29. Mainwaring RD, Reddy VM, Reinhartz O, Petrossian E, Punn R, Hanley FL. Surgical repair of anomalous aortic origin of a coronary artery. Eur J Cardiothorac Surg. 2014;46(1):20–6.

30. Osaki M, McCrindle BW, Van Arsdell G, Dipchand AI. Anomalous origin of a coronary artery from the opposite sinus of Valsalva with an interarterial course: clinical profile and approach to management in the pediatric population. Pediatr Cardiol. 2008;29(1):24–30.

31. Sachdeva S, Frommelt MA, Mitchell ME, Tweddell JS, Frommelt PC. Surgical unroofing of intramural anomalous aortic origin of a coronary artery in pediatric patients: single-center perspective. J Thorac Cardiovasc Surg. 2018;155(4):1760–8.

32. Yerebakan C, Ozturk M, Mota L, Sinha L, Gordish-Dressman H, Jonas R, Sinha P. Complete unroofing of the intramural coronary artery for anomalous aortic origin of a coronary artery: the role of commissural resuspension? J Thorac Cardiovasc Surg. 2019;158(1):208–217.e2.

33. Balasubramanya S, Mongé MC, Eltayeb OM, Sarwark AE, Costello JM, Rigsby CK, Popescu AR, Backer CL. Anomalous aortic origin of a coronary artery: symptoms do not correlate with intramural length or ostial diameter. World J Pediatr Congenit Heart Surg. 2017;8(4):445–52.

34. Doan TT, Zea-Vera R, Agrawal H, Mery CM, Masand P, Reaves-O'Neal DL, Noel CV, Qureshi AM, Sexson-Tejtel SK, Fraser CD Jr, Molossi S. Myocardial ischemia in children with anomalous aortic origin of a coronary artery with Intraseptal course. Circ Cardiovasc Interv. 2020;13(3):e008375.

35. Gaillard M, Pontailler M, Danial P, Moreau de Bellaing A, Gaudin R, du Puy-Montbrun L, Murtuza B, Haydar A, Malekzadeh-Milani S, Bonnet D, Vouhé P, Raisky O. Anomalous aortic origin of coronary arteries: an alternative to the unroofing strategy. Eur J Cardiothorac Surg. 2020;58(5):975–82.

36. Brothers JA, Kim TS, Fogel MA, Whitehead KK, Morrison TM, Paridon SM, Harris MA. Cardiac magnetic resonance imaging characterizes stenosis, perfusion, and fibrosis preoperatively and postoperatively in children with anomalous coronary arteries. J Thorac Cardiovasc Surg. 2016;152(1):205–10.

37. Mery CM, De León LE, Molossi S, Sexson-Tejtel SK, Agrawal H, Krishnamurthy R, Masand P, Qureshi

AM, McKenzie ED, Fraser CD Jr. Outcomes of surgical intervention for anomalous aortic origin of a coronary artery: a large contemporary prospective cohort study. J Thorac Cardiovasc Surg. 2018;155(1):305–319.e4.

38. Brothers JA, Gaynor JW, Jacobs JP, Caldarone C, Jegatheeswaran A, Jacobs ML; Anomalous Coronary Artery Working Group. The registry of anomalous aortic origin of the coronary artery of the congenital heart Surgeons' Society. Cardiol Young. 2010;20(Suppl 3):50–8.

39. Padalino MA, Franchetti N, Sarris GE, Hazekamp M, Carrel T, Frigiola A, Horer J, Roussin R, Cleuziou J, Meyns B, Fragata J, Telles H, Polimenakos AC, Francois K, Veshti A, Salminen J, Rocafort AG, Nosal M, Vedovelli L, Protopapas E, Tumbarello R, Merola A, Pegoraro C, Motta R, Boccuzzo G, Sojak V, Rito ML, Caldaroni F, Corrado D, Basso C, Stellin G. Anomalous aortic origin of coronary arteries: early results on clinical management from an international multicenter study. Int J Cardiol. 2019;291:189–93.

40. Bonilla-Ramirez C, Molossi S, Sachdeva S, Reaves-O'Neal D, Masand P, Mery CM, Caldarone CA, McKenzie ED, Binsalamah ZM. Outcomes in anomalous aortic origin of a coronary artery after surgical reimplantation. J Thorac Cardiovasc Surg. 2021;S0022-5223(20):33455–3.

41. Brothers J, Gaynor JW, Paridon S, Lorber R, Jacobs M. Anomalous aortic origin of a coronary artery with an interarterial course: understanding current management strategies in children and young adults. Pediatr Cardiol. 2009;30(7):911–21.

42. Poynter JA, Williams WG, McIntyre S, Brothers JA, Jacobs ML. Congenital heart surgeons society AAOCA working group. Anomalous aortic origin of a coronary artery: a report from the congenital heart surgeons society registry. World J Pediatr Congenit Heart Surg. 2014;5(1):22–30.

43. Poynter JA, Bondarenko I, Austin EH, WM DC, Jacobs JP, Ziemer G, Kirshbom PM, Tchervenkov CI, Karamlou T, Blackstone EH, Walters HL 3rd, Gaynor JW, Mery CM, Pearl JM, Brothers JA, Caldarone CA, Williams WG, Jacobs ML, Mavroudis C, Congenital Heart Surgeons' Society AAOCA Working Group. Repair of anomalous aortic origin of a coronary artery in 113 patients: a congenital heart surgeons' Society report. World J Pediatr Congenit Heart Surg. 2014;5(4):507–14.

44. Jegatheeswaran A, Devlin PJ, McCrindle BW, Williams WG, Jacobs ML, Blackstone EH, DeCampli WM, Caldarone CA, Gaynor JW, Kirklin JK, Lorber RO, Mery CM, St Louis JD, Molossi S, Brothers JA. Features associated with myocardial ischemia in anomalous aortic origin of a coronary artery: a congenital heart Surgeons' Society study. J Thorac Cardiovasc Surg. 2019;158(3):822–834.e3.

45. Law T, Dunne B, Stamp N, Ho KM, Andrews D. Surgical results and outcomes after reimplantation for the management of anomalous aortic origin of the right coronary artery. Ann Thorac Surg. 2016;102:192–8.

46. Jiang MX, Blackstone EH, Karamlou T, Ghobrial J, Brinza EK, Haupt MJ, Pettersson GB, Rajeswaran J, Williams WG, Saarel EV. Cleveland Clinic Adult AAOCA Working Group. Anomalous Aortic Origin of a Coronary Artery in Adults. Ann Thorac Surg. 2021;112(4):1299–305. https://doi.org/10.1016/j.athoracsur.2020.06.153. Epub 2020 Dec 4. PMID: 33279536.

M. Lo Rito, O. Raisky, and A. Frigiola

Introduction

Anomalous aortic origin of the coronary artery (AAOCA) is a rare congenital heart disease characterized by an ectopic connection of the main coronary arteries to the aorta. The anomalous origin of the right coronary artery (AAORCA) from the left sinus is the most common form, while the anomalous origin of the left coronary artery (AAOLCA) is less common but more lethal [1, 2]. AAOLCA is at higher risk of sudden cardiac death (SCD) than AAORCA, although the anatomical characteristics such as the course, the intramural segment, and the ostium morphology are among the most determinant risk factors [3, 4]. Clinical manifestations range from asymptomatic to angina or sudden cardiac death (SCD) during effort. The magnitude of the clinical presentation is associated with the severity of the AAOCA, although the SCD remains a stochastic and unpredictable event not dependent directly on the amount of effort. It is helpful to adopt a

structured approach while defining the AAOCA [4–6]. The risk is determined first by the type of anomalous coronary artery (LCA > RCA), second by the course (interarterial > subpulmonary infundibular, retroaortic, or prepulmonic), and third by the ostium morphology (round < oval < slit-like < pinhole) and the angle of take-off. Lastly, the presence of an intramural segment (IM) and its length > 10 mm are considered significant SCD risk factors [1, 2, 6]. Such anatomical risk classification can be obtained from coronary computed tomography (CT). Still, other provocative tests should be done, especially in asymptomatic subjects, to unmask myocardial perfusion alteration territory of the anomalous coronary artery.

The indications for surgical treatment are well accepted (Class 1 C) in symptomatic AAOCA or cases with stress-induced ischemia in the myocardium irrorated by the anomalous coronary [4, 7, 8]. The level of evidence to surgically intervene decreases in Class II for the asymptomatic cases or without inducible ischemia in the corresponding territory [4, 7, 8]. The AAOCA without surgical indication and no evidence of inducible ischemia return to physical/sport activity vary from complete restriction to participation in physical/sport activity after counseling [7].

There are various surgical techniques available, and each one has its specific field of application and ability to treat the ischemic mechanism. However, it must also be remembered that not all

M. Lo Rito (✉) · A. Frigiola
Department of Congenital Cardiac Surgery, IRCCS
Policlinico San Donato, San Donato Milanese,
Milan, Italy
e-mail: mauro.lorito@grupposandonato.it;
alessandro.frigiola@grupposandonato.it

O. Raisky
Pediatric Cardiac Surgery, Necker Sick Children's
Hospital and Paris University, Paris, France
e-mail: olivier.raisky@aphp.fr

© Springer Nature Switzerland AG 2023
G. Butera, A. Frigiola (eds.), *Congenital Anomalies of Coronary Arteries*,
https://doi.org/10.1007/978-3-031-36966-7_19

the techniques will allow restoring a typical origin. Therefore, in the following paragraphs, we will illustrate the specific indications, the technical pitfalls, and the possible complications of each technique, allowing the reader to plan the correct surgical repair and achieve the best long-term outcome possible.

Surgical Techniques for AAOCA

Patient Preparation

The patient's preparation depends on the surgical approach adopted to perform the operation. A standard sternotomy is preferred for complex AAOCA forms, because surgery may require extensive manipulation of the aortic and pulmonary roots. A minimally invasive approach has been proposed for adult patients either through a minimal sternotomy [9] or right anterior thoracotomy [10]. After pericardiotomy, careful examination of the epicardial coronary pattern may detect additional features useful for the following repair. The aorta is carefully separated from the pulmonary artery, and the periaortic fat is dissected to identify the abnormal coronary course and origin. The tissue dissection must be done gently to avoid damaging the unseen coronary segment. Heparin can be administered once the anomalous coronary origin and course are identified. Aortic cannulation needs to be performed slightly higher at about 1 cm below the emergency of the innominate artery, because the aortotomy has to be 1 cm distal to the sino-tubular junction or even higher to avoid coronary lesions and preserve a good portion of the aorta for the suturing after the repair. A dual-stage right atrial cannula is usually sufficient for central venous cannulation. However, a bicaval cannulation may be preferred in case of intracardiac repair, pulmonary artery translocation, or infundibular relief procedure [11–14]. A left atrial venting is recommended to maintain a bloodless field during the repair. When applying the aortic cross-clamp, avoid the anomalous coronary and leave adequate space for the high aortotomy. The choice of cardioplegia solution is based on center preference, but we found very useful single shot cold-blood antegrade del Nido solution, since it allows myocardial protection for any of the procedures planned, avoiding the need for repeated administration. The aortotomy needs to be done 1 cm distal to the sino-tubular junction, and in case of high take-off, even slightly higher. Before extending the initial aortotomy, the coronaries' ostium needs to be identified. This standard setup allows performing almost all repairs with some minor modifications that will be addressed in the dedicated paragraph.

Unroofing of Intramural Segment

The unroofing technique is one of the most frequent repair techniques used to treat AAOCA with intramural segment [14–18]. The intramural (IM) segment is the part of the anomalous coronary artery that runs within the aortic wall. By running within the aortic wall layers, the intramural segment acquired an oval shape [1, 2, 6, 19], and it can be reduced in lumen [20, 21] during effort due to dilatation of the aorta that "squeeze" such segment.

After the proximal aortic wall edges are suspended for better exposure, both coronary arteries' ostium needs to be identified. Usually, in the case of AAOLCA, a typical shape right coronary artery is found in the right sinus of Valsalva where it is possible to find also the ostium of the anomalous left coronary artery. For the AAORCA, in the left sinus of Valsalva, we will find a normal positioned and shaped ostium of the LCA with an oval or slit-like orifice of the RCA (insert Fig. 19.1). The anomalous ostium is usually placed in proximity aortic valve commissure, and it is fundamental to define if the IM segment runs above, at the level, or below the commissure pilar. The anomalous coronary needs to be gently inspected with a coronary probe or a small right angle. The maneuver also shows the exact point of coronary take-off from the aorta that represents the distal limit of the unroofing. It is possible to place a marking stitch in 6–0 Prolene passed from outside the aorta at the margin of the emergence of the anomalous coronary artery and backward inside outside the aorta. We

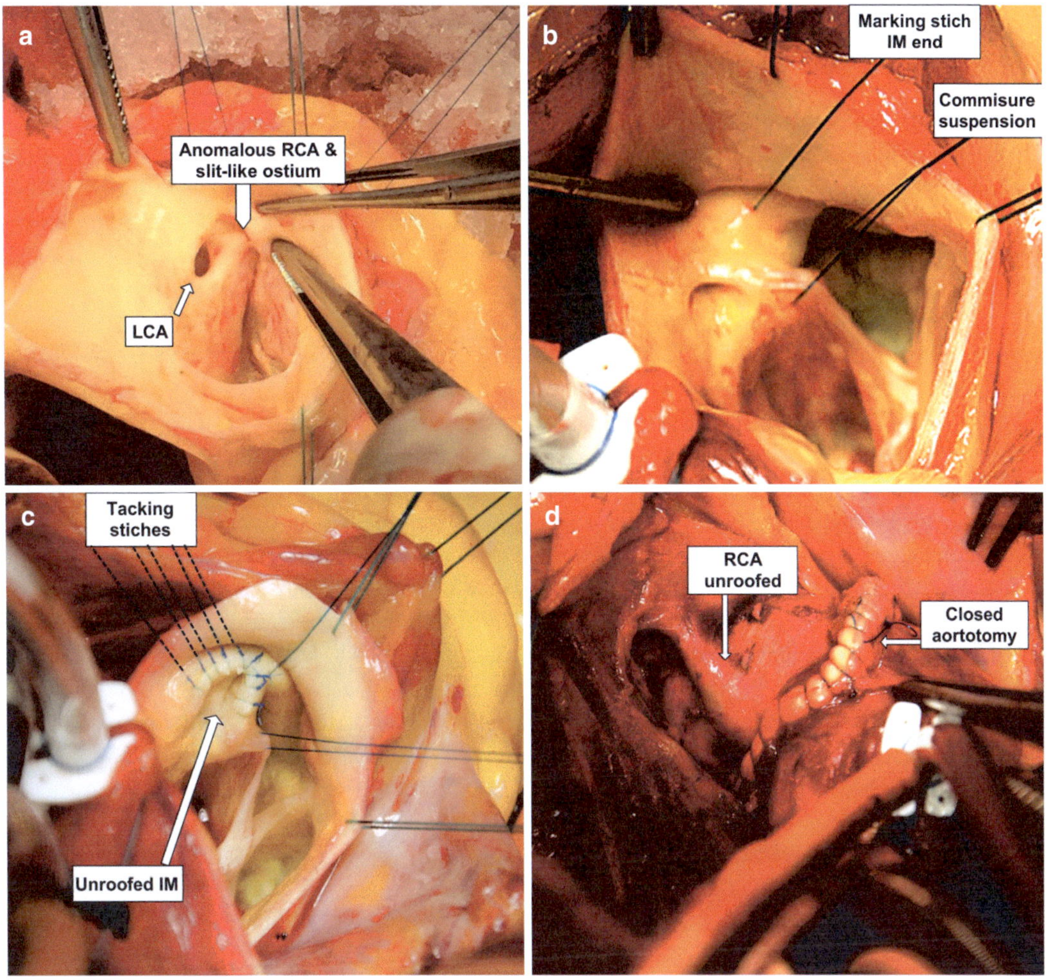

Fig. 19.1 Unroofing of Intramural Segment. (**a**) After transverse aortotomy, the origin of the anomalous coronary artery (RCA) is identified with its intramural segment (IM). (**b**) A marking stitch can be placed transfixing the aorta at the end of the IM segment. This marking stitch allows better visualization of the IM end and direction. A suspension stitch can be placed and the base of the aortic commissure pilar to improve exposure. (**c**) The IM is fully unroofed and several tacking sutures are placed to reinforce the incised aortic wall. (**d**) The aortotomy is closed and the anomalous RCA is inspected to assess the filling and check for bleeding points

recommended knotting the suture at the end of the procedure to avoid bleeding.

If the IM segment is above the aortic valve commissure, it is possible to proceed with the unroofing in three ways. Most commonly, the unroofing is done with Potts scissor angled, reverse, or straight depending on the IM orientation (AAOLCA or AAORCA). Another method is to leave the right angle inside the IM segment to protect the back wall and use a fine blade (n 15 or beaver blades) to incise the internal wall of the aorta and open the IM segment for its entire length.

The excessive aortic tissue can be removed with a fine blade or scissors to refine the margin. Such maneuver can be safely done in the superior margin of the incision, but it has to be carefully evaluated for the inferior aspect, considering the proximity of the aortic valve commissure.

The unroofing needs to be carefully evaluated if the IM segment runs at the aortic valve commissure level, because it may cause prolapse of both the leaflets [14, 22]. To preserve the commissure integrity, it may be partially detached and resuspended with pledgeted reinforced sutures after completing the unroofing [23].

If the IM runs below the commissure, other techniques such as anatomical repair, neo-ostium creation, and coronary translocation [18] should be chosen.

Once the unroofing is completed, the neo-ostium and the aortic cut wall can be reinforced with some interrupted figure of 8 tacking sutures using fine Prolene such 7–0. Tacking sutures prevent infiltration of blood within the aortic wall or coronary intima dissection. If possible, tight the suture with the knots directed outward the coronary lumen almost parallel to the aortic wall.

In conclusion, unroofing is a safe and easily reproducible operation that provides good results if adequately adopted. Significant advantages are the avoidance of coronary tissue manipulation, the impossibility of causing coronary distortion, and the reduced risk of bleeding. On the other hand, the disadvantages are mainly related to the impossibility of entirely correct the take-off direction of the coronary, especially in short IM segments, and the impossibility of enlarging the relative coronary hypoplasia immediately after the take-off from the aorta as described by some authors [11].

Neo-Ostium Creation or Partial Unroofing

The neo-ostium creation is indicated in the AAOCA, which presents an intramural segment that runs below the intercoronary pillar or aortic valve commissure [18, 22]. Technically consists of a partial unroofing of the distal intramural part that lays in the correct sinus of Valsalva [18, 22]. Firstly, the IM segment has to be identified with a right angle as for standard unroofing and then, leaving the right angle in place, an incision of the aortic wall above the instrument is carried out with a fine blade. Once the IM segment is opened, the right angle can be removed and the incision can be completed with Potts scissor. This maneuver creates a neo-ostium in the correct sinus of Valsalva without touching the aortic valve structures and the edges of the incision can be secured with a tacking suture as for the unroofing. This

technique prevents the risk of aortic regurgitation by relocating the anomalous coronary origin in the correct position, but it has the same limitations as the unroofing.

Ostioplasty or "Anatomical Repair"

Ostioplasty or anatomical repair is different from neo-ostium creation because it encompasses an incision of the anomalous coronary artery, the aorta, and an augmentation patch placement [18, 24–26]. The hospital Necker in Paris [11, 26, 27] popularized the technique developed for the ostial coronary stenosis developed after arterial switch operation [28, 29]. It can be used for AAOLCA or AAORCA and have the advantage of addressing any proximal hypoplasia of the coronary segment immediately after the aorta take-off. For AAOLCA the pulmonary trunk must be wholly separated from the aorta down to the annulus level. It may be necessary to transect it completely to visualize the anomalous LCA better. Pulmonary artery transection can also be done if a translocation is planned after the repair. Once the cardiopulmonary bypass is instituted, and cardioplegic arrest is achieved, the aortotomy has to be done at the level of the sinotubular region. The epicardial course of the anomalous coronary artery has to be dissected by removing any epicardial fat or connective tissue for about 1 cm or up to the first bifurcation. Then the anomalous coronary artery has to be open longitudinally, starting distally and ending proximally where the coronary leaves the aortic wall (insert Fig. 19.2). Then a vertical incision of the aorta in the proper sinus of Valsalva is carried out, directing it to join the longitudinal incision of the coronary artery at the point where it leaves the aortic wall. In case of IM absence, the two incisions have to be joined inferiorly together with some interrupted suture. At this point, a large neo-ostium is created and the repair is completed by suturing a fresh or treated autologous pericardial patch starting from the apex of the coronary incision and ending at the aortotomy edges [26]. The patch can also be done by harvesting a piece of the pulmonary artery wall [18]. The intramural segment is usually left intact without unroofing. The aortotomy is closed using the technique

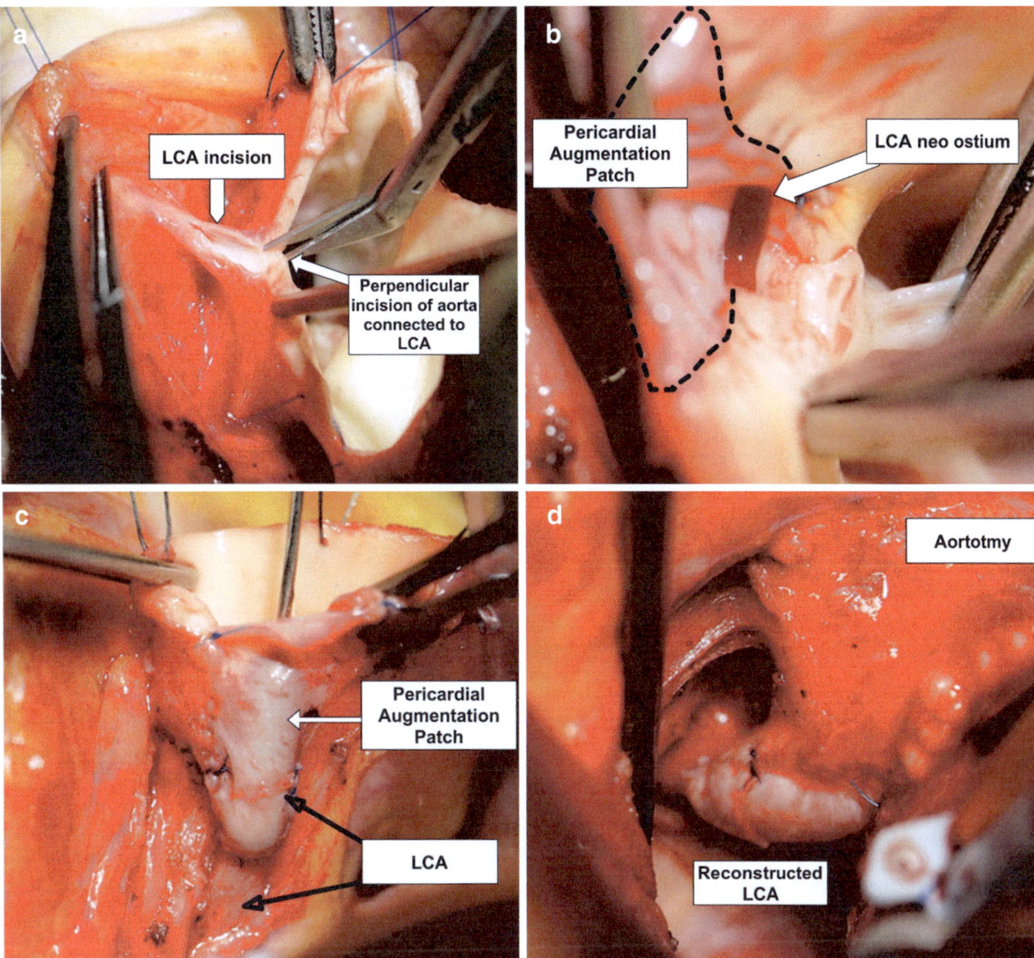

Fig. 19.2 Ostioplasty or Anatomical Repair. (**a**) The LCA is opened longitudinally from the distal segment before the bifurcation toward the aorta. The aorta is then opened vertically with the incision perpendicular to the coronary incision where the two openings need to join one to the other. (**b**) Inside vision of the new ostium with the autologous pericardial patch forming the superior roof for the repaired anomalous coronary artery. (**c**) The autologous pericardial patch is sutured starting from the apex of the LCA incision and continued to the edges of the aortic incision creating a roof for the new coronary ostium. (**d**) When the repair is completed, careful inspection is recommended to exclude coronary distortion

preferred and incorporating the patch in the suture line. If the MPA was transected, it will be resutured or translocated if a greater inter-arterial space is required. The advantage of this technique is that the neo-ostium is generally larger than the unroofing or osteoplasty. It also allows enlarging with the patch any relative proximal coronary hypoplasia. The major disadvantage is extensive manipulation of the coronary artery, the lumen may be distorted by an excessive long patch, and the patch can calcify or become aneu-rismatic in the long term. Despite the lack of large series of patients operated with such a technique, we can transfer some evidence of good outcomes from reoperation of coronary stenosis after arterial switch operation operated with the same method [28, 29].

Coronary Translocation and Reimplantation (TAR)

The coronary translocation and reimplantation (TAR) consist of detaching the anomalous coronary artery from the wrong sinus and the reimplantation in the appropriate sinus. This technique is indicated for those cases without intramural segment or in which the unroofing does not relocate the coronary artery in the appropriate sinus [14, 18, 22, 30]. It can also correct anomalous coronary with a very acute angle of take-off. The preparation of the patients is similar to the above-described techniques, although in particular cases, extensive mobilization of the anomalous coronary artery may need to be carried out to provide good coronary mobility [18, 30, 31]. After the aortotomy, the anomalous coronary artery needs to be inspected. If there is no intramural segment, and if the anomalous coronary artery is not closed to the aortic valve commissure, a coronary button can be prepared and reimplanted in the appropriate sinus using trap-door of punch techniques [14, 18, 30]. Next, the aortic wall needs to be reconstructed using a patch of the preferred material. In case of an intramural segment, its end needs to be identified and the coronary artery can be transected as it take-off from the aorta. Next, the coronary stump is closed by direct suture, and an opening in the aorta in the appropriate sinus is done using a punch. The coronary artery end is then sutured as a proximal bypass graft to the aorta [22, 30, 31], eventually with a proximal patch enlargement if the first millimeter of the coronary is narrow. Compared to the coronary button, this technique has been used more in adult patients. After reimplantation, the aortotomy is closed with the technique of preferences. TAR pitfalls are: a) avoid distortion and kinking of the coronary artery, b) properly select the reimplantation site, and c) keep the coronary adventitia layer intact to provide a stronger suture rim in case of TAR without an aortic wall button.

Transconal Repair or Septal Relief of Subpulmonary AAOLCA

The transconal unroofing [32, 33] and the septal relief [11] are similar surgical procedures that address one of the most challenging symptomatic or ischemic forms of AAOLCA, the subpulmonary or intraseptal course. Usually, these forms of AAOCA are at low risk of SCD, although few cases of symptomatic or ischemic presentation have been described [34]. Medical treatment with beta-blockers and restriction to sports activity is often sufficient to reduce the symptoms and the burden of adverse events. Transconal repair is a complex operation deemed only to the high-risk forms or not responsive to medical therapy. It includes an extensive mobilization of the pulmonary root that has to be detached from the right ventricle similarly to a Ross autograft harvesting [11, 32, 33] (insert Fig. 19.3). The RVOT needs to be incised 1 cm below the pulmonary valve plane on cardiopulmonary bypass and cardioplegic arrest. When detaching the posterior segment of the pulmonary root, the anomalous coronary usually lays 1–1.5 cm below the PV valve and it may be identified by an abnormal muscle bulging. After detaching the pulmonary root from the right ventricle, a careful division of the entire muscular bridge above the intraseptal course of the LMA needs to be carried out [11, 32, 33] up to the return of the LMA at the epicardial level. After complete unroofing, the pulmonary root has to be reconstructed with the interposition of a postero-lateral augmentation patch (autologous pericardium) to augment the distance between the RV and the pulmonary root to avoid compression of the relief anomalous coronary artery (insert Fig. 19.3). The pulmonary translocation can also be done during rewarming and on the beating heart [12, 13]. The result of such complex repair seems to be good in terms of symptoms and ischemia relief. Still, there are only a few case series [11, 33, 34] with short follow-up and it has not yet proven to be superior to medical therapy compared to the potential long-term complication of such complex repair.

Pulmonary artery Translocation

Pulmonary artery translocation has been proposed and successfully used by a few centers based on the concept that the compression of the coronary artery occurs, because the aorta and the pulmonary artery compress it. The procedure alone may be considered only in the cases without intramural segment, but it does not resolve the ostium morphology and does not restore the

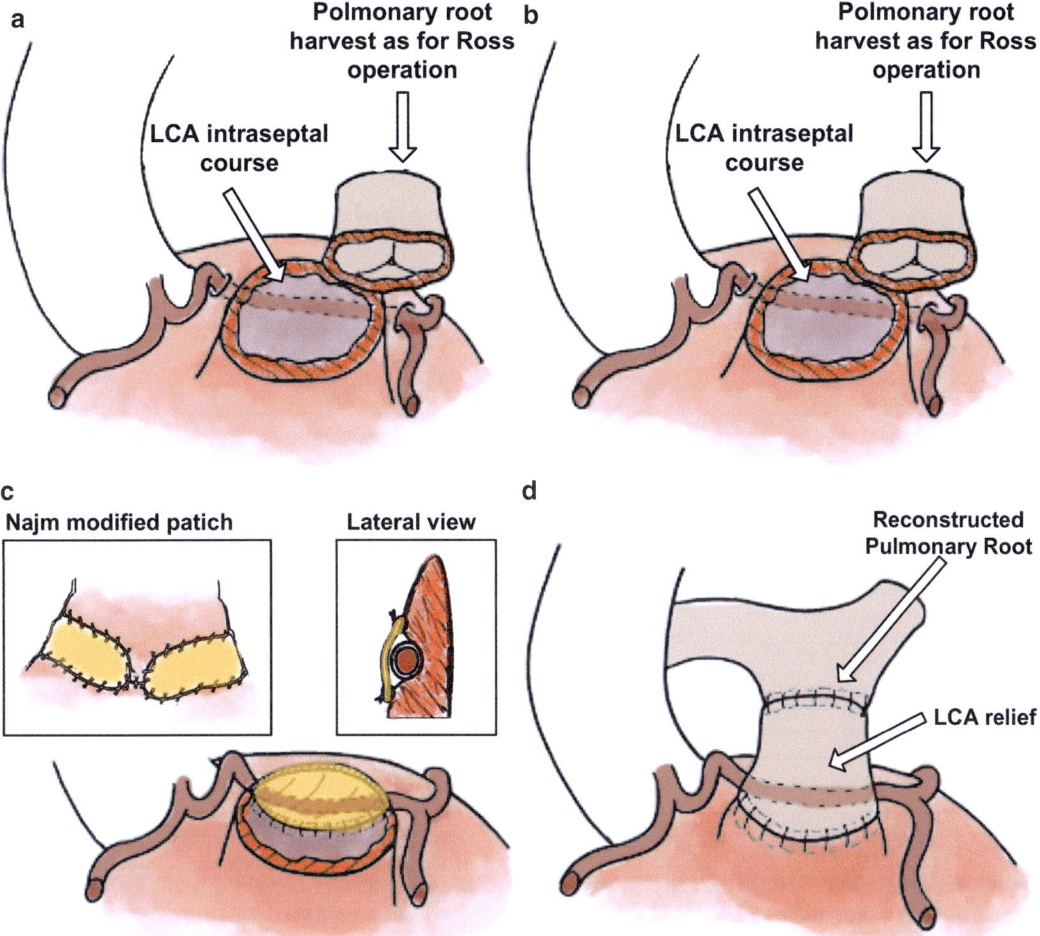

Fig. 19.3 Transconal Repair or Septal Relief of Subpulmonary AAOLCA. (**a**) Mobilization of the pulmonary root that has to be harvested as for a Ross operation; anomalous LCA has an intramyocardial course and may be appreciable as muscular bulging 1–1.5 cm below the pulmonary valve level. (**b**) Careful division of the entire LCA myocardial bridge. (**c**) Interposition of a posterior or postero-lateral (Najm modified patch) to augment the distance between the RV and the pulmonary root when reimplanted. (**d**) Final result with the complete relief of anomalous LCA and reconstructed pulmonary root. Figure modified from Gaillard M, Pontailler M, Danial P, Moreau de Bellaing A, Gaudin R, du Puy-Montbrun L, et al. Anomalous aortic origin of coronary arteries: an alternative to the unroofing strategy. Eur J Cardiothorac Surg [Internet]. 2020;58 (1):975–82. and Najm HK, Ahmad M. Transconal Unroofing of Anomalous Left Main Coronary Artery From Right Sinus With Transseptal Course. The Annals of Thoracic Surgery [Internet]. 2019 Dec;108 (2):e383–6

correct origin of the coronary artery. Different variations have been adopted but mainly consist of transecting the main pulmonary artery at the bifurcation level that is patch closed and resuture it more laterally toward the left pulmonary artery [12, 13, 35]. A Lecompte maneuver or anterior right pulmonary artery translocation can be done in case an anteriorization of the MPA is required [12]. In adolescence or adult patients, sometimes,

the adjunct of an augmentation patch or the interposition of the vascular graft may provide the mobilization or the space needed. The pulmonary translocation as a stand-alone procedure does not address the AAOCA pathogenetic mechanism and may leave behind residual lesions; therefore, it should be added to a primary repair technique listed above to create a larger distance between the two great vessels.

Coronary artery Bypass Grafting

Coronary artery bypass grafting (CABG) is a viable option to treat patients with AAOCA and diffuse atherosclerosis, severe ostial narrowing, and older age. The CABG is performed as each surgeon's preference, but an arterial graft with the mammary artery should be preferred. It is important to understand the degree of flow restriction when considering performing CABG, because a competitive antegrade flow in mild restricted lesions may jeopardize the graft durability and patency. Some anecdotal cases reported ligation of an anomalous coronary at its take-off from the aorta to reduce such competitive flow, but the patient's right or left coronary blood flow will rely only on the CABG. The CABG should not be used as primary repair unless for adult cases in which pathological atherosclerotic disease needs revascularization.

Conclusions

The surgical treatment of AAOCA remains a challenge for every surgeon and cardiologist, and a systematic approach should be recommended. There are several ways to manage AAOCA. Each one responds to a specific mechanism of ischemia or SCD that is often not demonstrated in provocative tests and depends on the experience of the surgical team. Therefore, defining the anatomical risk features is no longer a challenge, although those characteristics do not always correlate with symptoms or provocative positive tests. The surgical treatment in symptomatic patients is well established, because it prevents or resolves myocardial ischemia. However, the actual challenges remain for the majority of the patients that usually receive such diagnoses incidentally, do not present any provocative positive tests but have high-risk anatomical features and want to return to practice their active life. Knowing all possible surgical treatments and outcomes allows for correctly balancing surgical procedural risk with the benefit and the prevention of adverse events. A tailored approach using all the available techniques is the only way to provide the best care to such young patients who, most of the time, are otherwise healthy and asymptomatic.

Bibliography

1. Cheezum MK, Liberthson RR, Shah NR, Villines TC, O'Gara PT, Landzberg MJ, et al. Anomalous aortic origin of a coronary artery from the inappropriate sinus of Valsalva. J Am Coll Cardiol. 2017;69(12):1592–608.
2. Angelini P, Uribe C. Anatomic spectrum of left coronary artery anomalies and associated mechanisms of coronary insufficiency. Catheter Cardiovasc Interv. 2018;92(2):313–21.
3. Jegatheeswaran A, Devlin PJ, McCrindle BW, Williams WG, Jacobs ML, Blackstone EH, et al. Features associated with myocardial ischemia in anomalous aortic origin of a coronary artery: a congenital heart surgeons' society study. J Thorac Cardiovasc Surg. 2019;158(3):822–834.e3.
4. Brothers JA, Frommelt MA, Jaquiss RDB, Myerburg RJ, Fraser CD, Tweddell JS. Expert consensus guidelines: anomalous aortic origin of a coronary artery. J Thorac Cardiovasc Surg. 2017;153(6):1440–57.
5. Molossi S, Agrawal H. Clinical evaluation of anomalous aortic origin of a coronary artery (AAOCA). Congenit Heart Dis. 2017;12(5):607–9.
6. Agrawal H, Mery CM, Krishnamurthy R, Molossi S. Anatomic types of anomalous aortic origin of a coronary artery: a pictorial summary. Congenit Heart Dis. 2017;12(5):603–6.
7. Baumgartner H, De Backer J, Babu-Narayan SV, Budts W, Chessa M, Diller GP, et al. 2020 ESC guidelines for the management of adult congenital heart disease. Eur Heart J. 2021;42(6):563–645.
8. Stout KK, Daniels CJ, Aboulhosn JA, Bozkurt B, Broberg CS, Colman JM, et al. AHA/ACC guideline for the Management of adults with congenital heart disease: a report of the American College of Cardiology/American Heart Association task force on clinical practice guidelines. J Am Coll Cardiol. 2019;139:698–800.
9. Conway BD, Bates MJ, Hanfland RA, Yerkes NS, Patel SS, Calcaterra D, et al. A minimally invasive, algorithm-based approach for anomalous aortic origin of a coronary artery. Innovations: technology and techniques in cardiothoracic and vascular. Surgery. 2015;10(2):101–5.
10. Hinton ZW, Meza JM, Habermann AC, Andersen ND, Daneshmand MA, Turek JW. Right anterior mini-incision approach to anomalous right coronary artery repair. World J Pediatr Congenit Heart Surg. 2020;11(2):215–6.

11. Gaillard M, Pontailler M, Danial P, Moreau de Bellaing A, Gaudin R, du Puy-Montbrun L, et al. Anomalous aortic origin of coronary arteries: an alternative to the unroofing strategy. Eur J Cardiothorac Surg. 2020;58(5):975–82; http://www.ncbi.nlm.nih.gov/pubmed/32572445.

12. Said SM, Cetta F. Pulmonary root mobilization and modified Lecompte maneuver for Transseptal course of the left main coronary artery. World J Pediatr Congenit Heart Surg. 2020;11(6):792–6.

13. Mainwaring RD, Hanley FL. Surgical treatment of anomalous left main coronary artery with an intraconal course. Congenit Heart Dis. 2019;14(4):504–10.

14. Padalino MA, Jegatheeswaran A, Blitzer D, Ricciardi G, Guariento A. Surgery for anomalous aortic origin of coronary arteries: technical safeguards and pitfalls. Front Cardiovasc Med. 2021;8:1–12. https://doi.org/10.3389/fcvm.2021.626108/full.

15. Jegatheeswaran A, Devlin PJ, Williams WG, Brothers JA, Jacobs ML, DeCampli WM, et al. Outcomes after anomalous aortic origin of a coronary artery repair: a congenital heart surgeons' society study. J Thorac Cardiovasc Surg. 2020;160(3):757–771.e5.

16. Padalino MA, Franchetti N, Hazekamp M, Sojak V, Carrel T, Frigiola A, et al. Surgery for anomalous aortic origin of coronary arteries: a multicentre study from the European congenital heart surgeons association. Eur J Cardiothorac Surg. 2019;56(4):696.

17. Jiang MX, Blackstone EH, Karamlou T, Ghobrial J, Brinza EK, Haupt MJ, et al. Anomalous aortic origin of a coronary artery in adults. Ann Thorac Surg. 2021;112(4):1299–305.

18. Mavroudis C, Mavroudis CD, Jacobs JP. Repair techniques for anomalous aortic origins of the coronary arteries. Cardiol Young. 2015;25(8):1546–60.

19. Angelini P, Uribe C, Monge J, Tobis JM, Elayda MA, Willerson JT. Origin of the right coronary artery from the opposite sinus of Valsalva in adults: characterization by intravascular ultrasonography at baseline and after stent angioplasty. Catheter Cardiovasc Interv. 2015;86(2):199–208.

20. Lo Rito M, Romarowski RM, Rosato A, Pica S, Secchi F, Giamberti A, et al. Anomalous aortic origin of coronary artery biomechanical modeling: toward clinical application. J Thorac Cardiovasc Surg. 2021;161(1):191–201.e1.

21. Formato GM, Lo Rito M, Auricchio F, Frigiola A, Conti M. Aortic expansion induces lumen narrowing in anomalous coronary arteries: a parametric structural finite element analysis. J Biomech Eng. 2018;140(11):1–9.

22. Bonilla-Ramirez C, Molossi S, Caldarone CA, Binsalamah ZM. Anomalous aortic origin of the coronary arteries – state of the art Management and surgical Techniques. Semin Thorac Cardiovasc Surg Pediatr Card Surg Annu. 2021;24(Im):85–94. https://doi.org/10.1053/j.pcsu.2021.03.004.

23. Yerebakan C, Ozturk M, Mota L, Sinha L, Gordish-Dressman H, Jonas R, et al. Complete unroofing of the intramural coronary artery for anomalous aortic origin of a coronary artery: the role of commissural resuspension? J Thorac Cardiovasc Surg. 2019;158(1):208–217.e2. https://doi.org/10.1016/j.jtcvs.2019.01.140.

24. Alphonso N, Anagnostopoulos PV, Nölke L, Moon-Grady A, Azakie A, Raff GW, et al. Anomalous coronary artery from the wrong sinus of valsalva: a physiologic repair strategy. Ann Thorac Surg. 2007;83(4):1472–6; http://www.ncbi.nlm.nih.gov/pubmed/17383360.

25. Karl TR. Coronary artery from the wrong sinus of Valsalva: a physiologic repair strategy. Oper Tech Thorac Cardiovasc Surg. 2008;13(1):35–9; https://linkinghub.elsevier.com/retrieve/pii/S1522294208000044.

26. Gaudin R, Raisky O, Vouhe PR. Anomalous aortic origin of coronary arteries: "anatomical" surgical repair. Multimed Man Cardiothorac Surg. 2014;2014:mmt022; http://www.ncbi.nlm.nih.gov/pubmed/24586039.

27. Vouhé PR. Anomalous aortic origin of a coronary artery is always a surgical disease. Semin Thorac Cardiovasc Surg Pediatr Card Surg Annu. 2016;19(1):25–9. https://doi.org/10.1053/j.pcsu.2015.12.007.

28. Raisky O, Bergoend E, Agnoletti G, Ou P, Bonnet D, Sidi D, et al. Late coronary artery lesions after neonatal arterial switch operation: results of surgical coronary revascularization. Eur J Cardiothorac Surg. 2007;31(5):894–8; http://www.ncbi.nlm.nih.gov/pubmed/17344060.

29. Sepehripour AH, Harling L, Ashrafian H, Athanasiou T. Pediatric applications of surgical patch angioplasty of the main coronary trunks. World J Pediatr Congenit Heart Surg. 2014;5(2):283–90. https://doi.org/10.1177/2150135113508795.

30. Bonilla-Ramirez C, Molossi S, Sachdeva S, Reaves-O'Neal D, Masand P, Mery CM, et al. Outcomes in anomalous aortic origin of a coronary artery after surgical reimplantation. J Thorac Cardiovasc Surg. 2021;162(4):1191–9. https://doi.org/10.1016/j.jtcvs.2020.12.100.

31. Grau JB, Rahmouni K, Castillo J, Ruel M, Maharajh G. Reimplantation for anomalous right coronary artery. JTCVS Tech. 2021;7:226–8. https://doi.org/10.1016/j.xjtc.2021.01.033.

32. Najm HK, Ahmad M. Transconal unroofing of anomalous left main coronary artery from right sinus with trans-septal course. Ann Thorac Surg. 2019;108(6):e383–6. https://doi.org/10.1016/j.athoracsur.2019.04.021.

33. Najm HK, Karamlou T, Ahmad M, Hassan S, Salam Y, Majdalany D, et al. Early outcomes of Transconal repair of Transseptal anomalous left coronary artery from right sinus. Ann Thorac Surg.

2021;112(2):595–602; http://www.ncbi.nlm.nih.gov/pubmed/32822667

34. Doan TT, Zea-Vera R, Agrawal H, Mery CM, Masand P, Reaves-O'neal DL, et al. myocardial ischemia in children with anomalous aortic origin of a coronary artery with intraseptal course. Circ Cardiovas Interv. 2020;13(3):1–12.

35. Mainwaring RD, Reddy VM, Reinhartz O, Petrossian E, MacDonald M, Nasirov T, et al. Anomalous aortic origin of a coronary artery: medium-term results after surgical repair in 50 patients. Ann Thorac Surg. 2011;92(2):691–7. https://doi.org/10.1016/j.athoracsur.2011.03.127.

Impact and Management of Anomalous Aortic Origin of Coronary Arteries in Adult Patients Undergoing Cardiac Surgery for Acquired Heart Disease

Massimo Massetti, Maria Grandinetti, Federico Cammertoni, Piero Farina, and Piergiorgio Bruno

Outline of Epidemiology and Diagnostic Assessment Tools for Anomalous Aortic Origin of Coronary Arteries in the Adult Population

Anomalous aortic origin of a coronary artery (AAOCA) is a congenital anomaly in the origin and course of a coronary artery that arises from the aorta.

In the most common forms of AAOCA, the right coronary artery originates from the left sinus of Valsalva or the left main coronary artery (or one of its divisional branches: left anterior descending artery or circumflex artery) originates from the right sinus of Valsalva. Less frequently, a coronary artery may originate from the non-coronary sinus of Valsalva. Whatever the case, the anomalous coronary artery (ACA) may have either a separate or shared ostium with the normal coronary artery. As shown in Table 20.1, the course of an ACA may be interarterial, prepulmo-

Table 20.1 AAOCA classification according to anatomical and functional features

Classification of AAOCA according to the origin of the abnormal coronary artery
• Right coronary artery from the left sinus of Valsalva
• Left main coronary artery (or left anterior descending artery or circumflex artery) from the right sinus of Valsalva
• Either right coronary artery or left main coronary artery from the noncoronary sinus
Classification of AAOCA according to the course of the anomalous coronary artery
• Interarterial
• Retroaortic
• Prepulmonic
• Septal
High-risk anatomical features
• High take-off, ostial stenosis, slit-like/fish-mouth-shaped orifice, acute-angle take-off, intramural course and its length, interarterial course, and hypoplasia of the proximal coronary artery

AAOCA anomalous aortic origin coronary artery

nary, retroaortic, or septal. Finally, cases where one or both coronary arteries originate above the sinotubular junction should also be considered among AAOCAs [1, 2].

AAOCAs in the adult population have a clinical presentation ranging from occasional occurrence in asymptomatic patients to sudden cardiac

M. Massetti (✉) · M. Grandinetti · F. Cammertoni · P. Farina · P. Bruno
Catholic University of the Sacred Heart, University Policlinic "A. Gemelli" Foundation IRCSS, Rome, Italy
e-mail: massimo.massetti@unicatt.it

© Springer Nature Switzerland AG 2023
G. Butera, A. Frigiola (eds.), *Congenital Anomalies of Coronary Arteries*,
https://doi.org/10.1007/978-3-031-36966-7_20

death. In the United States of America, AAOCAs are the second leading cause of sudden cardiac death, after hypertrophic cardiomyopathy, in young, healthy adults such as athletes [1, 2].

The clinical impact depends on the site of origin of the anomalous coronary artery, the type of course, and whether there are any high-risk anatomical features (Table 20.1).

AAOCA is a rare disease, the exact prevalence of which in the adult population is difficult to ascertain.

In patients over 18 years of age, the available data come mainly from angiographic studies performed for ischemic heart disease due to atherosclerosis.

Although the true prevalence is unknown, many studies have reported data from 0.6% to 1.3% [3–8].

In a pioneering angiographic study of approximately 120,000 adult subjects between 1960 and 1988, Yamanaka and colleagues found an overall incidence of coronary anomalies of 1.3%, of which 87% were AAOCA [9].

The prevalence of AAOCA from autopsy studies in the adult population is generally lower than angiographic studies, probably due to the use of different autopsy diagnostic techniques and the enormous heterogeneity of the study population [8, 10].

In contrast, studies based on coronary computed tomography angiography (CCTA) have shown a higher incidence of coronary anomalies in the adult population than previous angiographic studies [11–13]. For example, in a recent retrospective CCTA study of approximately 6000 adult patients with a mean age of 52 ± 17 years (excluding patients with previous surgical revascularization or associated congenital heart disease), a 1.7% prevalence\of abnormal coronary artery origin from the opposite sinus of Valsalva (course: 39% interarterial; 38% retroaortic; 15% subpulmonic; 5% prepulmonic; 2% others) was found [11].

By providing a three-dimensional reconstruction of the coronary tree, CCTA allows the origin, course, and anatomical relationships of the abnormal coronary artery to be clearly defined. Due to its two-dimensional nature, coronary angiography does not provide this information. In addition, CCTA offers the possibility to investigate the presence of those anatomical features associated with the risk of sudden death, such as narrowed slit-like orifice, acute take-off angle, intramural, and/or interarterial course of the anomalous coronary segment. The use of CCTA to provide a comprehensive anatomical assessment of AAOCA may, when combined with clinical data, allows individualized treatment decisions for these complex patients. Therefore, the evaluation of coronary artery anomalies using CCTA may not only allow the detection of coronary abnormalities but also provide important prognostic information.

For these reasons, CCTA is the preferred diagnostic tool, so much so that the latest European guidelines for the management of adult patients with Congenital Heart Disease [14] recommend it as the reference method.

AAOCA and Adult Acquired Heart Disease

While the association of coronary artery anomalies with congenital heart disease is well known, the association of AAOCA with acquired valvular and aortic disease in the adult population is poorly investigated. The diagnosis of a coronary artery anomaly in adults may be an incidental finding during screening for acquired heart disease to be referred for surgery. In a recent retrospective study of 645 adult subjects diagnosed with a coronary artery anomaly, 167 were AAOCA cases. Among the latter, only 36 patients (21.6%) had undergone surgery to correct the coronary artery anomaly. In the subgroup of patients referred for correction of AAOCA, 36% had also undergone valve surgery, with aortic valve surgery being the most prevalent [15]. Similarly, in a large caseload study of over 3000 patients undergoing CCTA, 53 (1.5%) had an AAOCA. Of these, 4 patients (7.8%) underwent aortic valve replacement and coronary artery bypass, with no change in surgical strategy as a result of the coronary artery anomaly [13]. On the other hand, 4% of patients referred for elective aortic valve surgery had a coronary artery anomaly [16].

There is no specific evidence of the need to treat an anomalous coronary artery disease found occasionally as part of the preoperative screening of adult cardiac surgery candidates, and there is no agreed surgical strategy on which is the best treatment. Surgery for an acquired heart disease in the presence of an AAOCA raises important questions for the cardiac surgeon, first and foremost, the need to correct the anomaly. Indeed, unlike in children, a coronary artery anomaly found incidentally in adult patients who are candidates for other types of cardiac surgery would appear to have a low risk of sudden cardiac death. However, not correcting a coronary artery anomaly with risk characteristics could expose the patient to adverse clinical events in the future. Finally, it should be considered that during surgery, the abnormal coronary artery may be damaged, with severe short- and long-term complications.

When the decision is made to correct the coronary artery anomaly, the heart surgeon has to choose which strategy to adopt. The two options are anatomical correction (unroofing, ostioplasty, reimplantation, and others) and coronary artery bypass. In this regard, several aspects are considered: the analysis of the coronary artery anatomy and the technical feasibility for anatomical correction of the AAOCA, the age and comorbidities of the patient, and the possible presence of associated coronary artery stenosis.

Finally, it is essential to discuss the technical approach to preparing for cardiac surgery (cannulation sites for extracorporeal circulation, aortic clamping site, type of aortotomy, and cardiotomy), aiming to avoid all possible sources of iatrogenic injury that could involve the origin and abnormal course of the affected coronary artery.

Aortic Valve Surgery and AAOCA

As mentioned, an abnormal aortic origin of a coronary artery may be found in 4% of patients undergoing elective aortic valve replacement [16]. Bicuspid aortic valves are more often associated than tricuspid aortic valves (7% vs. 3%). In addition, the abnormal coronary artery is more frequently the right one [16]. According to a recent adult AAOCA registry, 39% of patients with an indication for abnormal coronary artery correction also undergo an associated cardiac surgical procedure, most commonly an aortic valve replacement [15].

There are four issues to be managed when performing an aortic valve replacement in a patient with an anomalous coronary artery origin and course: (1) direct coronary artery injury during aortotomy or dissection and suturing; (2) compression by the valve prosthesis; (3) myocardial protection; and (4) whether the coronary artery anomaly needs to be corrected.

An abnormal coronary artery may be directly injured during aortotomy or suture placement [17]. In addition, the ACA may be compressed by the sewing ring of the implanted valve prosthesis. In this sense, the interarterial and retroaortic courses are at greatest risk [18, 19]. On the contrary, in cases of a prepulmonic or septal course, the risk is low, because the anomalous coronary artery runs away from the aortic root and ring [19].

Myocardial protection can be challenging. An abnormal coronary artery with an intramural course may be compressed by persistent pressure increase in the aortic root when anterograde cardioplegia is used [20]. Similarly, the presence of a narrow, slit-like ostium may hinder the administration of selective anterograde cardioplegia. Finally, problems may arise if the aortic clamp is placed below a high take-off coronary artery or if the artery is inadvertently injured during aortotomy [21, 22].

Regarding the need for correction, an interarterial course exposes the patient to a risk of sudden cardiac death in itself; when we add an aortic valve replacement, this risk increases significantly and, therefore, corrective action seems reasonable during aortic valve surgery [8, 19]. A retroaortic course has not been associated with a high risk of sudden cardiac death. However, the patient undergoing aortic valve replacement may experience severe complications postoperatively or at some time in the future and, therefore, the problem should be addressed during surgery. The presence of a slit-like ostium, an intramural tract, and acute take-off are additional reasons to proceed with correction of the anomaly. Finally, septal and prepulmonic courses have rarely been described in patients undergoing aortic valve replacement: in these cases, the anomalous coronary artery is far from the aortic valve ring and the risk of periprocedural complications such as sudden cardiac death appears low.

Although patients with a coronary artery anomaly undergoing aortic valve replacement are at increased risk of ischemic complications in the postoperative period [16], there is no uniformity on when and how to treat this condition.

Retroaortic Course of an Anomalous Coronary Artery

The most common occurrence is an anomalous circumflex artery originating from the right sinus of Valsalva (or directly from the right coronary artery) and running retroaortically (Fig. 20.1). In this case, implantation of an aortic valve prosthesis may result in direct damage due to sutures or compression (Fig. 20.1 - insert), especially in cases of calcification of the mitral-aortic junction [23]. The typical clinical picture is characterized by myocardial ischemia with ST-segment changes, electrical or hemodynamic instability during weaning from cardiopulmonary bypass, or in the immediate postoperative period in the

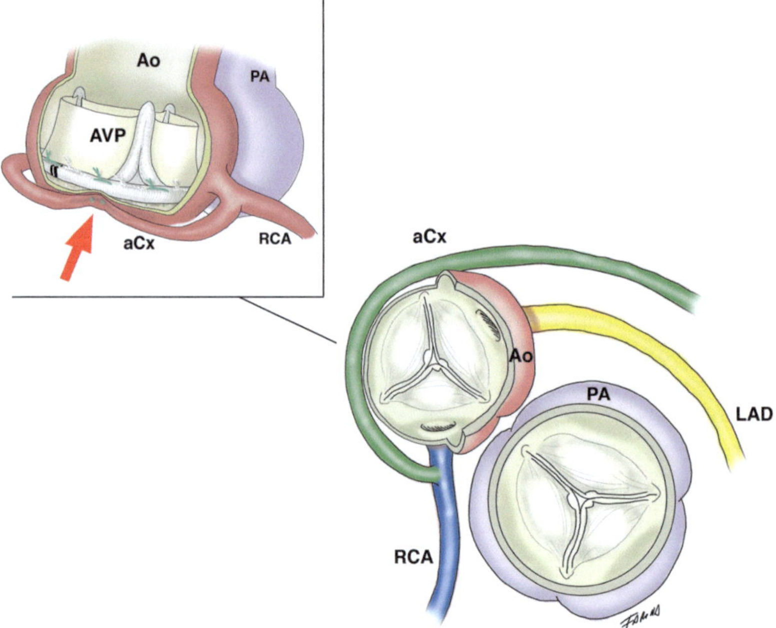

Fig. 20.1 Aortic Valve Replacement in the presence of an anomalous circumflex artery originating from the right sinus of Valsalva and with a retroaortic course. Most commonly, the anomalous coronary artery is the circumflex (aCx), which, originating from the right Valsalva sinus, assumes a retroaortic course, forming a close relationship with the aortic valve ring in the noncoronary artery portion of the Valsalva sinus. Implantation of an aortic valve prosthesis (AVP) can cause compression or constriction of the aCx due to the sewing ring or stitches, respectively (insert – red arrow). The two main approaches proposed to manage this condition have been the complete mobilization of the aCx or downsizing of the aortic valve prosthesis. *AO* aorta, *RCA* right coronary artery, *PA* pulmonary artery, *LAD* left anterior descending artery

intensive care unit [24, 25]. Serious complications may also occur at a considerable distance after surgery [26, 27].

Isolated Aortic Valve Replacement

Two approaches have been described to manage this situation: 1) mobilize the circumflex artery throughout its retroaortic course without undersizing the prosthesis [18, 28, 29] or 2) leave the circumflex in place and use an undersized prosthesis [30, 31], preferably stentless or homograft [17, 26, 31, 32]. In any case, it is preferable to implant the prosthesis in a supra-annular position and to use a noneverting, interrupted suture.

In a small study of 3 patients, Botta et al. [28] suggested completely skeletonizing the anomalous circumflex artery from the aortic root in order to implant a prosthesis of adequate size. Similarly, Liebrich et al. [29] reported the results of 6 patients, with an anomalous origin of the circumflex artery from the right sinus of Valsalva and a retroaortic course. In this case, too, the anomalous coronary artery was skeletonized and detached from the aorta down to the atrioventricular groove, only afterward performing a valve replacement with a stented prosthesis (4 patients), an isolated valve repair (1 patient – subcommissural plication + free margin reinforcement) or combined with a noncoronary sinus of Valsalva replacement (1 patient – modified Yacoub + central plication).

In contrast, Alameddine et al. [30] limited themselves to downsizing the prosthesis (5 patients) or to aortocoronary bypass without downsizing (2 patients). In their study, the need for aortocoronary bypass arose from the inability to mobilize the abnormal circumflex artery or in the case of a slit-like ostium of the coronary artery itself.

While Botta and Liebrich did not report any postoperative complications, Alameddine et al. described two cases of postoperative myocardial ischemia requiring urgent percutaneous coronary intervention in patients in whom downsizing alone had been chosen. Furthermore, the risk of patient-prosthesis mismatch is real, particularly for patients with a small aortic annulus.

Interestingly, Doty et al. [32] noted that, in cases of an anomalous circumflex artery associated with a bicuspid aortic valve, the rightward displacement of the anomalous circumflex and right coronary artery ostia causes the ACA to take an oblique course over the non-coronary sinus and a shorter relationship with the aortic annulus. Thus, in cases associated with a bicuspid aortic valve, they did not consider mobilization of the circumflex artery to always be necessary. Rather, Doty et al. pointed out that oblique aortotomy could be dangerous in this case and recommended transverse aortotomy. Umakanthan et al. described the case of a patient in whom a mechanical prosthesis was implanted tilted above the non-coronary annulus to prevent compression of the anomalous circumflex artery [33]. Although this approach was effective, there are concerns about the absence of perivalvular leaks at follow-up.

Sutureless prostheses have less radial force than a balloon-expandable transcatheter valve and reduce the number of stitches to be passed through the ring. Cerillo et al. reported favorable outcomes for 4 patients treated with sutureless prostheses without the need to undersize the prosthesis and without any special precautions against abnormal coronary artery disease [34].

Aortic Valve Replacement and Atrioventricular Valve Surgery

In the case of aortic valve replacement and a concomitant atrioventricular valve procedure, the risk of complications is higher. In a patient undergoing aortic valve replacement and tricuspid valve repair for endocarditis, Castillo et al. opted for simultaneous downsizing of the aortic valve prosthesis and mobilization of the anomalous circumflex artery [23]. To further reduce the risk of compression of the ACA between the two sewing rings, the tricuspid valve was repaired with a prosthetic band implanted only in the posterior and septal portion of the ring.

In cases of combined aortic and mitral valve replacement or aortic valve replacement in the presence of a calcified mitral annulus, undersizing the aortic valve prosthesis alone may be insufficient [35, 36]. In such cases, complete loosening of the abnormal circumflex and possibly aortocoronary bypass have been suggested [23, 31].

Aortic Valve Replacement and Aortic Root Enlargement

When a root enlargement procedure is necessary, the presence of an ACA course can be a problem. In these cases, a correct preoperative overview is even more important to choose the type of surgical approach. Anterior enlargement or reimplantation with posterior enlargement may be considered in cases of a retroaortic coronary artery [37]. Conversely, when the ACA has an interarterial course, the anterior approach should be avoided [38, 39].

Inter-Arterial Course of an Abnormal Coronary Artery

A coronary artery with an abnormal origin and interarterial course (Fig. 20.2) may require surgical treatment per se [8]. In fact, this condition has been associated with a high risk of sudden cardiac death due to compression of the anomalous coronary artery between the aorta and the pulmonary artery, especially during exercise. A slit-like orifice, an acute take-off angle, or the presence of an intramural tract increase the risk of myocardial ischemia. Although both an interarterial course of the right and left coronary artery have been associated with sudden cardiac death, the latter condition seems to be at greater risk [40].

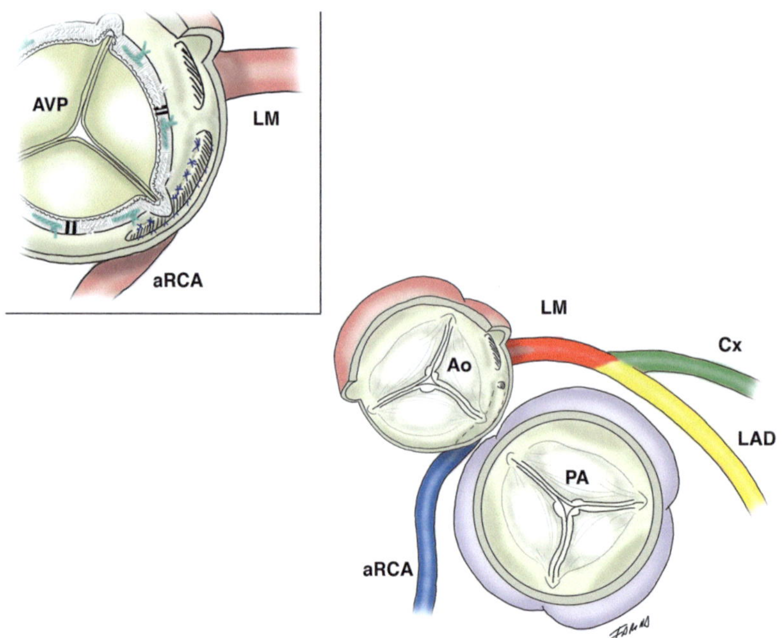

Fig. 20.2 Aortic Valve Replacement in the presence of an anomalous right coronary artery originating from the left sinus of Valsalva, and with an interarterial course and intramural tract. The anomalous interarterial course of a coronary artery represents a risk condition in itself, as the anomalous coronary artery can be compressed between the aorta (AO) and the pulmonary artery (PA), typically under stress conditions. The presence of a slit-like ostium, an acute take-off, or an intramural tract significantly increases the risk of complications. In the figure, an anomalous right coronary artery (aRCA), originating from the left Valsalva sinus and with an interarterial course, has an intramural tract (dashed line). In the case of aortic valve replacement with prosthesis (AVP), the risk of periprocedural complications is high and unroofing is highly recommended. *LM* left main coronary artery, *Cx* circumflex artery, *LAD* left anterior descending artery

In patients undergoing aortic valve replacement, complications related to compression of the abnormal interarterial vessel have been described and can be extremely severe [41, 42]. A strategy to manage this condition is mandatory in these cases. If the ACA has an intramural tract, unroofing has been the most widely used technique [43, 44] (Fig. 20.2 – insert). In their review, Davies et al. [43] described 36 patients with an ACA with an interarterial course. In 94% of the cases, the anomalous coronary artery also had an intramural course. Six patients (16.7%) also underwent associated procedures (replacement/repair of the aortic valve 4; mitral valve 1; or ascending aorta 1). Interestingly, 61% (22 patients) underwent unroofing, preferably when the anomaly involved the right coronary artery. The main risk of unroofing is distortion of the commissure between the right and left cusps, resulting in aortic valve failure. Obviously, in patients undergoing aortic valve replacement, this is not the case [15]. On the contrary, in patients in whom a valve repair is planned, the course of the intramural tract must be evaluated. If it lies above the commissure, the risk of distortion is minimal. If, however, it lies below the commissure, there are two possibilities: detach the commissure, unroof the intramural segment, and resuspend the commissure; or create a new ostium.

In cases where there is no intramural course, unroofing is not feasible, or there is associated atherosclerotic disease, coronary artery bypass has been the most popular alternative [43, 45, 46]. However, there are numerous concerns regarding the patency of a graft on an anomalous coronary artery without atherosclerotic disease [43, 47, 48], whether the anomalous coronary vessel should be ligated [49, 50], or what type of graft should be used (artery vs. vein).

Although pulmonary artery translocation [51] and reimplantation [52] are described as further options, there are no reports of patients undergoing aortic valve replacement. Although effective, these two procedures are technically demanding and do not fit well with the need to also perform aortic valve replacement.

Apart from anecdotal cases [53] in which correction of the anomalous coronary artery was not performed, complications have occurred during weaning from the extracorporeal circulation or in the intensive care unit, with the need to perform an urgent aortocoronary bypass [41, 42]. For this reason, this approach should be discouraged.

Abnormal Coronary Artery Originating above the Sinotubular Junction

In patients who are candidates for aortic valve replacement, the anomalous origin of one or both coronary arteries above the sinotubular junction is a potentially risky condition, especially when it has an intramural course [54, 55]. In these circumstances, the likelihood of injury to the anomalous coronary artery during aortotomy (Fig. 20.3) and the need for unplanned aortocoronary bypass are high [55]. To avoid this complication, a complete preoperative imaging that includes, in addition to coronarography, a CCTA

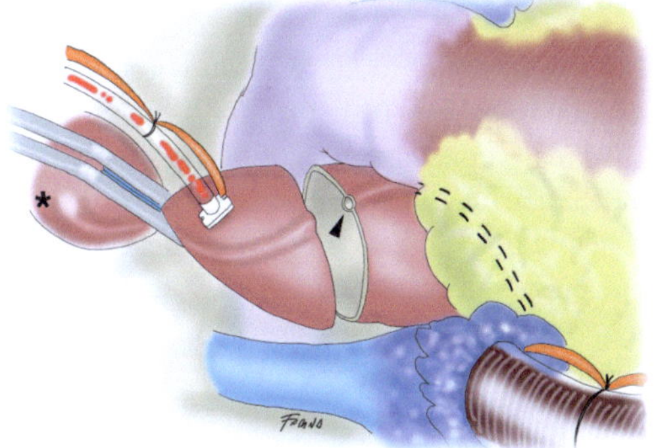

Fig. 20.3 Anomalous coronary artery originating above the sinotubular junction. In some cases, the anomalous coronary artery arises above the sinotubular junction. In these cases, myocardial protection can be compromised if the aortic clamp is placed below the ostium of the anomalous coronary artery (asterisk) or in the case of injury during aortotomy (black arrowhead). Comprehensive preoperative imaging allows, in most cases, the identification of the coronary artery anomaly and the taking of appropriate precautions (the dashed line describes the course of the right coronary artery in the atrioventricular sulcus.)

is essential [55, 56]. Indeed, coronarography alone may not be sufficient to clarify the origin and course of a coronary artery with high take-off [55–57]. When a high origin of the ACA is suspected or established, based on its course, it may be necessary to perform a right-sided transverse [22, 56] or vertical aortotomy [58]. When there is an intramural course, unroofing or reimplantation is not feasible, because there is a risk of excessively weakening the aortic wall and having to replace it [55]. Conversely, when there is no intramural course, prior isolation of the coronary artery has been proposed [22].

It is important to consider that in these circumstances, myocardial protection may be compromised [21]. Indeed, placement of the aortic cross-clamp below the ostium of an abnormal coronary artery or injury/disruption of the course may compromise the correct administration of cardioplegia (Fig. 20.3). In these cases, it is useful to consider retrograde administration, after excluding associated anomalies such as the presence of a persistent left superior vena cava [22].

Aortic Root Surgery and AAOCA

The risk of injury to an ACA during aortic root surgery is greater than that for isolated aortic valve replacement because of the need to free the aortic root from adjacent anatomical structures. In addition, the creation of the coronary buttons and their reimplantation on the vascular graft may be complex in the presence of an abnormal coronary artery origin or course.

In valve-sparing aortic root replacement, these critical issues may deter the surgeon from retaining the native valve [59–61]. However, even more so than in isolated aortic valve replacement, it is essential to know precisely the origin and course of the coronary arteries before planning an aortic root operation [59, 62, 63].

In the case of a circumflex artery with abnormal origin from the right sinus of Valsalva and retroaortic course, its complete mobilization, until it enters the oblique sinus and vanishes in the left atrioventricular groove just before the base of the left atrial appendage, is necessary to avoid damage during root skeletonization, during

packing of the proximal subannular suture line of the aortic graft at the ventricular-aortic junction (in case of reimplantation technique), and to prevent kinking after reimplantation [29, 60, 64, 65]. When preparation of the vessel is impossible or the vessel is damaged, it has been recommended to ligate the anomalous circumflex artery proximally and proceed to aortocoronary bypass [65]. Although they had successfully isolated the anomalous coronary artery from the root, Akiel et al. still packaged a graft with the left internal mammary artery on the obtuse marginal branch, but this occluded early due to competitive flow [64]. Systematic closure of the native anomalous coronary vessel has been proposed [60]. The ACA is reimplanted alone or together with the right coronary artery in a composite button in the right sinus of Valsalva [64, 66] or in the tubular portion of the vascular graft [65]. In Bentall's case, too, mobilization of an anomalous retroaortic circumflex artery is essential [63].

The management of an anomalous left coronary artery originating from the right sinus of Valsalva and with an interarterial course is complex in valve-sparing procedures. Kaczorowski and colleagues described an extended mobilization and translocation of an anomalous left coronary artery arising from the proximal right coronary artery. After the entire course between the pulmonary artery and aneurysmal aortic root of the left coronary artery had been freed, it was separated from the right coronary artery (the origin was oversewn) and reimplanted on the vascular graft [67].

In the case of a right coronary artery originating from the left sinus of Valsalva and with an intramural course behind the commissure between the right and left cusps, Zanotti et al. proposed mobilizing the right coronary artery from the point of emergence from the aorta (extramural segment of the anomalous artery) and creating a button at this level. This eliminated the intramural segment. However, the emergence of the right coronary artery from the aorta was extremely close to the commissure between the right and left cusps. To allow subsequent reimplantation, the aortic wall was left on the commissure and the incomplete button reconstructed with bovine pericardium before reimplantation.

The unknown of this solution is the fate of the pericardial patch [59].

Regardless of the course, an ACA often has a paracommissural ostium (misplaced very close to the commissure). In such cases, it is not possible to guarantee the simultaneous preparation of a button for reimplantation and the preservation of the commissure for resuspension in the vascular graft. A modified reimplantation technique has been proposed that involves leaving the anomalous coronary artery's ostium "in situ" (attached to the commissure) and shaping the vascular graft with a vertical slit to accommodate it [68, 69].

Similarly, Matsuda et al. described a modified remodeling technique that leaves the misplaced ostium attached to the commissure [61]. Should dilatation of the aortic annulus be a concern, Mazzitelli and colleagues suggested the addition of an internal annuloplasty aortic ring [62].

Whenever quality of reconstruction is a concern, the Bentall procedure should be considered, because proper coronary reconstruction should take precedence over valve preservation. Caceres et al. described a patient with aortic valve endocarditis and aortic root abscess who underwent the Bentall procedure. During the operation, they identified an anomalous right coronary artery, with its origin at the left sinus of Valsalva and an intramural course. In this case, as it was not necessary to preserve the aortic valve, it was possible to unroof the anomalous vessel and create a button that was reimplanted on a stentless prosthesis [70].

Finally, when the aortic root is normal and the patient is a candidate for ascending aorta replacement only, the high origin of one or both coronary arteries may be a problem. Recently, Urbanski and colleagues proposed an original coronary artery ostial slide plasty, which was used successfully in a series of 23 patients. The procedure involves leaving the aberrant ostium within a "tongue" of the ascending aorta wall. Then, a half-round piece of the aortic wall is resected below the ostium, which is subsequently moved proximally into the sinus of Valsalva and sutured to the aortic wall [71]. This technique is an alternative to reimplanting the anomalous coronary artery onto the vascular graft.

Mitral Valve Surgery and AAOCA

Cases of AAOCA found in patients who are candidates for surgical treatment of mitral valve stenosis or insufficiency are anecdotal.

Imori et al. described a case of severe mitral valve regurgitation due to myxomatous valve disease in which a right coronary artery originated from the left sinus of Valsalva with an interarterial course. After documenting the presence of ischemia on stress cardiac scintigraphy, a combined mitral valve replacement and aortocoronary bypass using a vein graft was performed [72].

Bakker et al., on the other hand, described a case of severe mitral valve regurgitation due to myxomatous valve disease associated with an anomalous left coronary artery originating from the right coronary sinus with a retroaortic course (course close to the anterior mitral annulus). In this case, the Authors did not treat the ACA, but simply used an open flexible annuloplasty ring to minimize the risk of iatrogenic compression injury [73].

In a case of mitral valve stenosis associated with an anomalous right coronary artery originating from the left sinus of Valsalva with an interarterial course and a very short intramural course, Refattlari et al. described a combined operation of mitral valve replacement with mechanical prosthesis and a saphenous vein by-pass. Their surgical choice was explained by the technical infeasibility of unroofing due to the presence of a too short intramural course and the presence of coronary stenosis at the ostium of the right coronary artery. The use of the venous conduit was justified by the small caliber of the right internal mammary artery [74].

The lack of data in the literature on the association between AAOCA and mitral valvulopathy still leaves much room for debate on whether coronary artery disease should be treated at all times during mitral valve repair/replacement. However, there is agreement that adequate preoperative screening with coronary angiography or CCTA should be performed in all mitral surgery candidates, as with aortic surgery, regardless of age or risk factors, to exclude the presence of possible coronary artery anomalies.

Conclusions

In the adult population, the finding of an anomalous coronary artery aortic origin in conjunction with other cardiac surgery is rare, and presents a controversial scenario for cardiac surgeons operating on adults.

The literature on this subject is scarce and heterogeneous, and no treatment algorithms are defined. Both the need to correct the anomaly and the type of correction must be weighted and "tailored" to the individual patient, considering the type of coronary artery anomaly (origin, course), the surgical risk, and, last but not least, the risk of developing periprocedural or future complications due to the coronary artery anomaly itself (Fig. 20.4). Indeed, a coronary artery anomaly,

which remains silent until adulthood, could create numerous problems following aortic/mitral valve or aortic surgery. In this sense, accurate preoperative imaging and a multidisciplinary approach by the Heart Team are absolutely necessary.

Of no less importance is the possibility to perform the surgery in a hybrid operating theatre. In fact, this solution makes it possible to verify angiographically, already at the end of the procedure, the patency of the anomalous coronary artery, both in cases where it has been corrected and in cases where the conservative approach has been chosen.

An international registry that could unify data on AAOCA in the context of adult-acquired heart disease is highly desirable.

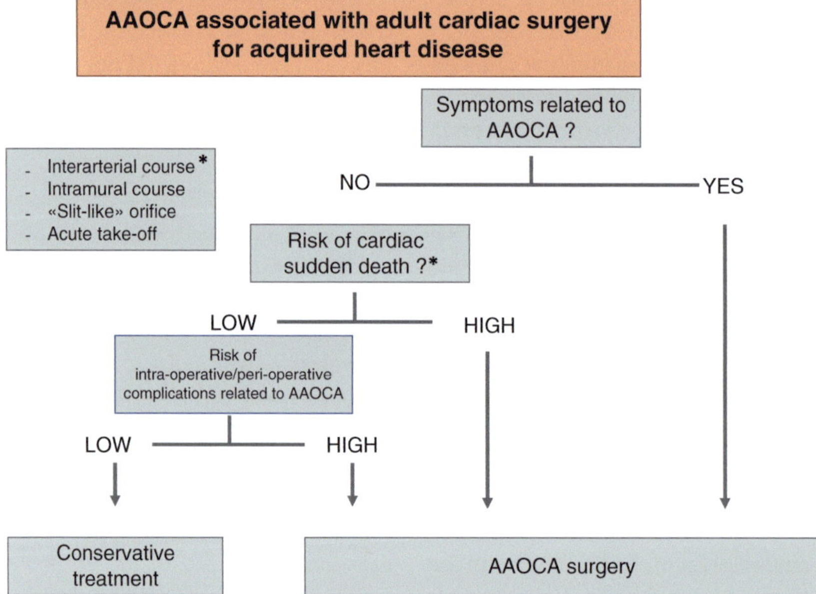

Fig. 20.4 Algorithm for the management of AAOCA associated with acquired adult cardiac surgery. Although the evidence is too limited to allow the drafting of a shared algorithm, it is still possible to trace a decision-making process based on the principles of good clinical practice. The first element to be clarified is whether the patient presents, or has presented, symptoms attributable to the coronary artery anomaly. Establishing whether a certain symptom is due to the cardiac defect for which the patient is a candidate for cardiac surgery rather than the coronary artery anomaly is not always easy. In such circumstances, it may be necessary to resort to specific diagnostic tests. In the absence of symptoms referable to the coronary artery anomaly, it is necessary to evaluate whether those anatomical features (*) associated with the risk of sudden cardiac death are present. Finally, in cases of asymptomatic patients without features that expose them to a significant risk of sudden death, it is necessary to consider the specific procedure for which the patient is a candidate and the specific risk of developing complications induced by the anomalous coronary artery

References

1. Brothers J, Gaynor JW, Paridon S, Lorber R, Jacobs M. Anomalous aortic origin of a coronary artery with an interarterial course: understanding current management strategies in children and young adults. Pediatr Cardiol. 2009;30:911–21. https://doi.org/10.1007/s00246-009-9461-y.
2. Poynter JA, Williams WG, McIntyre S, Brothers JA, Jacobs ML. Congenital heart surgeons society AAOCA working group. Anomalous aortic origin of a coronary artery: a report from the congenital heart surgeons society registry. World J Pediatr Congenit Heart Surg. 2014;5:22–30. https://doi.org/10.1177/2150135113516984.
3. Angelini P, Velasco JA, Flamm S. Coronary anomalies: incidence, pathophysiology, and clinical relevance. Circulation. 2002;105:2449–54. https://doi.org/10.1161/01.cir.0000016175.49835.57.
4. Engel HJ, Torres C, Page HL Jr. Major variations in anatomical origin of the coronary arteries: angiographic observations in 4,250 patients without associated congenital heart disease. Catheter Cardiovasc Diagn. 1975;1:157–69. https://doi.org/10.1002/ccd.1810010205.
5. Wilkins CE, Betancourt B, Mathur VS, Massumi A, De Castro CM, Garcia E, Hall RJ. Coronary artery anomalies: a review of more than 10,000 patients from the Clayton cardiovascular laboratories. Tex Heart Inst J. 1988;15:166–73.
6. Pelliccia A. Congenital coronary artery anomalies in young patients: new perspectives for timely identification. J Am Coll Cardiol. 2001;37:598–600. https://doi.org/10.1016/s0735-1097(00)01122-0.
7. Topaz O, DeMarchena EJ, Perin E, Sommer LS, Mallon SM, Chahine RA. Anomalous coronary arteries: angiographic findings in 80 patients. Int J Cardiol. 1992;34:129–38. https://doi.org/10.1016/0167-5273(92)90148-v.
8. Brothers JA, Frommelt MA, Jaquiss RDB, Myerburg RJ, Fraser CD Jr, Tweddell JS. Expert consensus guidelines: anomalous aortic origin of a coronary artery. J Thorac Cardiovasc Surg. 2017;153:1440–57. https://doi.org/10.1016/j.jtcvs.2016.06.066.
9. Yamanaka O, Hobbs RE. Coronary artery anomalies in 126,595 patients undergoing coronary arteriography. Catheter Cardiovasc Diagn. 1990;21:28–40. https://doi.org/10.1002/ccd.1810210110.
10. Yildiz A, Okcun B, Peker T, Arslan C, Olcay A, Bulent VM. Prevalence of coronary artery anomalies in 12,457 adult patients who underwent coronary angiography. Clin Cardiol. 2010;33:E60–4. https://doi.org/10.1002/clc.20588.
11. Cheezum MK, Ghoshhajra B, Bittencourt MS, Hulten EA, Bhatt A, Mousavi N, et al. Anomalous origin of the coronary artery arising from the opposite sinus: prevalence and outcomes in patients undergoing coronary CTA. Eur Heart J Cardiovasc Imaging. 2017;18:224–35. https://doi.org/10.1093/ehjci/jev323.
12. Cademartiri F, La Grutta L, Malagò R, Alberghina F, Meijboom WB, Pugliese F, et al. Prevalence of anatomical variants and coronary anomalies in 543 consecutive patients studied with 64-slice CT coronary angiography. Eur Radiol. 2008;18:781–91. https://doi.org/10.1007/s00330-007-0821-9.
13. Amado J, Carvalho M, Ferreira W, Gago P, Gama V, Bettencourt N. Coronary arteries anomalous aortic origin on a computed tomography angiography population: prevalence, characteristics and clinical impact. Int J Card Imaging. 2016;32:983–90. https://doi.org/10.1007/s10554-016-0849-5.
14. Baumgartner H, De Backer J, Babu-Narayan SV, Budts W, Chessa M, Diller GP, et al. 2020 ESC guidelines for the management of adult congenital heart disease. Eur Heart J. 2021;42:563–645. https://doi.org/10.1093/eurheartj/ehaa554.
15. Jiang MX, Blackstone EH, Karamlou T, Ghobrial J, Brinza EK, Haupt MJ, et al. Anomalous aortic origin of a coronary artery in adults. Ann Thorac Surg. 2020;S0003-4975(20):32042–7. https://doi.org/10.1016/j.athoracsur.2020.06.153.
16. Naito S, Petersen J, Reichenspurner H, Girdauskas E. The impact of coronary anomalies on the outcome in aortic valve surgery: comparison of bicuspid aortic valve versus tricuspid aortic valve morphotype. Interact Cardiovasc Thorac Surg. 2018;26:617–22. https://doi.org/10.1093/icvts/ivx396.
17. Misawa Y, Saito T, Oki S, Fuse K. Management of anomalous right coronary arteries encountered during aortic valve surgery. Eur J Cardiothorac Surg. 2002;21:102–4. https://doi.org/10.1016/s1010-7940(01)01053-3.
18. Flores RM, Byrne JG. Aortic valve replacement with an anomalous left circumflex coronary artery encircling the aortic anulus. J Thorac Cardiovasc Surg. 2001;121:396–7. https://doi.org/10.1067/mtc.2001.110179.
19. Hamamoto M, Futagami D. Aortic valve replacement for a patient with anomalous left coronary artery from the right sinus of Valsalva. Gen Thorac Cardiovasc Surg. 2013;61:46–50. https://doi.org/10.1007/s11748-012-0101-8.
20. Jadoon MA, Graham AN. Alternative myocardial protection strategies are necessary in patients with intramural aortic course of anomalous coronary artery. BMJ Case Rep. 2012;2012:bcr2012007448. https://doi.org/10.1136/bcr-2012-007448.
21. Ogino H, Miki S, Ueda Y, Tahata T, Morioka K. High origin of the right coronary artery with congenital heart disease. Ann Thorac Surg. 1999;67:558–9. https://doi.org/10.1016/s0003-4975(98)01293-4.
22. Morimoto H, Mukai S, Obata S, Furukawa T, Hiraoka T. High anomalous origin of both coronary arteries in a patient with aortic valve disease. Ann Thorac Surg. 2011;92:731–3. https://doi.org/10.1016/j.athoracsur.2011.01.103.

23. Castillo JG, Sanz J, Fischer GW, Bowman K, Filsoufi F. Management of anomalous left circumflex artery encircling the aortic annulus in a patient undergoing multivalvular surgery. J Card Surg. 2009;24:667–9. https://doi.org/10.1111/j.1540-8191.2009.00930.x.

24. Alsaddique AA, Elsaegh MM, Fouda MA. Aortic valve replacement in a patient with an aberrant left coronary artery. Asian Cardiovasc Thorac Ann. 2003;11:169–70. https://doi.org/10.1177/021849230301100220.

25. Pellicano M, Toth G, Di Gioia G, Rusinaru D, Wijns W, Barbato E, et al. Unrecognized anomalous left circumflex coronary artery arising from right sinus of Valsalva: a source of perioperative complication. J Cardiovasc Med (Hagerstown). 2016;17(Suppl 2):e228–30. https://doi.org/10.2459/JCM.0000000000000251.

26. Veinot JP, Acharya VC, Bedard P. Compression of anomalous circumflex coronary artery by a prosthetic valve ring. Ann Thorac Surg. 1998;66:2093–4. https://doi.org/10.1016/s0003-4975(98)01082-0.

27. de Marchena EJ, Russo CD, Wozniak PM, Kessler KM. Compression of an anomalous left circumflex coronary artery by a bioprosthetic valve ring. J Cardiovasc Surg. 1990;31:52–4.

28. Botta L, Amodio C, Pagano V, Di Marco L, Leone A, Loforte A, et al. AVR in patients with anomalous course of the circumflex artery without prosthetic downsizing. J Card Surg. 2020;35:3125–7. https://doi.org/10.1111/jocs.14927.

29. Liebrich M, Tzanavaros I, Scheid M, Voth W, Doll KN, Hemmer WB. Aortic valve/root procedures in patients with an anomalous left circumflex coronary artery and a bicuspid aortic valve: anatomical and technical implications. Interact Cardiovasc Thorac Surg. 2015;21:114–6. https://doi.org/10.1093/icvts/ivv063.

30. Alameddine AK, Binnall BJ, Conlin FT, Broderick PJ. Aortic valve replacement in 8 adults with anomalous aortic origin of coronary artery. Tex Heart Inst J. 2019;46:189–94. https://doi.org/10.14503/THIJ-17-6473.

31. Yokoyama S, Takagi K, Mori R, Aoyagi S. Aortic valve replacement in patients with an anomalous left circumflex artery: technical considerations. J Card Surg. 2012;27:174–7. https://doi.org/10.1111/j.1540-8191.2011.01365.x.

32. Doty DB. Anomalous origin of the left circumflex coronary artery associated with bicuspid aortic valve. J Thorac Cardiovasc Surg. 2001;122:842–3. https://doi.org/10.1067/mtc.2001.118043.

33. Umakanthan R, Brewer ZE, Byrne JG, Ahmad RM. Use of the hybrid operating room for aortic valve replacement in a patient with anomalous left circumflex artery. J Thorac Cardiovasc Surg. 2010;139:e123–5. https://doi.org/10.1016/j.jtcvs.2009.04.048.

34. Giuseppe Cerillo A, Haxhiademi D, Berti S, Solinas M. Sutureless aortic valve replacement: an easy and safe approach for patients with anomalous left circumflex coronary artery. J Heart Valve Dis. 2016;25:145–8.

35. Vaishnava P, Pyo R, Filsoufi F, Sharma S. Compression of an anomalous left circumflex artery after aortic and mitral valve replacement. Ann Thorac Surg. 2011;92:1887–9. https://doi.org/10.1016/j.athoracsur.2011.04.095.

36. Roberts WC, Morrow AG. Compression of anomalous left circumflex coronary arteries by prosthetic valve fixation rings. J Thorac Cardiovasc Surg. 1969;57:834–8.

37. Inan K, Ucak A, Onan B, Tamtekin B, Temizkan V, Yilmaz AT. Posterior root enlargement for aortic valve replacement associated with unexpected anomalous right coronary artery. J Card Surg. 2010;25:92–5. https://doi.org/10.1111/j.1540-8191.2009.00952.x.

38. Schang SJ, Pepine CJ, Bemiller CR. Anomalous coronary artery origin and bicuspid aortic valve. Vasc Surg. 1975;9:67–72.

39. Ayusawa M, Sato Y, Kanamaru H, Kunimasa T, Sumitomo N, Matsumoto N, et al. MDCT of the anomalous origin of the right coronary artery from the left sinus of Valsalva associated with bicuspid aortic valve. Int J Cardiol. 2010;143:e45–7. https://doi.org/10.1016/j.ijcard.2008.12.032.

40. Taylor AJ, Byers JP, Cheitlin MD, Virmani R. Anomalous right or left coronary artery from the contralateral coronary sinus: "high-risk" abnormalities in the initial coronary artery course and heterogeneous clinical outcomes. Am Heart J. 1997;133:428–35. https://doi.org/10.1016/s0002-8703(97)70184-4.

41. Roughneen PT, Al-Dossari GA. The anomalous coronary artery in aortic valve replacement: a case for caution. Ann Thorac Surg. 2016;102:e113–5. https://doi.org/10.1016/j.athoracsur.2016.01.020.

42. Benedetti M, Pratali S, Scioti G, Petronio AS, Balbarini A. Solitary coronary ostium and aberrant coursing left coronary arteries: unfavorable anatomic anomaly in a case of aortic valve replacement. J Thorac Cardiovasc Surg. 1995;109:1259–62. https://doi.org/10.1016/S0022-5223(95)70220-2.

43. Davies JE, Burkhart HM, Dearani JA, Suri RM, Phillips SD, Warnes CA, et al. Surgical management of anomalous aortic origin of a coronary artery. Ann Thorac Surg. 2009;88:844–7. https://doi.org/10.1016/j.athoracsur.2009.06.007; discussion 847-8.

44. Nader J, Labont BA, Houpe D, Caus T. "killer coronary artery" and aortic valve stenosis: a tricky case. Asian Cardiovasc Thorac Ann. 2015;23:1079–82. https://doi.org/10.1177/0218492314533685.

45. Koyama S, Itatani K, Kyo S, Aoyama R, Tubokou Y, Fujimoto H, et al. Aortic valve replacement and concomitant coronary artery bypass grafting in a patient with infective endocarditis and anomalous origin of the right coronary artery from the opposite sinus of valsalva. Ann Thorac Cardiovasc Surg. 2013;19:386–9. https://doi.org/10.5761/atcs.cr.12.01901.

46. Yanagawa B, Alghamdi AA, Chen RB, Amankwaa A, Verma S. Coronary artery bypass graft for anoma-

lous right coronary artery. J Card Surg. 2011;26:44–6. https://doi.org/10.1111/j.1540-8191.2010.01116.x.

47. Fedoruk LM, Kern JA, Peeler BB, Kron IL. Anomalous origin of the right coronary artery: right internal thoracic artery to right coronary artery bypass is not the answer. J Thorac Cardiovasc Surg. 2007;133:456–60. https://doi.org/10.1016/j.jtcvs.2006.10.011.

48. Tavaf-Motamen H, Bannister SP, Corcoran PC, Stewart RW, Mulligan CR, DeVries WC. Repair of anomalous origin of right coronary artery from the left sinus of Valsalva. Ann Thorac Surg. 2008;85:2135–6. https://doi.org/10.1016/j.athoracsur.2007.07.006.

49. Reul RM, Cooley DA, Hallman GL, Reul GJ. Surgical treatment of coronary artery anomalies: report of a 37 1/2-year experience at the Texas heart institute. Tex Heart Inst J. 2002;29:299–307.

50. Imamura Y, Kin H, Goto T, Koizumi J. Coronary artery bypass grafting for an anomalous origin of the right coronary artery: is it a valid surgical procedure? Gen Thorac Cardiovasc Surg. 2021;69:1125. https://doi.org/10.1007/s11748-021-01614-4.

51. Rodefeld MD, Culbertson CB, Rosenfeld HM, Hanley FL, Thompson LD. Pulmonary artery translocation: a surgical option for complex anomalous coronary artery anatomy. Ann Thorac Surg. 2001;72:2150–2. https://doi.org/10.1016/s0003-4975(01)03208-8.

52. Di Lello F, Mnuk JF, Flemma RJ, Mullen DC. Successful coronary reimplantation for anomalous origin of the right coronary artery from the left sinus of Valsalva. J Thorac Cardiovasc Surg. 1991;102:455–6.

53. Ponsiglione A, Spagnuolo G, Spagnuolo G, Stanzione A, Nappi C, Dell'Aversana S, et al. Aberrant right coronary artery in a grown up congenital cardiac patient, successfully treated 46 years earlier with a double Starr-Edwards silastic ball valve replacement: a case report. BMC Cardiovasc Disord. 2020;20:37. https://doi.org/10.1186/s12872-020-01351-1.

54. Lentini S, Specchia L, Gregorini R. Aortic valve surgery and an anomalous origin of the intramural right coronary artery from the ascending aorta. Eur J Cardiothorac Surg. 2013;43:e199. https://doi.org/10.1093/ejcts/ezt087.

55. Tarhan A, Kehlibar T, Yilmaz M, Arslan Y, Pancaroglu C, Yigit S, et al. Right coronary artery with high take-off. Ann Thorac Surg. 2007;83:1867–9. https://doi.org/10.1016/j.athoracsur.2006.11.032.

56. Nishi H, Mitsuno M, Tanaka H, Ryomoto M, Fukui S, Miyamoto Y. High anomalous origin of the right coronary artery associated with aortic stenosis: a word of caution. Ann Thorac Surg. 2010;89:961–3. https://doi.org/10.1016/j.athoracsur.2009.07.055.

57. Shi H, Aschoff AJ, Brambs HJ, Hoffmann MH. Multislice CT imaging of anomalous coronary arteries. Eur Radiol. 2004;14:2172–81. https://doi.org/10.1007/s00330-004-2490-2.

58. Singh D, Darbari A, Sharma MK, Parikh N. Anomalous high origin of right coronary artery above the sinotubular junction: rarely diagnosed anomaly. BMJ Case Rep. 2010;2010:bcr1220092537. https://doi.org/10.1136/bcr.12.2009.2537.

59. Zanotti G, Gupta R, Reece TB, Campbell DN, Jaggers J, Babu A. Aortic valve sparing root replacement with Unroofing and reconstruction of an anomalous right coronary artery. Ann Thorac Surg. 2016;101:1980–2. https://doi.org/10.1016/j.athoracsur.2015.07.065.

60. Nezic DG. The left internal thoracic artery to bypass an abnormal circumflex artery arising from the right coronary sinus in a patient scheduled for root aneurysm. Interact Cardiovasc Thorac Surg. 2014;19:885. https://doi.org/10.1093/icvts/ivu285.

61. Matsuda H, Ichikawa H, Iwai S, Takahashi T. Modified aortic root remodeling for annuloaortic ectasia with abnormal coronary take-off. Ann Thorac Surg. 2002;74:1687–9. https://doi.org/10.1016/s0003-4975(02)03956-5.

62. Mazzitelli D, Nöbauer C, Rankin JS, Schreiber C, Lange R. Valve-sparing aortic root replacement in the presence of coronary anomalies. Ann Thorac Surg. 2014;98:1858–9. https://doi.org/10.1016/j.athoracsur.2014.03.058.

63. O'Blenes SB, Feindel CM. Aortic root replacement with anomalous origin of the coronary arteries. Ann Thorac Surg. 2002;73:647–9. https://doi.org/10.1016/s0003-4975(01)03116-2.

64. Akiel R, Guihaire J, Isorni MA, Deleuze P. Valve-sparing aortic root replacement in a patient with retroaortic course of the left circumflex artery. J Card Surg. 2020;35:2817–20. https://doi.org/10.1111/jocs.14740.

65. Siepe M, Rylski B, Kari FA, Beyersdorf F. Detection of abnormal circumflex artery from the right coronary sinus in a patient scheduled for root aneurysm repair. Interact Cardiovasc Thorac Surg. 2014;19:883–4. https://doi.org/10.1093/icvts/ivu222.

66. Gasparovic I, Artemiou P, Kiss M, Hulman M. Bentall operation in a patient with an anomalous left circumflex artery: case report and review. J Saudi Heart Assoc. 2017;29:305–7. https://doi.org/10.1016/j.jsha.2017.03.003.

67. Kaczorowski DJ, Woo YJ. Valve-sparing aortic root replacement with translocation of anomalous left coronary artery. Ann Thorac Surg. 2013;96:1466–9. https://doi.org/10.1016/j.athoracsur.2013.01.090.

68. Sheikh AM, David TE. Aortic valve-sparing operations: dealing with the coronary artery that is too close to the aortic annulus. Ann Thorac Surg. 2009;88:1026–8. https://doi.org/10.1016/j.athoracsur.2008.10.074.

69. Hechadi J, De Kerchove L, Tamer S, El Khoury G. Modified valve-sparing reimplantation technique for Para-commissural coronary ostia. Eur J Cardiothorac Surg. 2014;45:937–8. https://doi.org/10.1093/ejcts/ezt466.

70. Caceres J, Sood V, Farhat L, Yang B. Aortic valve endocarditis with anomalous origin of the right coronary artery and unknown infected thrombus in the dissected descending thoracic aorta. Aorta (Stamford). 2020;8:76–9. https://doi.org/10.1055/s-0040-1714715.

71. Urbanski PP, Irimie V, Diegeler A, Morka A, Thamm T, Lehmkuhl L. Ascending aorta replacement in patients with coronary ostia localized above the sinotubular junction. Eur J Cardiothorac Surg. 2021;59:758–64. https://doi.org/10.1093/ejcts/ezaa414.

72. Imori Y, Murakami M, Tanaka M, Saito S. Anomalous origin of the right coronary artery with concomitant myxomatous mitral valve disease: a rare coexistence. BMJ Case Rep. 2014;2014:bcr2014206351. https://doi.org/10.1136/bcr-2014-206351.

73. Bakker RC, Bouma W, Wijdh-den Hamer IJ, Natour E, Mariani MA. Mitral valve repair in a patient with an anomalous left coronary artery. J Card Surg. 2014;29:782–4.

74. Refatllari A, Likaj A, Dumani S, Hasimi E, Goda A. Surgical treatment of anomalous origin of right coronary artery in a patient with mitral stenosis. Open Access Maced J Med Sci. 2016;4:131–4.

Giuseppe Isgrò

Introduction

The postoperative care of patients undergoing surgery with cardiopulmonary bypass (CPB) requires expertise in intensive care, as well as a thorough understanding of congenital heart disease (CHD) pathophysiology. Significant challenges are management of the low cardiac output (LCO) syndrome, pulmonary hypertension management, systemic inflammatory response, and bleeding following CPB. Another major challenge is the postoperative care of premature and low-weight infants (2.5 kg) with complex CHD who have a higher mortality risk when compared with children of normal weight with similar defects.

The type of surgical procedure, as well as age and weight and preoperative clinical conditions, will greatly impact the postoperative care. Neonates with ALCAPA and severe left ventricle (LV) dysfunction undergoing surgery procedure are at high risk of postoperative LCO syndrome. Extracorporeal Membrane Oxygenation (ECMO) support in this case should be considered as a first therapeutic choice, to avoid the use of high doses of catecholamines [1].

G. Isgrò (✉)
Department of Cardiothoracic and Vascular
Anaesthesia and Intensive Care, IRCCS Policlinico
San Donato, San Donato Milanese, Milan, Italy
e-mail: Giuseppe.Isgro@grupposandonato.it

Anesthesia

Preoperative Consideration

Preoperative clinical evaluation is mandatory to assess the general condition of the patient and the type of cardiac disease and make plans for postoperative care.

Routine preoperative tests (ECG, chest X-ray, and lab investigations) are usually required and evaluated by the anesthesiologist and, in some cases, review of echocardiography and other diagnostic tests (i.e., angiography, CT scan, and MRI). An assessment should include scrutiny of previous anesthetic records and prior premedication.

Certain patients, including chronically cyanotic patients, are at risk of postprocedural bleeding, so that packed red cell units, fresh frozen plasma, and concentrated platelet units should be quickly available according to the procedure.

Strict attention to intercurrent illness, mainly infections, is required, and if necessary, according to patient clinical condition, the surgical procedure should be postponed till this resolves.

Fasting should be planned according to the age, clinical condition, and related laboratory investigations.

Psychological counseling aimed at adult patients and healthy teenagers at the first diagnosis should be considered prior scheduling surgery

© Springer Nature Switzerland AG 2023
G. Butera, A. Frigiola (eds.), *Congenital Anomalies of Coronary Arteries*,
https://doi.org/10.1007/978-3-031-36966-7_21

in order to reduce anxiety and allow patients to be collaborative with ICU staff for postoperative care.

Premedication

Drugs for premedication are administered to reduce anxiety and promote cooperation. Additional benefits include induction of anesthesia without memory of this stressful time and reduced adrenergic stimulation that can be deleterious, particularly certain anomalies (i.e., tetralogy of Fallot, uncompensated ventricular septal defect with pulmonary hypertension, and anomalous origin of left coronary artery arising from the pulmonary artery).

Children under 6 months of age or those that are very sick often can be managed without premedication as this can be deleterious under some circumstances.

Many drugs are available for premedication; the most commonly used are ketamine, midazolam, fentanyl, and morphine. Dexmedetomidine, a new centrally acting alpha 2-adrenoceptor agonist, has been used in the setting of cardiac operations safely with good results.

The choice of the drug alone or in combination must be decided by the anesthesiologist after assessment of the patient and according to local experience and protocols.

Sedation and Anesthesia

General anesthesia and invasive monitoring is the only choice for cardiac surgical procedures and can be administered according to the preoperative condition [2].

Pathophysiology of any cardiac lesion should be discussed beforehand with the cardiac surgeons to reduce the risk of anesthesia delivery, although modern anesthesia drugs have reduced impact on cardiovascular system (Table 21.1). Sevoflurane, a volatile anesthetic, has very little effects on systemic pressure and heart rate.

Midazolam is safely used to maintain sedation, usually in combination with fentanyl or morphine.

The use of muscle relaxants that permit to keep the patient ventilated under general anesthesia is nowadays safe, because the introduction of many newer agents with low rate of adverse effects, as well as the combination of modern volatile anesthetics and modern muscle relaxants, has reduced to very rare event the incidence of malignant hyperthermia.

Cisatracurium, a non-depolarizing muscle relaxant, a cis-isomer of atracurium, is indicated in pediatric anesthesia because of the absence of histamine release; its half-life is 22–29 min and it is eliminated through the Hoffman metabolism, so it can be used safely in patients with poor renal function.

Table 21.1 Anesthetic drugs

Drug	Induction	Maintenance
Ketamine	0.5–2 mg/kg	0.01–0.05 mcg/kg/min
Midazolam	0.1–0.3 mg/kg	1–3 mcg/kg/min
Propofol	1–2 mg/kg	3–5 mg/kg/h
Sevoflurane	3–5%	1–2%
Fentanyl	3–5 mcg/kg	1–2 mcg/kg/min
Morphine	0.1 mg/kg	1–2 mcg/kg/min
Cisatracurium	0.1–0.2 mg/kg	1–2 mcg/kg/min
Rocuronium	0.6–1.2 mg/kg	1–1.2 mcg/kg/min
Dexmedetomidine	1 mcg/kg	0.2–1.4 mcg/kg/h

Rocuronium, as cisatracurium, is indicated also in pediatric anesthesia: it has a short onset (1–2 min), while the half-life is longer (60–70 min).

Rocuronium can be antagonized by Sugammadex (not indicated in children under 2 years age).

Monitoring in ICU

Electrocardiogram

Electrocardiogram is used for continuous monitoring of heart rate, rhythm, and ST changes throughout the pre-, intra-, and postoperative period.

Blood Pressure

Systemic blood pressure may be monitored noninvasively during the most common procedures by an automated oscillometric technique.

During cardiac operations, it is necessary to monitor invasive blood pressure by arterial cannulation.

Central venous lines insertion and arterial cannulations can be technically difficult or impossible to perform in particular in those patients that are submitted to multiple procedures in their clinic history, so that is important to consider the use of Ultrasonogaphy-guide approaches to vascular access to reduce the risk of vessels demage and related complications (i.e., pseudoaneurysm, arterial on venous occlusion, arterial dissection).

Pulse Oximetry

It provides a continuous and noninvasive monitor of oxygen saturation, which is mandatory during both sedation and general anesthesia in pediatric cardiac patients, who are at risk of developing hypoxia.

Capnometry

Is a continuous and noninvasive method of measurement of expired carbon dioxide and is very useful to monitor the adequacy of ventilation during general anesthesia or to detect malfunction or failure of the anesthesia machine. Moreover, it provides a useful information related to the quality of pulmonary perfusion and can reflect hemodynamic changes.

Temperature Monitoring

Temperature monitoring is extremely important especially in the newborns, who are at risk for hypothermia because of their relatively large surface area and the inefficiency of their thermoregulatory mechanisms. Cutaneous temperature may be monitored by adequate probes. Central temperature, if required, can be measured using a nasogastric probe.

In order to avoid hypothermia in children, it is important to warm the environment and the inhalatory gases by a humidifier. Warming of intravenous fluids may be needed. The use of heating blankets is also recommended especially in the newborn [3].

ScvO$_2$ (Continuous Mixed Venous Oxygen Saturation) Monitoring

Pediatric and adult patients with severe cardiac disease, who undergo cardiac operations, can be monitored with respect to cardiac output. In congenital heart disease patients, it is usually either not possible or desirable to insert a pulmonary artery catheter designed for output measurement. Currently central venous catheters with oximetry are available to continuously monitor venous saturations. These catheters are usually inserted into the right jugular internal vein like a normal central venous line, with the same dimension and length (PediaSat and PreSep catheters—Edwards Lifesciences, Irvine, CO) (Fig. 21.1).

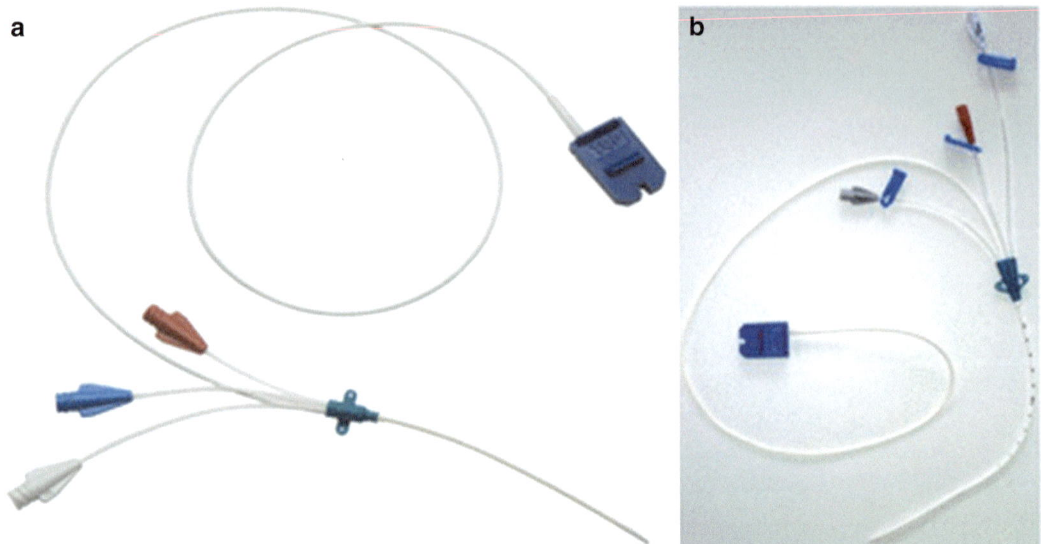

Fig. 21.1 (**a**, **b**) PediaSat catheter (pediatric) (**a**) and PreSep catheter (adult) (**b**) (Courtesy of Edwards Lifesciences)

The continuous monitoring of venous saturation can help to identify sudden changes in hemodynamic status, rapidly changing when cardiac output decreases or increases.

This parameter is included also in the management of the early goal-directed therapy (EGDT) for critically ill patients [4, 5].

Near-Infrared Spectroscopy (NIRS) Monitoring

Another tool of hemodynamic monitoring is near-infrared spectroscopy (NIRS) (Fig. 21.2). NIRS is used in many clinical situations to continuously monitor cerebral and splanchnic perfusion and has the potential to provide information on the adequacy of systemic oxygen delivery. Some authors have demonstrated a good correlation between NIRS and $ScvO_2$, but NIRS cannot precisely predict $ScvO_2$ value, though it can be used for trend monitoring.

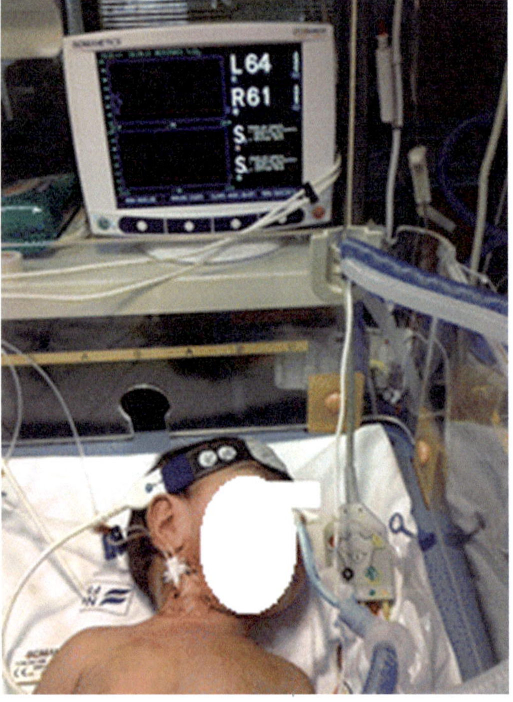

Fig. 21.2 NIRS monitoring

Pulmonary Artery Pressure Monitoring

Bedside inserted pulmonary artery Swan-Ganz catheter gives the physician the capability of direct intracardiac measurements in adult patients. Pulmonary artery catheters allow direct, simultaneous measurement of right atrial, right ventricular, pulmonary arterial, and pulmonary capillary wedge pressure. Moreover, pulmonary artery catheters can be used to estimate the cardiac output via thermodilution technique. It also allows the diagnosis of oximetric fluctuations and the monitoring of mixed venous oxygen saturation.

Cardiac Output (CO) Monitoring

Adequate tissue oxygen delivery (DO2) must be ensured in any intensive care patient [6]. The components of DO2 include cardiac output, blood hemoglobin concentration, and the s of oxygen saturation of the hemoglobin molecule.

DO2 = Cardiac output × 1.34 × hemoglobin concentration × oxygen saturation

There are several methods of CO monitoring based on thermodilution, Fick's principle, Doppler, pulse contour analysis, and bioimpedance. CO monitoring methods are classified as invasive (pulmonary artery thermodilution), minimally invasive (pulse contour analysis or lithium dilution and esophageal Doppler), or noninvasive (thoracic bioimpedance, transthoracic Doppler, and plethysmography).

Postoperative Management

Ventilation Strategies

General anesthesia with positive pressure ventilation provides a secure airway and control of $Paco_2$, but increased intrathoracic pressure may alter hemodynamic parameters.

However, general anesthesia or deep sedation in ICU with positive pressure ventilation requires a correct approach to the patient and to the pathophysiology of the underline cardiac disease; in some particular case is better to avoid high PEEP (Positive End Expiration Pressure), and use correct I:E time (Inspiration/Expiration ratio) is necessary to have a less impact on venous return, mainly in patients with right heart failure, hypovolemia, or Fontan physiology.

The effect of pulmonary pressure on pulmonary venous flow depends on the relative filling state of the pulmonary circulation.

During hypovolemic condition lung volume increase reduces venous return to the left ventricle, while in a condition of fluid overload, lung volume increase would shift blood, thus increasing pulmonary venous flow to the left ventricle.

Change in lung volume can alter the diastolic compliance of the left ventricle because of direct compression of the chamber and also due to elevated right ventricular pressure that results in a conformational change of the interventricular septum.

As well as good ventilator setting is fundamental, the optimal Endotracheal Tube placement is very important: displacement in right or left main bronchus or placement upon the Tracheal Carina can alter the hemodynamic parameters.

Fluid Management

Appropriate fluid resuscitation is perhaps the most important hemodynamic intervention in the immediate postoperative period and should be first-line therapy for early hemodynamic instability.

Hypovolemia might be present at the beginning of the procedure, particularly in small infants and children, secondary to dehydration occurring during prolonged periods of preoperative fasting (NPO).

Hypovolemia is particularly important in very young, cyanotic, erythrocytotic, or shunt-dependent patients.

In these circumstances, it is preferable to administer intravenous (IV) isotonic fluids to maintain hydration during the fasting period prior to operations.

Careful attention to blood loss is particularly important in neonates who have a small blood volume and in cyanotic patients.

Blood transfusion is mandatory to maintain normal level of hematocrit that should be 40–45% in newborn.

Cyanotic patients that experience blood loss may require red cell transfusions despite relative normal level of hematocrit.

In this case, it is very important to asses DO_2 (Oxygen Delivery) and Lactates levels to address the best fluid therapy.

Volume overload can occur during ICU stay and is less tolerated in patients with congestive heart failure or shunt lesions.

Fluids restriction and diuretics administration is required in this case.

Hemodynamic Management

Hemodynamic lability is the rule in the early postoperative period. Virtually, all patients have postoperative myocardial dysfunction and decreased ventricular compliance, intravascular hypovolemia, and vasodilation. It is critical to appropriately manipulate preload, afterload, and inotropic support.

Causes of functional impairment include microcirculatory disturbances, hypertensive heart disease, congestive heart failure due to coronary artery disease, hypertrophic obstructive and non-obstructive cardiomyopathy, and dilative cardiomyopathy.

The following surrogate parameters are possible indicators of a cardiocirculatory failure:

- ScvO2 < 60% with SaO2 98%.
- Mean arterial pressure < 60 mmHg.
- Urine output <0.5 mL/h, existing for longer than an hour.
- Plasma lactate >2.0 mmol/L.
- Peripheral vasoconstriction, delayed capillary refill and cool extremities.

Desired hemodynamic goals are a key element of the OR to ICU handover and may be adapted to individual patient characteristics or clinical scenarios. Commonly targeted hemodynamic variables include blood pressure, indices of pre-load (cardiac filling pressures), and assessments of cardiac function and output. The overall goal of hemodynamic management is to maintain adequate organ perfusion and oxygen delivery. There is increasing interest in "goal-directed therapy" (GDT) protocols, which place a premium on optimizing cardiac output and systemic oxygen delivery to meet patient-specific perfusion goals.

Hemodynamic management of postoperative cardiac patients requires integration of hemodynamic, clinical, and laboratory data and interpretation of those data within the overall clinical context.

Inotrope and Vasopressor Support

Ventricular and vascular dysfunctions are frequent after cardiac surgery, and many patients require inotropic or vasopressor support upon separation from CPB [7].

There are few data guiding choice of vasoactive agents, and huge variability exists in their use.

Inotropes and vasopressors are included in different drug classes, together with catecholamines, phosphodiesterase inhibitors (PDEIs), and hormonal analogs, each with specific characteristics.

Commonly used inotropic catecholamines include epinephrine, norepinephrine, dopamine, and dobutamine.

PDEIs have attractive systemic and pulmonary vasodilatory properties and may be particularly useful in the settings of right heart failure and pulmonary hypertension. PDEIs are inodilators and frequently require a concomitant vasopressor to maintain adequate MAP.

PDEIs have longer half-lives than catecholamines, ranging from 30 to 60 min (milrinone) to 3.5 h (amrinone).

This long half-life, along with well-described effects on platelet function and number, is an important consideration with PDEIs, in particular Enoximone. There is emerging interest in the calcium sensitizer levosimendan. However, available data do not yet support a beneficial effect of levosimendan on mortality.

Vasopressors are useful either in the face of excessive vasodilation or inodilator-induced hypotension. Typical agents are norepinephrine and the hormone vasopressin. At low doses (0.02–0.04 U/min), vasopressin is effective at treating postoperative vasodilation and vasoplegia.

Despite their invaluable role in the management of postoperative cardiac patients, caution is required with inotropes and vasopressors. Inotropes increase myocardial oxygen demand and are arrhythmogenic; dopamine seems to be the worst drug in this regard. The use of inotropes after cardiac surgery may be independently associated with postoperative myocardial infarction, stroke, renal dysfunction, and increased mortality.

Titrating vasopressors to achieve a higher MAP does not necessarily indicate an increase in cardiac output. Indeed, the increase in afterload may be at the expense of stroke volume and systemic perfusion. Furthermore, high doses can cause ischemia in peripheral and splanchnic vascular beds. Thus, the use of inotropes and vasopressors should be judicious.

Vasodilators are commonly used to control blood pressure, reduce cardiac preload (venodilators) or afterload (arterial vasodilators), maximize stroke volume, and prevent native and graft coronary vasospasm. Vasodilators are frequently used in combination with inotropes to minimize afterload and optimize cardiac output. In a hypertensive or normotensive patient, reduction of afterload can dramatically increase cardiac output and spare inotropic agents.

Intra-Aortic Balloon Counterpulsation

The intra-aortic balloon counterpulsation (IABP) is today routinely used in cardiac surgery for cardiovascular support in left ventricular failure. Its employment in postoperative low cardiac-output syndrome due to an intra-

or postoperative myocardial infarction following aorto-coronary bypass operation or heart valve intervention is the classic indication in heart surgery patients. The IABP is usually implanted intraoperatively to facilitate weaning from the CPB or postoperatively in the intensive care unit when the hemodynamic situation is deteriorating, and revascularization is not optimal.

The classic indications for the implantation of an IABP include a persistent or worsening LCOS, despite treatment with high-dose inotropes or vasoactive substances, ST- elevation, or new hypokinesia in the TEE, where surgical or interventional reversal is not possible and/or where surgical anastomoses are known to be problematic and coronary revascularization was not complete.

IABP should only be used after cardiac surgery when hemodynamic stabilization is not possible despite the use of high-dose positive inotropic agents and catecholamines.

Venoarterial ECMO

ECMO support has become the preferred device for short-term hemodynamic support in patients with cardiogenic shock or difficult weaning from cardiopulmonary bypass (CPB), in particular in neonates and children (Fig. 21.3).

Nowadays, ECMO is increasing also in adult population.

VA-ECMO is used to restore adequate systemic perfusion. Pump flow depends on the size of the vascular accesses, venous circuit resistance, and the pump itself.

The blood is diverted from the systemic venous circulation to a pump that generates the suction and the propelling force. An external drive unit, controlled by a console, drives the pump that pushes blood inside a membrane oxygenator.

Centrifugal pumps are the most widely employed: they are preload and afterload dependent as native heart, they act in a self-controlled

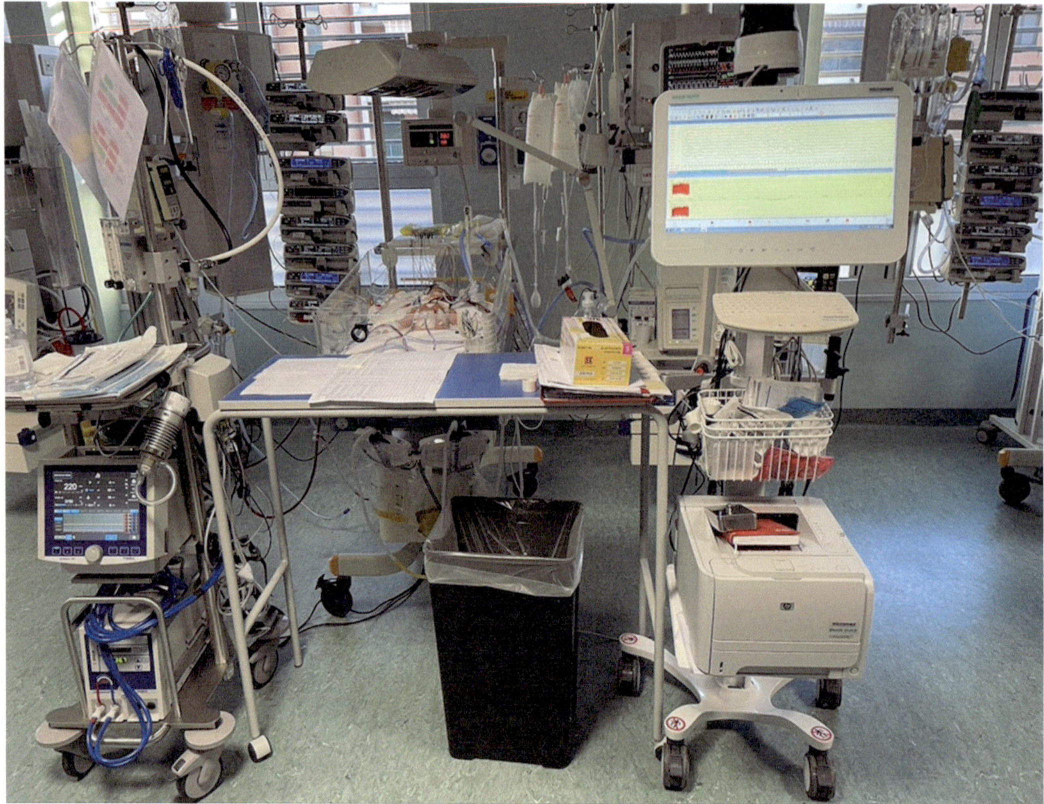

Fig. 21.3 A patient on ECMO with full monitoring

mode, and they have been implemented in the easy-to-use and easy-to-transport characteristics.

Membrane oxygenator is an artificial lung made of micro-fenestrated hollow fibers: blood flows outside the fibers, while, inside, an air mixture allows gas exchange. Blood is rich in oxygen and removed by carbon dioxide (moved by a partial pressure gradient) as normally happens inside alveolar-capillary membrane.

V-A ECMO provides both cardiac and lung functions so that native ventilation must be adjusted to trans-pulmonary flow: protective ventilation (4–6 mL/kg) could be safely used, preventing ventilator-induced lung injury (VILI).

ECMO requires anticoagulation, and bleeding and thrombosis are both faces of the same coin. Balancing these two aspects is large part of the ECMO job.

Unfractioned heparin (UFH) is the most widely used anticoagulant: empowering anti-

thrombin (AT) activity, it slows thrombin formation.

Direct Thrombin Inhibitors (DTI), as Bivalirudin and Argatroban, are going to be the first-choice anticoagulant in some large volume ECMO centers, to treat or prevent heparin-induced thrombocytopenia (HIT), a rare form of thrombosis.

Management of Bleeding and Transfusion Strategies

Bleeding is expected after cardiac surgery, but some patients experience significant hemorrhage [8, 9].

Perioperative bleeding in patients undergoing cardiac surgery is common. It may be insignificant and not require treatment or may be serious and life threatening.

Bleeding is frequently treated with allogeneic blood product transfusion: packed red blood cells (PRBCs), fresh frozen plasma (FFP), or platelet concentrates (PC).

Although transfusion is recognized to adversely affect early and late outcomes, it remains common after cardiac surgery despite improvements in transfusion medicine and system-based protocols.

Although allogenic blood products transfusions account for about 60% of cardiac surgical patients, there is an increasing use of plasma-derived pro-coagulant factors (i.e., fVIIa, fibrinogen, prothrombin complex concentrate) according to different point-of-care tests (i.e., thromboelastography, platelet function tests) to minimize the side effects of multiple blood products transfusions, among witch stands out for gravity the Transfusion Related Lung Injury (TRALI) that is correlated to longer mechanical ventilation time, ICU stay and hospital stay, and increased mortality rate.

Management of postoperative bleeding and transfusions should be done according to international specific guidelines and internal protocols, to minimize excessive bleeding damage and related huge transfusions.

Postoperative Outcome

Surgery for coronary anomalies is safe with a low incidence of operative deaths and morbidity and usually is related to bad preoperative conditions.

Increased risk of heart failure, LCOS, and death is highly correlated to ALCAPA syndrome, in particular in those neonates with severe preoperative LV failure.

In this case, it is desirable to shift from CPB directly on ECMO those patients in operating room, to reduce the possible systemic adverse effects of high-dose catecholamines to treat LCOS.

V-A ECMO support, in fact, allows the possible recovery from surgery of LV dysfunction, using high dose of inodilators as Milrinone or Levosimendan reducing the risk of excessive vasodilatation enabling excellent perfusion of the splanchnic organs and the brain; in this way, the risk of kidney failure and brain damage should be minimized as these are the most critical adverse events correlated to LCOS.

Kidney failure alone, with the necessity of any kind of renal replacement therapy (RRT), accounts up to 50% of mortality risk in ICU.

Brain damage as consequence of LCOS can become a severe form of disability in the future of patients, especially for infants and children [10].

References

1. Bianchi P, Carboni G, Pesce G, Isgrò G, Carlucci C, Frigiola A, Giamberti A, Ranucci M. Cardiac catheterization and postoperative acute kidney failure in congenital heart pediatric patients. Anesth Analg. 2013;117(2):455–61. Epub 2013 Jun 18
2. Odegard KC, Vincent R, Baijal RG, Daves SM, Gray RG, Javois AJ, Love JA, Moore P, Nykanen D, Riegger LQ, Walker SG, Wilson EC. (2016) SCAI/CCAS/SPA expert consensus statement for anesthesia and sedation practice: recommendations for patients undergoing diagnostic and therapeutic procedures in the pediatric and congenital cardiac cathcterization laboratory. Anesth Analg. 2016;123:1201–9.
3. Sessler DI. Temperature monitoring and perioperative thermoregulation. Anesthesiology. 2008;109(2):318–38.
4. Ranucci M, Isgrò G, Carlucci C, De La Torre T, Enginoli S, Frigiola A, Surgical and Clinical Outcome Research Group. Central venous oxygen saturation and blood lactate levels during cardiopulmonary bypass are associated with outcome after pediatric cardiac surgery. Crit Care. 2010;14(4):R149; Epub 2010 Aug 4.
5. Ranucci M, Isgrò G, De La Torre T, Romitti F, De Benedetti D, Carlucci C, Kandil H, Ballotta A. Continuous monitoring of central venous oxygen saturation (Pediasat) in pediatric patients undergoing cardiac surgery: a validation study of a new technology. J Cardiothorac Vasc Anesth. 2008;22(6):847–52; Epub 2008 Jun 20.
6. Ofori-Amanfo G, Cheifetz IM. Pediatric postoperative cardiac care. Crit Care Clin. 2013;29:185–202.
7. Rizza A, Bignami E, Belletti A, Polito A, Ricci Z, Isgrò G, Locatelli A, Cogo P. Vasoactive drugs and hemodynamic monitoring in pediatric cardiac intensive care: an Italian survey. World J Pediatric Congenit Heart Surg. 2016;7(1):25–31.
8. Boer C, et al. 2017 EACTS/EACTA guidelines on patient blood management for adult cardiac surgery. J Cardiothorac Vasc Anesth. 2018;32(1):88–120.

9. Pagano D, Milojevic M, Meestersa MI. The task force on patient blood management for adult cardiac surgery of the European Association for Cardio-Thoracic Surgery (EACTS) and the European Association of Cardiothoracic Anaesthesiology (EACTA). Eur J Cardiothorac Surg. 2018;53:79–111.

10. Peyvandi S, Kim H, Lau J, Barkovich AJ, Campbell A, Miller S, Xu D, McQuillen P. The association between cardiac physiology, acquired brain injury, and postnatal brain growth in critical congenital heart disease. J Thorac Cardiovasc Surg. 2018;155(1):291–300.

Anusha Jegatheeswaran

Introduction

A variety of coronary artery anomalies exist, categorized as anomalies of the origin, course, or termination of the coronary artery. The variants of anomalous aortic origin of a coronary artery (AAOCA), while primarily categorized by their origin, often also include anomalies in the course of the vessel. Fortunately, the majority of these variants do not have any clinical implications. The challenge that clinicians face is in predicting which of the many variants of AAOCA do not fit this general paradigm and can have adverse outcomes, such as unexpected sudden cardiac arrest or death. In those where the risk of adverse events is felt to be greater than the risk of surgery (something which still remains difficult to predict), surgeons are given the task of repairing these lesions in order to mitigate these risks. Historically, the impression was that many of these repairs were relatively simple low-risk cases, with the primary benefits of surgery considered to be eliminating the risks of sudden cardiac events and putting at ease both the families and patients who are often diagnosed incidentally.

The purpose of this chapter is to provide a current understanding of the complications that can arise from surgery and the longer-term outcomes of repair for AAOCA. In recent years, as AAOCA has continued to be a hot topic, we are finally beginning to accrue adequate outcomes data, from both single center and multi-institutional cohorts, to not only have a clearer understanding of risk stratification, but to analyze and understand the complications and outcomes of the various repairs for AAOCA.

Anatomy

AAOCA occurs when one or more coronary arteries arise from their non-usual sinus, or even an abnormal position within their usual sinus, or from a location above the sinotubular junction. Variations are defined based on which coronary artery is anomalous (most frequently right AAOCA (AAORCA), left AAOCA (AAOLCA), but may also more rarely be the left anterior descending, circumflex, or multiple vessels), the details of the origin (high, slit-like, stenotic, hypoplastic, and intramural), and the course the vessel takes (interarterial, intraconal (intraseptal), prepulmonic, retroaortic, or retrocardiac). The anatomical variants of AAOCA result in heterogeneous risk profiles, which lead to a lack of clarity regarding how individual variants should be managed. A recent evolution in the perception of the anatomy, is that an interarterial course is no longer felt to be one of the main culprits of

A. Jegatheeswaran (✉)
Department of Cardiothoracic Surgery, Great Ormond Street Hospital for Children, London, UK
e-mail: anusha.jegatheeswaran@utoronto.ca

© Springer Nature Switzerland AG 2023
G. Butera, A. Frigiola (eds.), *Congenital Anomalies of Coronary Arteries*,
https://doi.org/10.1007/978-3-031-36966-7_22

ischemia, as the majority of patients with AAOCA in the CHSS study evaluating features of ischemia were found to have this anatomical variant [1].

Balancing the Risk of Surgery with the Risk of Complications

One of the reasons why there has been interest in evaluating the complications resulting from AAOCA repair and the outcomes related to these repairs, was that it was thought to be simple and benign. This resulted in many patients rightly or wrongly undergoing surgery, with little understanding of the implications of repair. Especially when little was understood about the natural history of leaving these patients unrepaired. It remains that there is a significant amount of institutional and surgeon preference regarding how to proceed when presented with a patient with AAOCA. While the indication for repair is clear when a patient has presented with a sudden cardiac event, it is less clear when a patient presents incidentally. The current expert consensus guidelines recommend that those who have had chest pain or syncope due to ventricular arrhythmias, or aborted sudden cardiac death, be activity restricted and undergo surgery (Class I), in addition to those with AAOLCA with an interarterial course (Class I), while those with an AAORCA should be evaluated for inducible ischemia prior to determining whether to undergo surgery [2]. While this recommends that essentially all patients with AAOLCA undergo surgery, in comparison, the protocol from Texas Children's recommends that all patients undergo rigorous testing, and that asymptomatic AAOLCA patients only undergo surgery if they have high-risk anatomy, while for AAORCA patients with high-risk anatomy, the decision should be made in conjunction with the family [3]. Finally, the ACC/AHA adult congenital heart disease guidelines give a Class I indication for AAOLCA or AAORCA to undergo surgery in the setting of ischemic symptoms or ischemia, but this drops to IIa in AAOLCA patients without this, and IIa in AAORCA patients without this who have ventricular arrhythmia, and IIb in AAORCA patients without ventricular arrhythmia [4].

Postoperative Complications

At present, there is still very little data examining the complications and outcomes of patients following AAOCA repair. One of the issues is that most of the studies in the literature are single center and have minimal follow-up. Complications following AAOCA repair from both short- and mid-term studies include those pertaining to all cardiac surgery, and those specific to the AAOCA repair itself. General complications reported in the literature include postoperative bleeding, wound infection, and pericardial effusions [5, 6]. Surgery specific complications include new or residual coronary ostial stenosis, new aortic insufficiency, new abnormal ejection fraction, and new arrhythmias or sudden cardiac death. The rate of complications reported in the literature has varied widely ranging from 4% to 67% depending on the patient group or study [5–11]. However, this large range is likely secondary to numerous factors including small sample sizes, lack of standardization in post operative assessment, lack of follow-up, and the definitions used for specific complications (e.g., the degree of aortic insufficiency considered to be a new finding).

Surgery-Specific Complications

One of the primary studies evaluating complications following AAOCA repair is the study by Jegatheeswaran and colleagues using the Congenital Heart Surgeons' Society (CHSS) AAOCA cohort [5]. This study evaluated 395 patients who underwent surgery from a cohort of 682 patients from 45 centers, with a median age of surgery of 12.9 years (range 0.01–30.6 years), and a median follow-up of 2.8 years. Primary repairs in this study were dominated by unroofing in 87% (344/395). Repair types also included 6% each of patch ostioplasty (25/395), reimplantation (24/395), and pulmonary artery translocation (22/395). This was followed by neo-ostial creation in 3% (11/395), and both aortocoronary window creation and bypass grafting in 1% (3/395) each. Note that this does not add to 100% (total = 122%), as multiple strategies may have been used to address an individual patients' anatomy. For example, this is often the case for patients with an intramural segment, where unroofing may be used in addition to another strategy such as reimplantation or an aortocoronary window if unroofing alone does not relocate the vessel to the proper sinus. Of note, 26% (104/395) of all repairs included commissural manipulation as an adjunct.

This study evaluated a range of surgery specific morbidities. It found that 2% of patients developed new abnormal ejection fraction, that 2–8% developed new aortic insufficiency (2% if moderate, 8% if mild), and that 2–4% developed new postoperative ischemia (2% if at their last investigation, or 4% if at any investigation following surgery). Of note, new mild or greater postoperative aortic insufficiency was associated with commissural manipulation during surgery. This suggests that techniques, which avoid commissural takedown and/or resuspension, may decrease the risk of developing aortic insufficiency postoperatively. Overall, when all surgical adverse events were considered, 7–13% of patients had one or more of coronary-related reoperations, new abnormal ejection fraction, new abnormal aortic insufficiency, new postoperative ischemia, and/or death. The range is due to whether one considers the occurrence of mild or moderate aortic insufficiency, in addition to whether one considers postoperative ischemia at any time or at the last evaluation.

Figure 22.1 demonstrates this data in a format useful to clinicians evaluating specific patient subgroups. The subgroups evaluated included patients with AAOLCA, AAORCA, those with patients with preoperative ischemia, those without preoperative ischemia, those who underwent isolated unroofing, those who underwent unroofing with commissural manipulation, and those who underwent strategies other than unroofing. It demonstrates that subgroups with a higher adverse event rate in comparison to the overall cohort rate of 7–13% include those with unroofing with commissural manipulation (7–15%), surgical repair other than unroofing (12–19%), left AAOCA (14–20%), and most importantly those with preoperative ischemia (21–33%). In comparison, those subgroups with a decreased adverse event rate in comparison to the entire cohort include those without preoperative ischemia (4–9%), those undergoing isolated unroofing without commissural manipulation (5–9%), and those with right AAOCA (4–10%). It should be noted that these are rough numbers, which do not incorporate a time-dependent component, but should simply be used as a rough guide to see trends. These data suggest that risk increases dramatically when all but a straightforward unroofing without commissural manipulation is done in a patient with AAORCA who does not have preoperative ischemia. It should also be noted that risk depends on a combination of features specific to an individual patient, and patients may have one or more of the features described above, which would alter these estimates.

Other studies have reported varying rates of postoperative aortic insufficiency. Nees et al. reported that during follow-up of 54/60 patients with a median of 1.6 years, it was found that 8/54 (17%) patients had mild or greater AI, while 1 also had moderate supravalvar aortic stenosis [6]. Wittlieb-Weber and colleagues reported that in their series of 24 patients with a median follow-up of 63 months (range 12–110 months), 4 (17%) developed mild aortic insufficiency [8].

The Columbia group also reported that, of 53/60 (88%) patients with symptoms preoperatively, only 34/53 (64%) had complete postoperative resolution of symptoms [6]. In comparison, when this was evaluated in the multi-institutional study by Jegatheeswaran and colleagues, it was found that a large proportion of patients did not undergo pre- or postoperative testing (which would be required to truly evaluate this), but that of 64 patients with confirmed ischemia preoperatively, 13 remained positive, and 23 did not have postoperative evaluation at the time of last follow-up. It should also be noted that of 130 patients who were negative preoperatively, 7

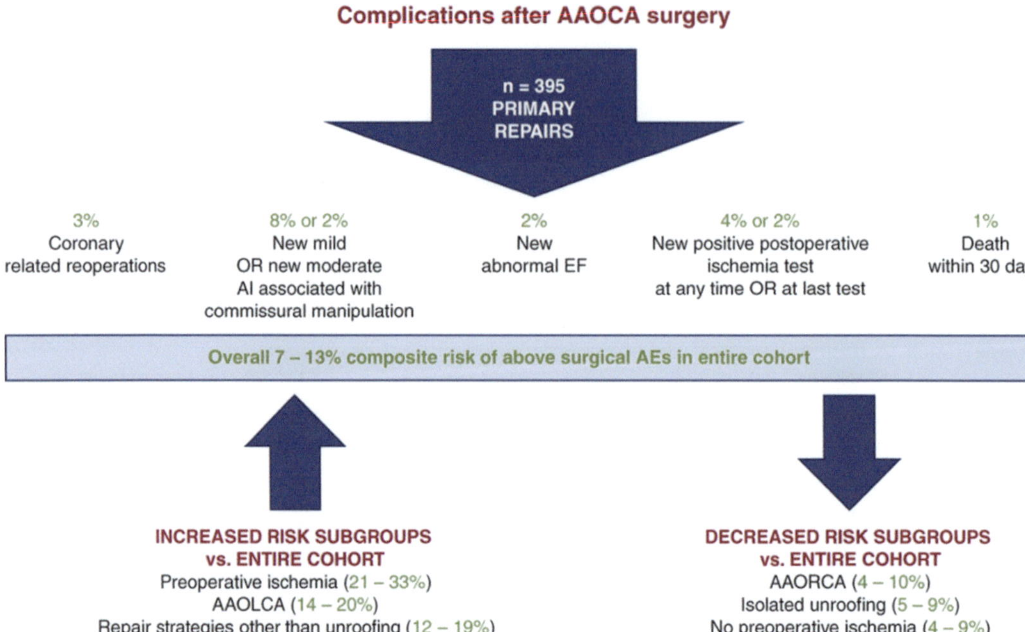

Fig. 22.1 Primary findings related to the surgical risks of AAOCA repair from the Congenital Heart Surgeons' Society Study of outcomes following repair. Ranges for surgical adverse events based on calculation using occurrence of new mild or new moderate AI associated with commissural manipulation and new postoperative ischemia based on any or last postoperative ischemia test. *AAOCA* anomalous aortic origin of a coronary artery, *AI* aortic insufficiency, *EF* ejection fraction, *AE* adverse event, *AAOLCA* anomalous aortic origin of a left coronary artery, *AAORCA* anomalous aortic origin of a right coronary artery. Figure 3 reprinted from The Journal of Thoracic and Cardiovascular Surgery, Volume 160 (3), from the article by Jegatheeswaran A, Devlin PJ, Williams WG, Brothers JA, Jacobs ML, DeCampli WM, Fleishman CE, Kirklin JK, Mertens L, Mery CM, Molossi S, Caldarone CA, Aghaei N, Lorber RO, McCrindle BW titled Outcomes after anomalous aortic origin of a coronary artery repair: A Congenital Heart Surgeons' Society Study, pages 757–771, copyright 2020 with permission from Elsevier [5]

were positive postoperatively. In this evaluation, the presence of ischemia could have been due to symptom-based criteria, the occurrence of a coronary reoperation, or death after elective surgery. See Fig. 22.2.

General Complications and Surgical Outcomes

In addition to the surgery specific complications described above, the study by Jegatheeswaran and colleagues also reported non-AAOCA surgery-specific complication rates including 1% stroke (3/395), 1% wound infection requiring antibiotics (3/395), 4% post-pericardiotomy syndrome requiring medical therapy (14/395), 1%
chest tube insertion for pleural effusion (2/395), and 2% chest tube insertion for pneumothorax (6/395) [5]. It should be noted that these numbers were obtained from documents sent to the CHSS Data Centre by individual sites, including discharge summaries and clinic notes, as opposed to primary data collection. As such, these rates may be an underestimation. Nees and colleagues similarly reported low rates of general complications including transient arrhythmia in 7% (4/60), superficial wound infection in 2% (1/60), pneumothorax requiring chest tube placement in 2% (1/60), and eventual wound revision in 3 patients (5%). Following discharge, they also reported that 18% (11/60) developed post-pericardiotomy syndrome (2 required pericardiocentesis). Wittlieb-Weber and colleagues reported that a

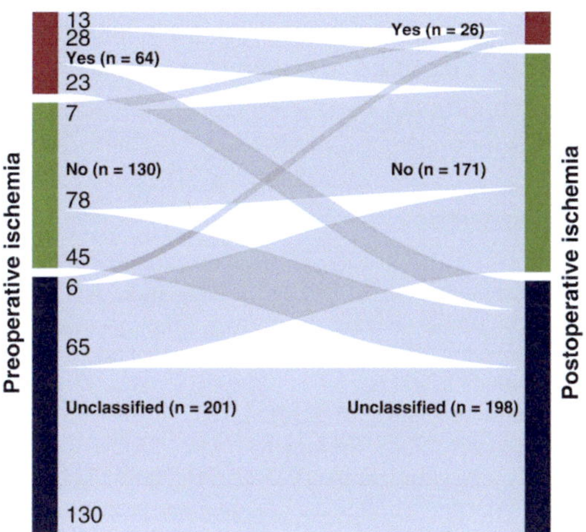

Fig. 22.2 Sankey diagram of preoperative and postoperative ischemia status from the Congenital Heart Surgeons' Society study of outcomes following repair. Presence of ischemia is based on ischemia testing, symptom-based criteria, coronary reoperation, or death following an elective surgery. To be classified as negative for ischemia, patients need to have undergone ischemia testing with a negative result. Unclassified patients did not undergo ischemia testing. Figure 1-A reprinted from The Journal of Thoracic and Cardiovascular Surgery, Volume 160 (3), from the article by Jegatheeswaran A, Devlin PJ, Williams WG, Brothers JA, Jacobs ML, DeCampli WM, Fleishman CE, Kirklin JK, Mertens L, Mery CM, Molossi S, Caldarone CA, Aghaei N, Lorber RO, McCrindle BW titled Outcomes after anomalous aortic origin of a coronary artery repair: A Congenital Heart Surgeons' Society Study, pages 757–771, copyright 2020 with permission from Elsevier [5]

total of 16/24 patients experience one or more postoperative morbidities, with 1 patient requiring reoperation for aortic dehiscence, 11 (46%) patients had pericardial effusion (1 with tamponade), and 2 (8%) had wound infection managed with antibiotics [8]. Finally, a thorough summary presented by Penalver et al. in 2012 reviewed the complications in 15 studies of both children and adults, which included additional complications such as complete heart block, heart failure, and even heart transplantation [11].

Mortality has generally been reported to be low, with 3/395 deaths following elective surgery (2 asymptomatic, 1 symptomatic), and an additional patient death after surgery following presentation in extremis in the paper from the CHSS [5]. In addition, there was a larger than expected number of coronary-related reoperations.

However, it was found that of the 13/395 (3%) surgical patients underwent 15 coronary-related reoperations. This is in comparison to no mortality at last follow-up as reported by Nees and colleagues (however 1 patient had aborted sudden cardiac death), with 5% (3/60) reoperation (all patients had AAOLCA, 1 underwent reoperation for moderate AI with left ventricular dilation and 2 had restenosis) [6].

Problems Understanding Outcomes and Guidelines

One of the primary unexpected findings from the CHSS study evaluating surgical complications was that a significant number of patients were not managed based on the most recent guidelines and did not have the required follow-up investigations both before and after surgery to determine whether they had ischemia [5]. Understanding whether patients have preoperative ischemia in the setting of an incidental diagnosis, and residual ischemia is extremely important as it allows us to understand whether surgical therapy has had the desired outcome. The current expert consensus recommendations include having a follow-up appointment with cardiology at 7–10 days and at 4–6 weeks, at which times patients have both an electrocardiogram (ECG) and an echocardiogram, in addition to an appointment at 3 months for activity clearance at which time patients undergo exercise stress testing with imaging [2]. This evaluation for activity clearance is extended to 12 months if patients presented with sudden cardiac arrest, and in both cases, patients should only resume competitive athletics following this. Lastly, at 6 months, patients should again have a follow-up with an ECG and cardiac magnetic resonance imaging (MRI) (where available). Cardiac MRI is often favored as a form of follow-up for patients due to the lack of radiation. With respect to long-term follow-up, patients should be seen annually by Cardiology, and undergo an ECG, echocardiogram, and exercise stress test every 1–3 years based on activity level (often annually if involved in competitive or high-level recreational sports). This should be accompanied by nuclear perfusion, stress echocardiogram, and Holter testing if the patient has new symptoms. With respect to medication, the expert consensus guidelines recommend indefinite therapy with baby aspirin following surgery [2]. For patients undergoing repairs, which include the coronary orifice such as unroofing and direct reimplantation, this follows the logic used in adult coronary procedures. For patients undergoing repairs such as reimplantation with a button (as in transposition of the great arteries) and pulmonary artery translocation, the indication may not be as clear.

Conclusions

A diagnosis of AAOCA can create significant anxiety and fear, not only for the patient and their family, but also for the practitioner tasked with providing a recommendation regarding the best course of action. This recommendation, is in what at times seems to be an unpredictable lesion even when there are no high-risk markers. Despite all the advances we have made with respect to improved imaging, provocative testing modalities, and even computational models that evaluate various physiologic scenarios, there are many gaps in our knowledge regarding which patients should proceed to surgery, because the risk of a sudden event is greater than the risk of surgery. This is especially true in those with incidental presentations or rare anatomic variants. The evidence presented demonstrates that surgery is not without risk, and could perhaps even be extrapolated to suggest that these repairs should be performed at Centers of Excellence well versed in the nuances of these lesions and the subtleties of the repair techniques. Due to the occurrence of postoperative complications and the lack of resolution of ischemia or its recurrence, patients should be counseled that they require lifelong follow-up. While we are still awaiting long-term follow-up data from multicenter initiatives and single centers with large cohorts of patients, patients and families need to be aware that what was once thought to be an innocuous procedure no longer appears to be benign. This should be a consider-

ation of paramount importance when taking incidentally diagnosed asymptomatic patients to the operating room.

References

1. Jegatheeswaran A, Devlin PJ, McCrindle BW, et al. Features associated with myocardial ischemia in anomalous aortic origin of a coronary artery: a congenital heart Surgeons' Society study. J Thorac Cardiovasc Surg. 2019;158:822.
2. Brothers JA, Frommelt MA, Jaquiss RDB, Myerburg RJ, Fraser CD Jr, Tweddell JS. Expert consensus guidelines: anomalous aortic origin of a coronary artery. J Thorac Cardiovasc Surg. 2017;153:1440–57.
3. Molossi S, Martinez-Bravo LE, Mery CM. Anomalous aortic origin of a coronary artery. Methodist Debakey Cardiovasc J. 2019;15:111–21.
4. Stout KK, Daniels CJ, Aboulhosn JA, et al. 2018 AHA/ACC guideline for the Management of Adults with Congenital Heart Disease: executive summary: a report of the American College of Cardiology/American Heart Association task force on clinical practice guidelines. J Am Coll Cardiol. 2019;73:1494–563.
5. Jegatheeswaran A, Devlin PJ, Williams WG, et al. Outcomes after anomalous aortic origin of a coronary artery repair: a congenital heart Surgeons' Society study. J Thorac Cardiovasc Surg. 2020;160:757–771 e755.
6. Nees SN, Flyer JN, Chelliah A, et al. Patients with anomalous aortic origin of the coronary artery remain at risk after surgical repair. J Thorac Cardiovasc Surg. 2018;155:2554.
7. Brothers JA, Gaynor JW, Jacobs JP, et al. The registry of anomalous aortic origin of the coronary artery of the congenital heart Surgeons' Society. Cardiol Young. 2010;20(Suppl 3):50–8.
8. Wittlieb-Weber CA, Paridon SM, Gaynor JW, Spray TL, Weber DR, Brothers JA. Medium-term outcome after anomalous aortic origin of a coronary artery repair in a pediatric cohort. J Thorac Cardiovasc Surg. 2014;147:1580–6.
9. Gulati R, Reddy VM, Culbertson C, et al. Surgical management of coronary artery arising from the wrong coronary sinus, using standard and novel approaches. J Thorac Cardiovasc Surg. 2007;134:1171–8.
10. Mainwaring RD, Reddy VM, Reinhartz O, et al. Anomalous aortic origin of a coronary artery: medium-term results after surgical repair in 50 patients. Ann Thorac Surg. 2011;92:691–7.
11. Penalver JM, Mosca RS, Weitz D, Phoon CK. Anomalous aortic origin of coronary arteries from the opposite sinus: a critical appraisal of risk. BMC Cardiovasc Disord. 2012;12:83.

Correction to: Congenital Anomalies of Coronary Arteries

Gianfranco Butera and Alessandro Frigiola

Correction to:
G. Butera, A. Frigiola (eds.), *Congenital Anomalies of Coronary Arteries*,
https://doi.org/10.1007/978-3-031-36966-7

This book was inadvertently published without the introduction in the Front Matter and with the following missing authors in Chapter 11.

Chapter 11—Authors' list has been updated as follows:
  Mauro Agnifili
  Luca Arzuffi
  Omar Alessandro Oliva
  Miriam Deamici

The updated version of the chapters can be found at
https://doi.org/10.1007/978-3-031-36966-7
https://doi.org/10.1007/978-3-031-36966-7_11

G. Butera, A. Frigiola (eds.), *Congenital Anomalies of Coronary Arteries*,
https://doi.org/10.1007/978-3-031-36966-7_23